◆

CHILD
MALTREATMENT

A COMPREHENSIVE
PHOTOGRAPHIC REFERENCE
IDENTIFYING POTENTIAL
CHILD ABUSE

SECOND EDITION

G. W. Medical Publishing, Inc.
St. Louis

TO PATTY, PATRICK, LISA,
GABRIEL AND DACEY

◆

CHILD
MALTREATMENT

A COMPREHENSIVE
PHOTOGRAPHIC REFERENCE
IDENTIFYING POTENTIAL
CHILD ABUSE

SECOND EDITION

JAMES A. MONTELEONE, M.D.

Professor of Pediatrics and Gynecology
Saint Louis University School of Medicine
Director of the Division of Child Protection
Cardinal Glennon Children's Hospital
St. Louis, Missouri

G. W. Medical Publishing, Inc.
St. Louis

Publisher: Glenn E. Whaley

Design Director: Glenn E. Whaley

Developmental Editor: Elaine Steinborn

Production Manager: William R. Anderson

–Book Design/Page Layout: Sue E. White
–Print/Production Coordinator: William R. Anderson
–Cover Design: G.W. Graphics
–Production: Christine Bauer

Indexer: Linda Caravelli

Printed in the United States of America

Publisher:
G. W. Medical Publishing, Inc.
2601 Metro Blvd., St. Louis, Missouri 63043 U.S.A.
ph (314) 298-0330 fax (314) 298-2820
http://www.gwmedical.com

Library of Congress Cataloging in Publication Data
    Child maltreatment / [edited by] James A. Monteleone. -- 2nd ed.
        p.   cm.
        Includes bibliographical references and index.
        Contents: [v. 1]. A clinical guide and reference -- [v. 2]. A
    comprehensive photographic reference identifying potential child abuse.
        ISBN 1-878060-22-8 (casebound : v. 1 : alk. paper). -- ISBN
    1-878060-23-6 (casebound : v. 2 : alk. paper)
        1. Child abuse--Diagnosis. 2. Battered child syndrome--Atlases.
    3. Battered child syndrome--Diagnosis. 4. Child abuse--Reporting.
    I. Monteleone, James A.
        [DNLM: 1. Child Abuse. 2. Child Abuse--atlases. 3. Wounds and
    Injuries--in infancy & childhood--atlases. WA 320 C53483 1997]
    RA1122.5.C49 1998
    618.92'858223--dc21
    DNLM/DLC
    for Library of Congress   97-41395
                                                                  CIP

CONTRIBUTORS

Joan M. Boyer
President, STOP IT!, Inc.
St. Louis, Missouri

John R. Brewer, M.D.
Associate Clinical Professor of Pediatrics
Saint Louis University School of Medicine
Medical Director of Grace Hill Neighborhood
Health Clinics
St. Louis, Missouri

**Armand E. Brodeur, M.D., M.Rd., L.L.D.,
F.A.C.R., F.A.A.P.**
Professor Emeritus of Radiology and Pediatrics
Saint Louis University School of Medicine
Emeritus Director of Pediatric Radiology
Cardinal Glennon Children's Hospital
Director of Radiology
Shriners Hospital for Crippled Children
St. Louis Unit
St. Louis, Missouri

Phillip M. Burch, M.D.
Deputy Chief Medical Examiner
St. Louis, Missouri

Mary E. Case, M.D.
Associate Professor of Pathology
Saint Louis University Health Sciences Center
Chief Medical Examiner
St. Louis, St. Charles, Jefferson and
Franklin Counties, Missouri

Oscar A. Cruz, M.D.
Associate Professor of Ophthalmology
Saint Louis University School of Medicine
Director of Pediatric Ophthalmology
Cardinal Glennon Children's Hospital
St. Louis, Missouri

Timothy J. Fete, M.D.
Associate Professor of Pediatrics
Saint Louis University School of Medicine
Director of the Division of General
Academic Pediatrics
Cardinal Glennon Children's Hospital
St. Louis, Missouri

Jane B. Geiler
Assistant Circuit Attorney
St. Louis, Missouri

Michael Graham, M.D.
Professor of Pathology
Co-director, Division of Forensic &
Environmental Pathology
Saint Louis University School of Medicine
Chief Medical Examiner,
City of St. Louis, Missouri
Deputy Medical Examiner,
St. Louis and Jefferson Counties, Missouri

Detective Gary W. Guinn
St. Louis County Police Department
Family Crime Unit/Child Abuse Section
Clayton, Missouri

Sgt. Milton Jones, Ret.
Metropolitan St. Louis Police Department
Sex Crimes and Child Abuse Unit
Missouri Police Juvenile Officers Association
St. Louis, Missouri

Vicki McNeese, M.S.
Staff Psychologist
Cardinal Glennon Children's Hospital
Adjunct Instructor of Psychology
Saint Louis University
St. Louis, Missouri

James A. Monteleone, M.D.
Professor of Pediatrics and Gynecology
Saint Louis University School of Medicine
Director of the Division of Child Protection
Cardinal Glennon Children's Hospital
St. Louis, Missouri

**Lynn Douglas Mouden, D.D.S., M.P.H.,
F.I.C.D., F.A.C.D.**
Associate Chief, Bureau of Dental Health,
Missouri Department of Health
Jefferson City, Missouri

Christian E. Paletta, M.D.
Associate Professor of Surgery
Division of Plastic Surgery
Saint Louis University School of Medicine
St. Louis, Missouri

Colette M. Rickert, LPCC, A.T.R.-BC
American Art Therapy Association
American Counseling Association

Anthony J. Scalzo, M.D.
Professor of Pediatrics
Division of Emergency Medicine
Medical Toxicologist and Director,
Division of Toxicology
Saint Louis University School of
Medicine
Medical Director, Missouri Regional
Poison Center at Cardinal Glennon
Children's Hospital
St. Louis, Missouri

Elaine C. Siegfried, M.D.
Associate Professor of Dermatology
and Pediatrics
Department of Dermatology
Saint Louis University School of
Medicine
St. Louis, Missouri

George F. Steinhardt, M.D.
Professor of Surgery and
Associate Professor Pediatrics
Department of Surgery
Division of Urology
Saint Louis University School of
Medicine
Director of Pediatric Urology
Cardinal Glennon Children's Hospital
St. Louis, Missouri

Detective Gary L. Thompson
Metropolitan St. Louis Police
Department
Sex Crimes and Child Abuse Unit
St. Louis, Missouri

FOREWORD

Why is an atlas of child abuse needed? What is the advantage of showing color photographs of children who have been abused?

The author has been involved with child protection since the early 1960s. He was a member of the Child Protection Team established by Cardinal Glennon Children's Hospital and served on the early committee to address child abuse issues. It was the policy of this team to document evidence of abuse with photographs, and this extensive collection is a part of the files depicting both abuse and situations mistaken for abuse over the years. To accomplish the purpose of educating clinicians in this important area, the author felt that it was important to share these photographs along with their histories.

The topics for this atlas represent the broad spectrum of areas seen in child abuse. Although the majority of cases involve sexual abuse and trauma, it is important to examine the various manifestations of abuse that may present in the emergency room. This collection is truly comprehensive and will serve as an important reference for those in general practice, pediatricians, emergency room personnel, radiologists, lawyers, psychiatrists, police and safety personnel, state agencies, psychologists, and forensic specialists.

Preface to the Second Edition

The first edition of *Child Maltreatment: A Comprehensive Photographic Reference Identifying Potential Child Abuse* offered the practitioner extensive photographic evidence of what is and what is not child abuse. It dealt with the areas of physical abuse, radiologic investigations, sexual abuse, cases involving the police, neglect, and drawings. Hundreds of color photographs documented cases of abuse as well as accidental injury, and the textual descriptions noted pertinent details that helped in the identification of each injury mechanism.

This second edition contains two new chapters, The Medical Examiner in a new part titled Forensics and Art Therapy in the existing Drawings part, as well as over 180 new photographs. In these new chapters, we have followed the same format of offering a complete case description of the photographs so that the reader can understand the context in which the abusive or accidental injury occurred.

In the chapter on art therapy, drawings made by abused children both during the time of their abuse and later in their adult lives give the reader insights into the phenomenon of child maltreatment from the viewpoint of the victim. This is particularly dramatic material that should prove enlightening to the medical practitioner.

The chapter on the medical examiner is divided into two parts, one written by Dr. Mary Case and the other by Dr. Michael Graham. The photographs and case histories in this chapter focus on children who have suffered fatal injury and have come to autopsy with suspicious or unconvincing histories.

Along with its companion volume, *Child Maltreatment: A Clinical Guide and Reference,* this atlas presents a comprehensive source of information covering all areas of child maltreatment. It is hoped that these volumes will prove useful in educating readers about the face of child abuse and neglect and in furthering efforts to prevent this national tragedy.

James A. Monteleone, M.D.

THE G.W. MEDICAL PUBLISHING MISSION

To become the world leader in publishing and information services

on child abuse, maltreatment and diseases, and domestic violence.

We seek to heighten awareness of these issues and provide relevant

information to professionals and consumers.

A portion of our profits is contributed to non-for-profit
organizations dedicated to the prevention of child abuse
and the care of victims of abuse and other children
and family charities.

REVIEWS OF THE FIRST EDITION

"I've been in this business for over 20 years, and this is the first time I can honestly say a reference work has surpassed our expectations. **Child Maltreatment** *is an invaluable tool to make accurate assessments of child abuse."*

Lloyd Malone, Administrator
El Paso County
Department of Social Services
Colorado Springs, CO

"The photographic atlas is extremely helpful in evaluation of suspected child abuse injuries. We are not doctors, but we must recognize retinal hemorrhages and long bone and other skeletal injuries caused by abuse." "It's the most comprehensive child abuse reference we've ever seen."

Deborah Gelb
Manhattan District Attorney
Child Abuse Bureau
New York, NY

"The picture atlas provides valuable photos." "We only have one two-volume set and we guard it with our lives, it's that valuable. It's a great training aid for our new people. Great resource!"

Phill Setter
Child Protection Supervisor
Colorado Springs, CO

"This two-volume set of comprehensive and very valuable material on Child Maltreatment and Abuse is a welcome and timely addition to our understanding of this global problem. Every chapter is an excellent reference for all health care professionals, social services, law enforcement, hospitals, attorneys and anyone who cares for victims of child abuse."

Ranjit N. Ratnaike, M.D.,
F.R.A.C.P., F.A.F.P.H.M. Director,
International Health Programs,
Department of Medicine,
Queen Elizabeth Hospital
South Australia

"The books are a state-of-the-art comprehensive text that clearly explains the multiple aspects of child maltreatment. It should serve as an excellent reference source."

Allan D. Friedman, M.D.
Department of Pediatrics
Saint Louis University School of Medicine
St. Louis, MO

"I feel that these that two books will soon be the pre-eminent references on the issues of child abuse and neglect; and they should be required reading for all health care professionals who work with children and families."

Lynn Douglas Mouden, DDS, MPH
Associate Chief
Bureau of Dental Health
State of Missouri

"This two-part book **(Child Maltreatment)** *provides a comprehensive understanding of the issues raised in child maltreatment cases. It is critical reading for all professionals in the child protection field–attorneys, social workers, law enforcement officers and health care professionals."*

Clire Sandt
American Bar Association
Center on Children and the Law
Washington, D.C.

"Most comprehensive set of books available on child abuse." "Excellent resource for physicians who care for victims of child abuse. An excellent reference for hospital emergency rooms, physicians, medical students and residents in training!"

Mark Bugnitz, M.D.
LeBonheur Hospital
Division of Pediatric Critical Care
University of Tennessee
Memphis, TN

". . . This product is a most valuable reference work for all persons who are involved in the care of children. I have strongly recommended it to concerned colleagues, students, residents and nurses."
"You have provided an important service to child advocacy with these books!"

C. George Ray, M.D.
Professor and Chairman of Pediatrics
Saint Louis University
Health Sciences Center
St. Louis, MO

". . . An issue truly important to the child's and its family's welfare."
★★★★★ *"A must-have reference for police, paramedics, school administrators and any officials who must confront and deal with this issue!"*

Wayne Hill, Sr., BCFE, FACFE
Book Review
Forensic Examiner / Mar-Apr '96

"The Atlas provides the type of high quality detailed photographs of abuse-related injuries that front-line professionals need to understand the complexities of child abuse. We have found this two-volume set particularly valuable to the non-medical professionals to gain a better understanding of injuries children have received and the implications of any related medical diagnoses. The quality of the publication is outstanding."

Charles Wilson, MSSW
Executive Director
National Children's Advocacy Center
Huntsville, Alabama

". . . The book's (volume one) accessibility and relevance make it a fine reference for clinical personnel dealing with child abuse. . . The book of photographs (volume two) addresses an important need in the field of pediatrics . . . these are worthwhile books. Busy clinicians will find the book of photographs especially useful."

The New England Journal of Medicine
April 6, 1995, Vol. 332, No. 14

*"**Child Maltreatment** is a wonderful addition to the core reference shelf of professionals who work with children . . . each chapter is written clearly, with carefully edited consistency . . . Each section begins with definitions and an overview. The approach to each problem is established clearly . . . This very comprehensive work will meet most needs for both the new learner and the experienced professional."*

Archives of Family Medicine
American Medical Association
Vol. 4, October 1995

PREFACE TO THE FIRST EDITION

Over the years, the author has had extensive experience in teaching the subject of child abuse to medical students, house staff, attending physicians, and other interested groups. Such educational endeavors demand quality visual presentations to reinforce these teachings and clarify the injuries being discussed. The Child Protection Team established by Cardinal Glennon Children's Hospital has been confronted by nearly every form of abuse and has adopted the practice of documenting their findings with photographs. The author feels strongly that it is important to share this information with other professionals and has prepared this atlas to accomplish this goal.

Pictures of abused children are not pleasant. It is impossible to make child abuse palatable. Yet for education to be effective, the effects of abuse must be shown clearly and understood for what they are. Therefore, the author has sought to provide the clearest, most instructive cases in this book.

It is difficult to relate to the statistics that millions of children are abused, just as it is hard to cite the numbers of needy children in the world and feel that any one individual is capable of making an impact on the problem. As a result, little may be done. Yet when one child falls down a well, the whole world can be drawn together in an effort to rescue that one child. In the same way that this one child becomes real, it is hoped that the readers will be able to relate to one or more of the children presented in this atlas and truly experience compassion for these victims. It is to the millions of nameless, faceless abused children that this book is dedicated. May those who see the faces of these abused children be moved to continue our efforts in valuing and protecting all children from mistreatment.

ACKNOWLEDGMENTS

*We would like to thank the personnel in the Record Room, Cardinal Glennon
Children's Hospital:*

Dorothy S. Strasser, R.R.A., Director

Cecily R. Curry, R.R.A., Medical-Legal Coordinator

Elizabeth Mullen

Carolyn Vogler

Without their immense help and cooperation, this atlas would not have been possible.

TABLE OF CONTENTS

◆

CHILD
MALTREATMENT

A COMPREHENSIVE
PHOTOGRAPHIC REFERENCE
IDENTIFYING POTENTIAL
CHILD ABUSE

SECOND EDITION

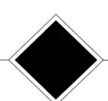

PART ONE

Physical Abuse

TRAUMA

JAMES A. MONTELEONE, M.D.

Differentiating accidental injuries from inflicted injuries is important in the management of injured children. A caretaker rarely reports to an emergency room or physician's office stating that he or she has abused the child. He will try to convince the staff that the injury resulted from an accident initiated by the child. To diagnose abuse you must first believe that abuse is a possibility and then effectively eliminate the potential that an accident produced the presenting injury(ies).

This chapter presents a spectrum of injuries caused by trauma, whether abusive or accidental. There are instances of natural pigmentation masquerading as injury, folk medicine producing injury in the course of treatment, and innocent sources of injury such as tight elastic socks. However, the majority of cases illustrate the types of injuries seen in child abuse. The stories offered by the caregivers are detailed to account for the most obvious injuries, but upon investigation by medical personnel, child abuse was apparent in most of these cases.

The evaluator must ask two questions when presented with these types of cases:

1. Could the injury have occurred as described?
2. Is this child developmentally mature enough to have caused the injury?

If the evaluator determines that the injury is nonaccidental and the history offered is false, the case must be considered abuse and a report made to child protective services.

The diagnosis of the classic battered child who presents with multiple injuries in differing stages of healing is easy for the experienced physician. However, determining, with certainty, whether a single injury is accidental or intended is difficult. Inflicted injury is diagnosed when the physician is certain that a single injury in a child could not have been the result of the circumstances described by the caregiver, a decision based on the physician's clinical experience and reliance on studies in the literature.

The following cases were selected as examples of physical abuse or are cases that were mistaken for abuse. It is not always possible to ascertain how an injury happened. It is only necessary to determine that the history given (if any is given) does not adequately explain the situation. Guidelines to help in this process are offered in the accompanying tables.

Table 1-1. Situations that are Child Abuse and Dictate a Report to the Authorities

Severe neglect
Abandonment
Long periods with no supervision, infant to 8-year-old left unattended
Long delay in obtaining medical help for a serious condition
Maternal deprivation and/or failure to thrive

Head injury
Evidence of shaken infant syndrome
Altered level of consciousness
Closed head injury
CNS hemorrhaging
Retinal hemorrhages

Skeletal injuries
Rupture of the costovertebral junction
Posterior rib fractures
Metaphyseal avulsion fracture
Two or more fractures in different stages of healing
Multiple skull fractures
Long bone fracture in a nonambulating child

Bruises
Bilateral black eyes without broken nose
Skin bruises and lacerations in recognizable shapes, such as a whip, belt, stick, fist, fingers, buckle, rope, or teeth
Circumferential injuries (burns, bruises, lacerations, or scars) of the wrists, arms, ankles, legs, and neck
Multiple bruises in inaccessible places, in different stages of healing
Injury resulting from discipline in a child less than 1 year of age

Trauma
Blunt trauma to the abdomen or chest with inappropriate or no history

Table 1-2. Caregiver Indicators

Indicators strongly suggesting abuse

Explanation of injury not believable

Explanations that are inconsistent or changing

Paramour in the home

Previously suspected of abuse

Caregiver understates the seriousness of the child's condition

Caregiver projects blame to third party

Caregiver has delayed bringing the child to the hospital

Caregiver cannot be located

History of substance abuse

Caregiver unable to function

Child not up to date on immunizations

Child has severe diaper rash, is poorly kept, is dirty

Caregiver is psychotic

Nonspecific indicators

Caregiver is hostile and aggressive

Caregiver is compulsive, inflexible, unreasonable, and cold

Caregiver is passive and dependent

Father is unemployed

History of unwanted baby

Caregiver has unrealistic expectations of child

Caregiver is hospital shopper

Frequent visits to the pediatrician without a medical reason

Caregiver overreacts to child's misbehavior

Table 1-3. Situations that are Possibly Child Abuse and Dictate a Report to the Authorities

Death of an infant with unknown cause and poor or questionable history

Evidence of emotional abuse

Hair loss

Suicide

Runaway

Drug use

Child perpetrator

Child has flat affect, is passive, and/or exhibits failure to thrive

Neglect is obvious

Medical treatment delayed (depending on the seriousness of the condition)

Failure to thrive with no medical condition to explain it

First drug or toxin ingestion with suspicious history

Repeated drug or toxin ingestion

Small child(ren) supervised by child under 12 years of age

Severe dehydration, underweight with no medical condition to explain it

Head injury

Subdural hematoma without appropriate history

Fracture of the skull with suspicious or no history

Skeletal injuries

Fractured long bone with no appropriate history

Bruises

Multiple bruises

Injuries suggesting the use of an instrument

Injuries resulting from discipline in child over 1 year of age

Figure 1-1. This 12-year-old boy was taken to the emergency room by the police after a domestic argument. The child's father had disciplined the boy, injuring his lower lip (**a**) and ear (**b**).

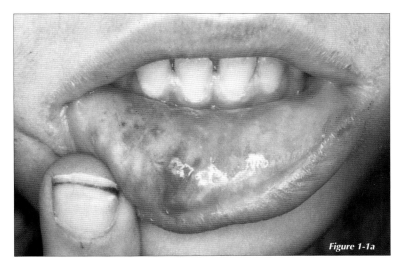

Figure 1-1a

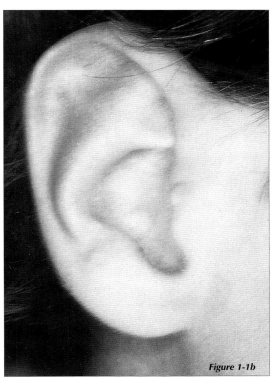

Figure 1-1b

Figure 1-2. This 13-month-old boy had bruises to his face (**a**) and buttocks (**b**). The injuries were found on routine examination.

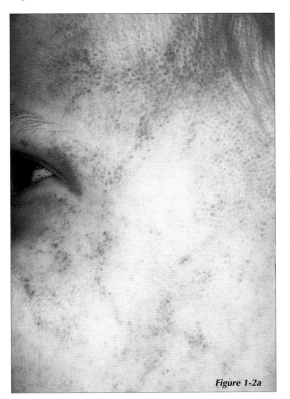

Figure 1-2a

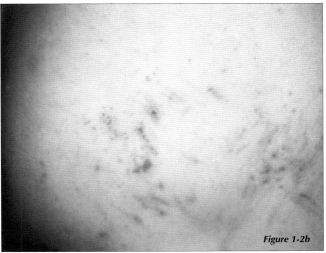

Figure 1-2b

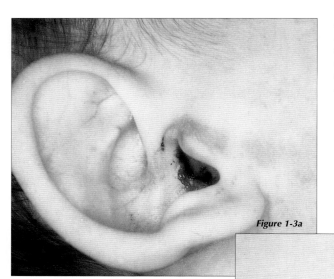

Figure 1-3a

Figure 1-3. *This 2-year-old boy's parents noted "blood coming out of his ear, after he had fallen out of his high chair"* **(a)**. *Abuse was suspected and reported. The child had a perforated right eardrum. Note the bruising to the right cheek* **(a)** *and left eye* **(b)**. *The child also had circumferential markings to his arm where he was restrained* **(c)**. *Other old and fresh bruises were noted on his forehead.*

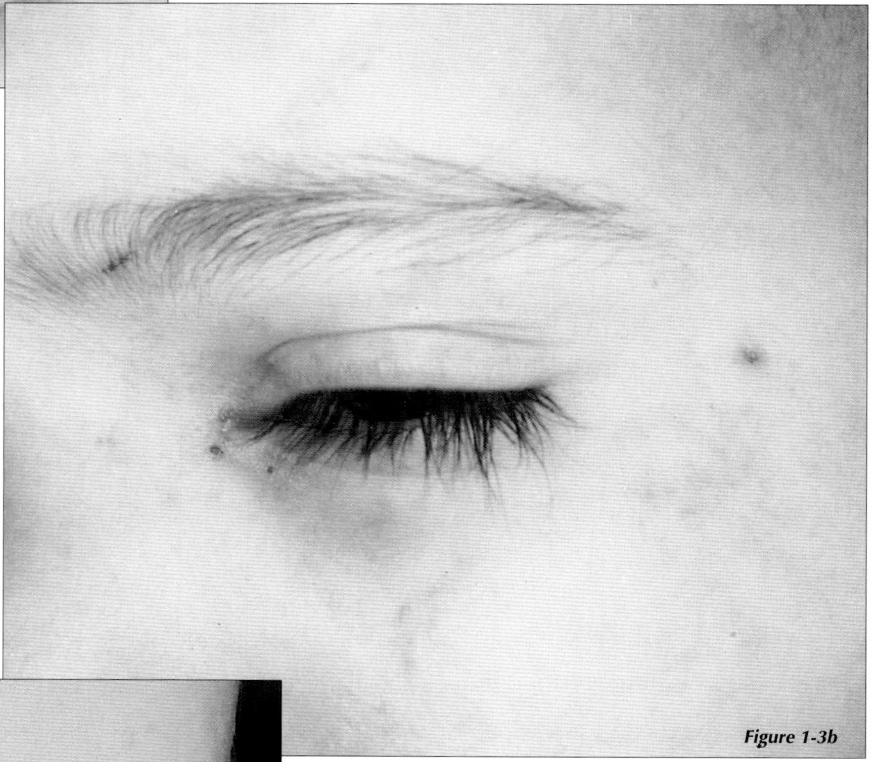

Figure 1-3b

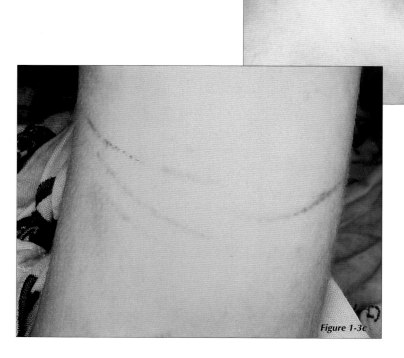

Figure 1-3c

Figure 1-4. a, *Lateral view and* **b**, *frontal view of attempted strangulation of a 12-year-old. Note the small petechial hemorrhages above the injury.*

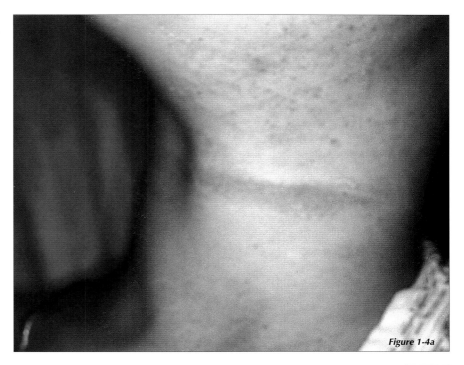

Figure 1-4a

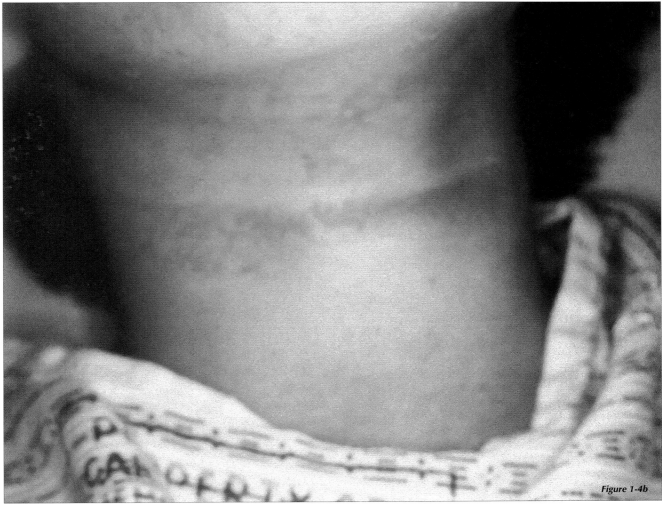

Figure 1-4b

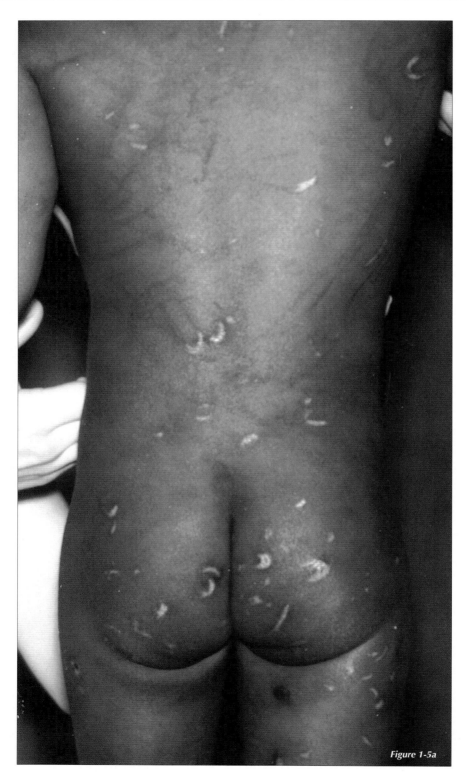

Figure 1-5a

Figure 1-5. *This 3-year-old girl was seen in the emergency room for an upper respiratory infection. The child was found to have numerous old loop and linear marks, some leaving scars, on both the back (a) and the front (b) of her body. She was also developmentally delayed and deaf.*

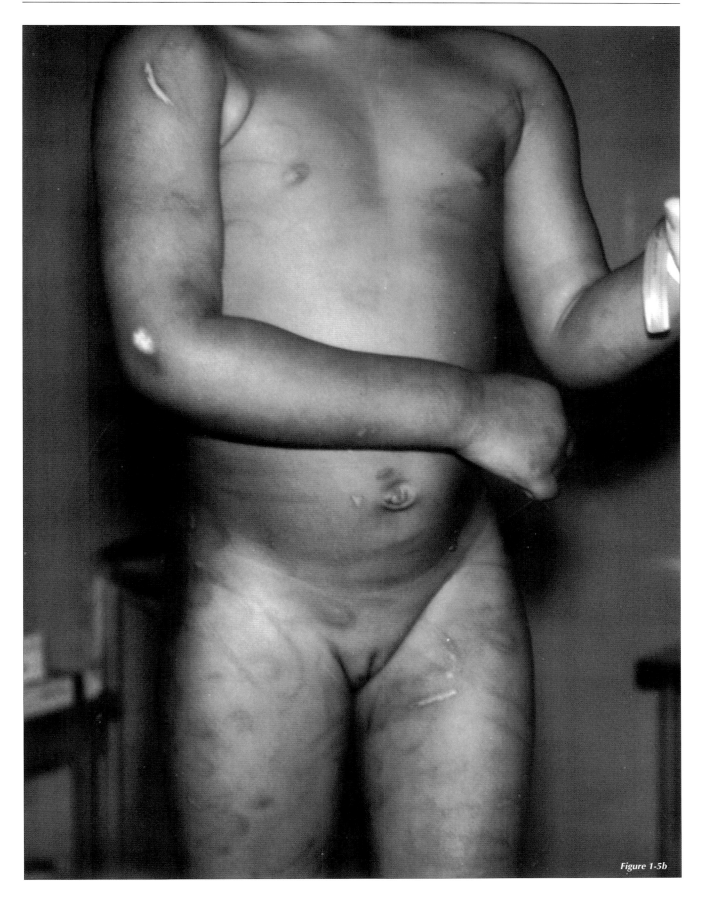

Figure 1-5b

Figure 1-6. *Evidence of a recent beating of a 6-year-old boy with a belt (linear marks) and fist (round marks). Shown here are the boy's back (a), right side (b), and left upper leg and hip (c). There was no evidence of old lesions.*

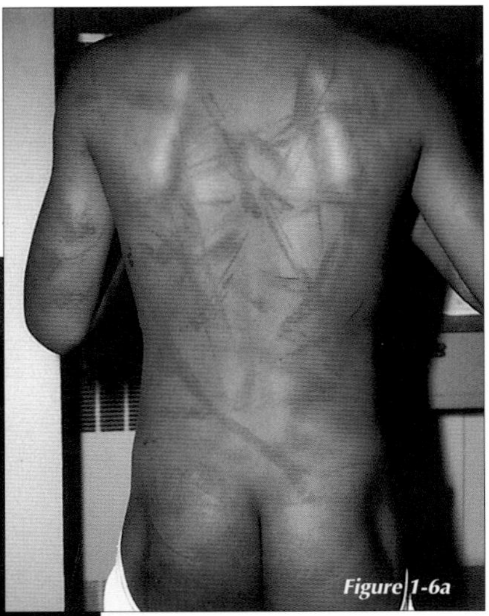

Figure 1-6a

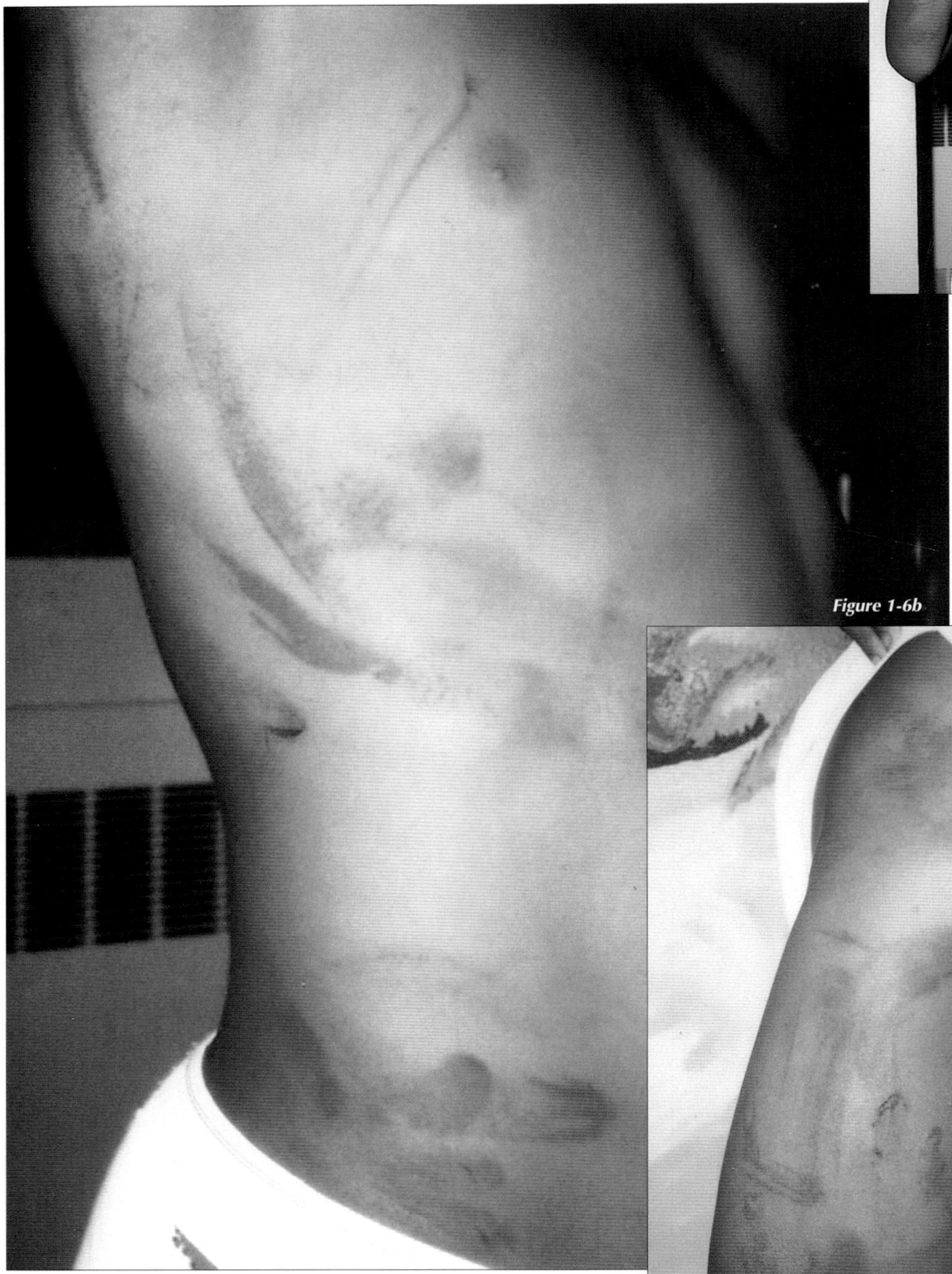

Figure 1-6b

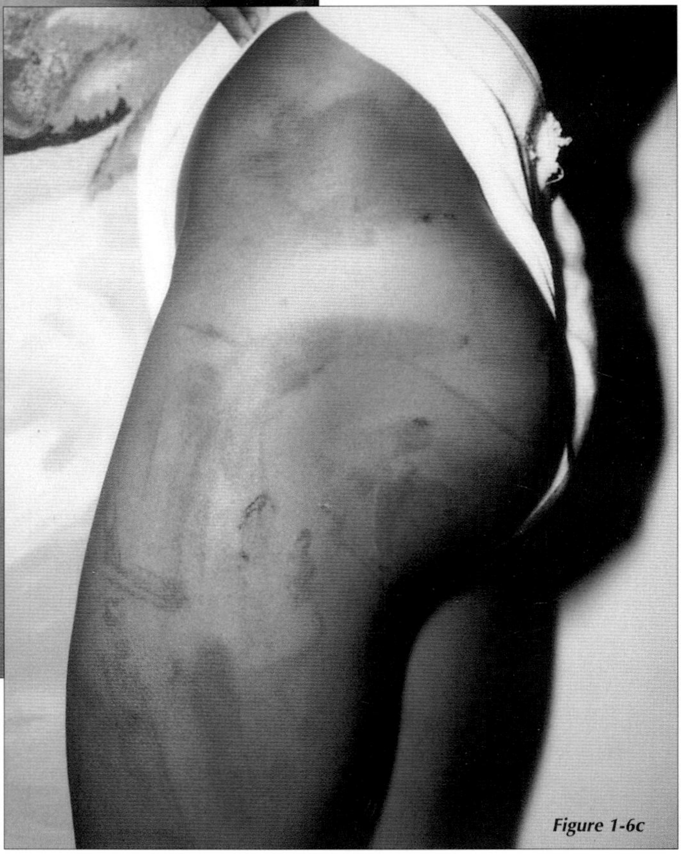

Figure 1-6c

Figure 1-7. *This 11-month-old biracial boy was reported to the hotline by a new daycare employee for bruising on his buttocks. The child was healthy and happy. The mother said that the discoloration was present from birth. The staff determined that the discoloration was a mongolian spot. It involves the buttocks (**a**) and part of the left thigh (seen better on **b**).*

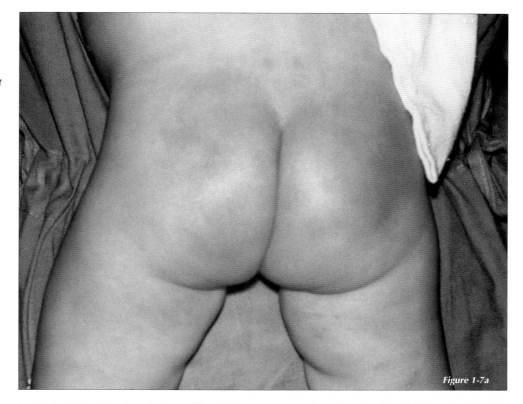

Figure 1-7a

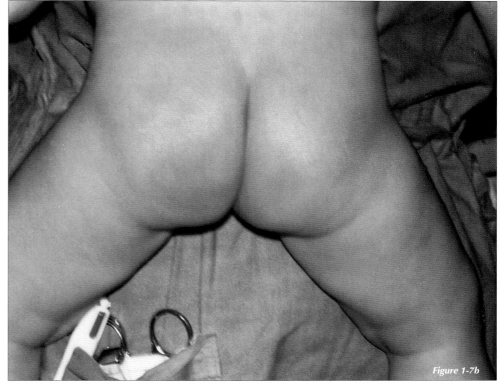

Figure 1-7b

Figure 1-8. *This 2-year-old boy was taken to the emergency room because of a swollen prepuce **(a)**. The mother did not know how he had suffered the injury. The child was found to have several other lesions, including a loop mark on his right thigh **(b)**, linear marks on his left thigh and lower abdomen **(c and d)**, and a small rounded, healed burn scar on his left shoulder that resembled a cigarette burn. The prepuce lesions were thought to be due to pinching or clamping as punishment for soiling himself.*

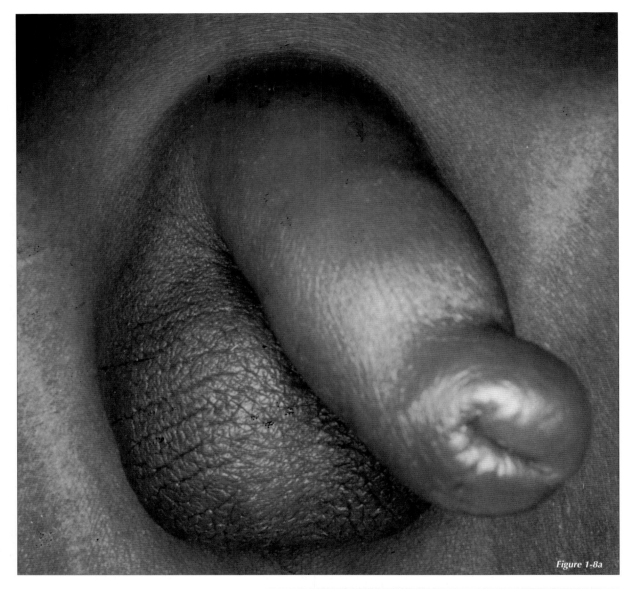

Figure 1-8a

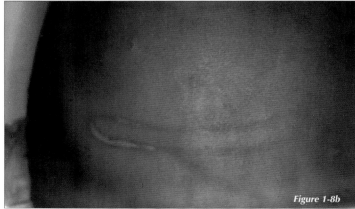

Figure 1-8b

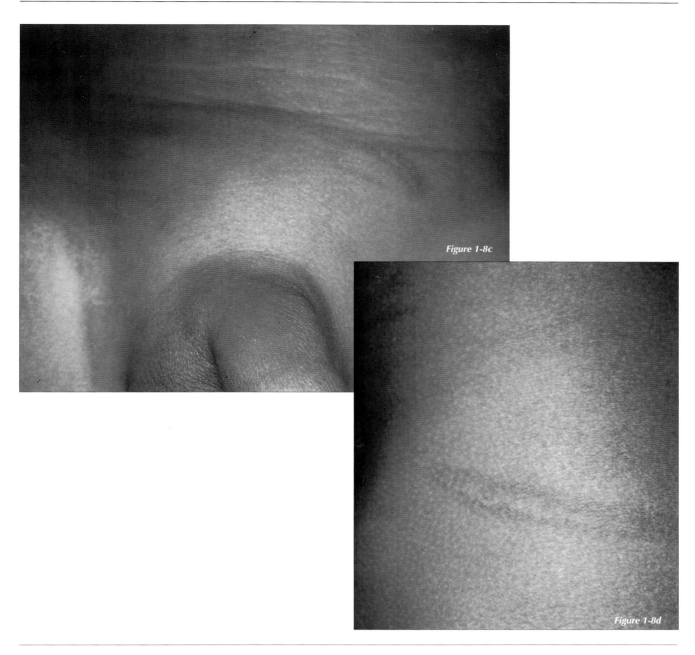

Figure 1-8c

Figure 1-8d

Figure 1-9. Seventeen-month-old boy with a human bite mark on his right arm.

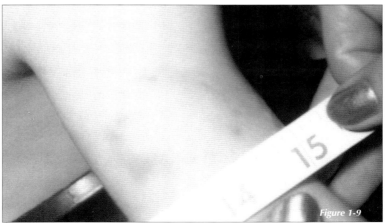

Figure 1-9

Figure 1-10. This 11-month-old child was taken to the emergency room by his mother. She had been at work when the babysitter dropped him off saying that he had just fallen out of his crib and injured his right eye. The child's older sibling, a 6-year-old, corroborated that the child had fallen out of his crib.

On examination, the emergency room physician noted an ecchymotic area involving the right upper lid and temporal area (**a**). The left eye showed no injury. Also noted were an injury to the left side of the head with an abrasion (**b**), a band of punctate, petechial-looking lesions across the side of the left leg (**c**), a bite mark behind the left leg (**d**), an ecchymotic area behind the right ear with punctate ecchymotic lesions on the ear itself (**e**), rudimentary bite marks to the buttocks (**f**), a pinch lesion of the glans penis (**g**), and a band of bruising across the back of the right forearm (**h**). The child was admitted to the hospital and reported to the Division of Family Services as a case of suspected child abuse. The following morning the child showed changes with marked bilateral periorbital edema and ecchymosis (**i** and **j**) and now had bruising of the left cheek. The child did not have a bleeding disorder, and bleeding and clotting studies were normal.

The Division of Family Services investigated the case. The sibling revealed that he had lied and the child did not fall out of his crib but was beaten with a paddle by the babysitter. **I** and **j** demonstrate how there can be a delay in the development of ecchymotic changes and that blood can follow fascial planes and surface in distal areas. The blood accumulation in the left eye originated from the injury of the left side of the head (**b**).

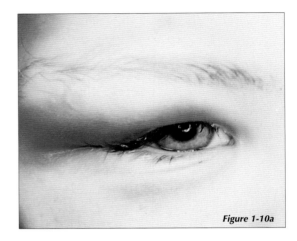

Figure 1-10a

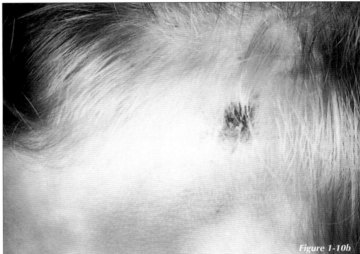

Figure 1-10b

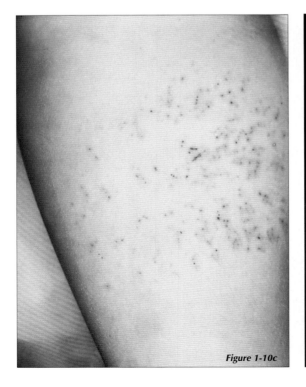

Figure 1-10c

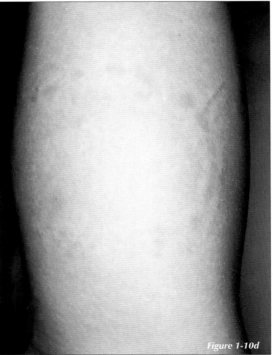

Figure 1-10d

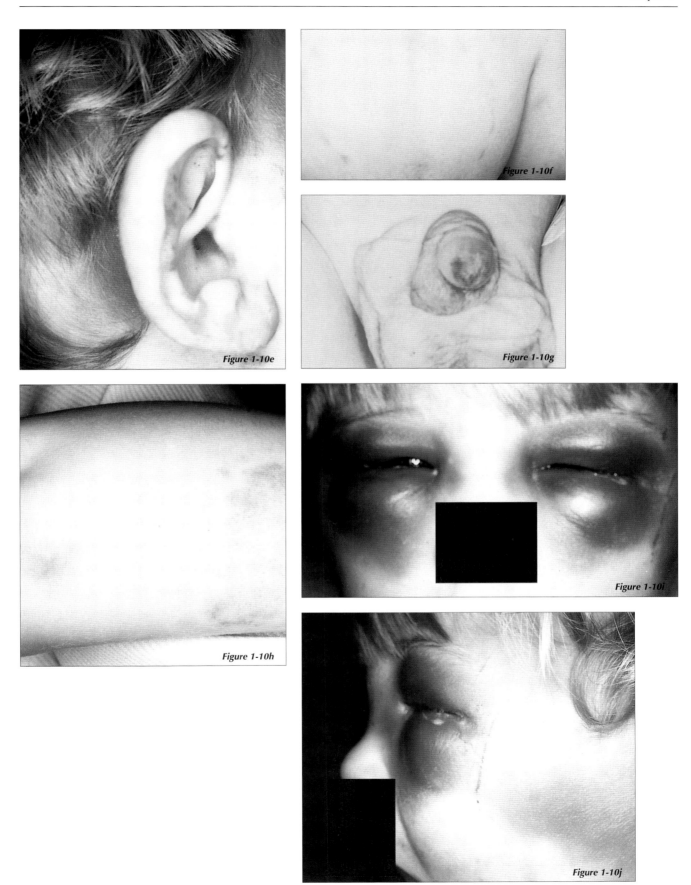

Figure 1-10e

Figure 1-10f

Figure 1-10g

Figure 1-10h

Figure 1-10i

Figure 1-10j

Figure 1-11. This 4-year-old boy was seen in the emergency room with the history of having fallen down the stairs. He had bruising on multiple surface areas in various stages of healing. He also had an ecchymotic area on the right cheek with a five-pointed abrasion (**a** and **c**), which is repeated lateral to the right eye and on the chin (**b**). These were believed to be left by a ring. He had perioral ecchymosis with older lip injuries and conjunctival hemorrhages in the right eye (**d**). Other findings included scrotal ecchymosis and an ecchymotic area on the upper right thigh (**e**), scalp injury, and injuries to his arms and legs. The child had a past history of spiral fracture of the humerus, lead toxicity, and hearing deficiency. He was developmentally delayed and considered a behavioral problem.

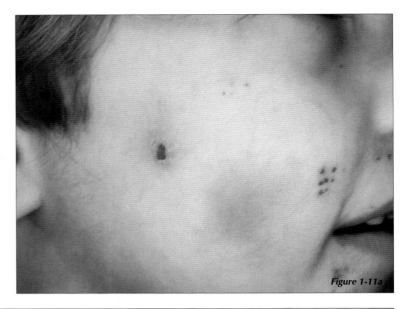

Figure 1-11a

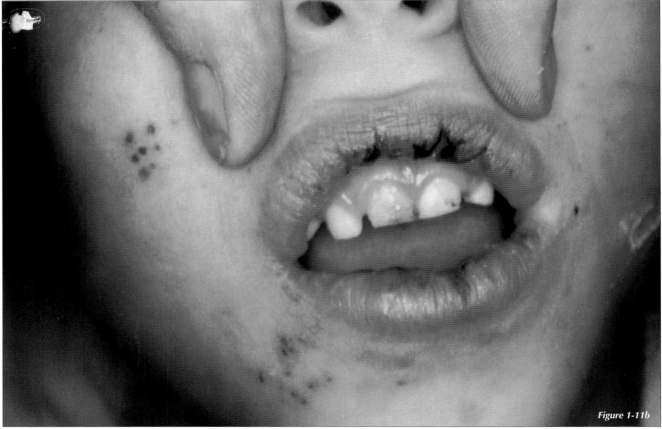

Figure 1-11b

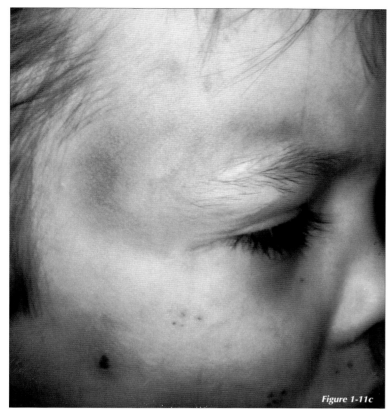

Figure 1-11c

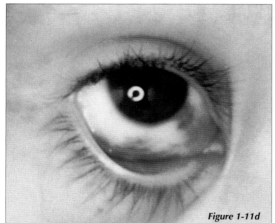

Figure 1-11d

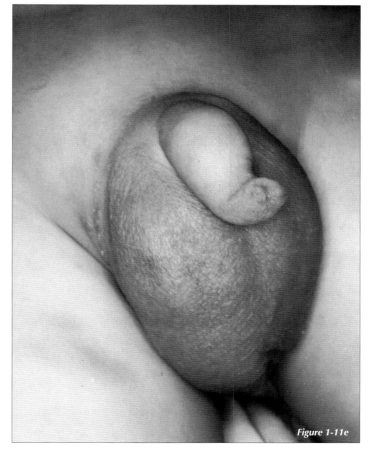

Figure 1-11e

Figure 1-12. *Multiple fresh loop and linear marks on a 12-year-old girl.*

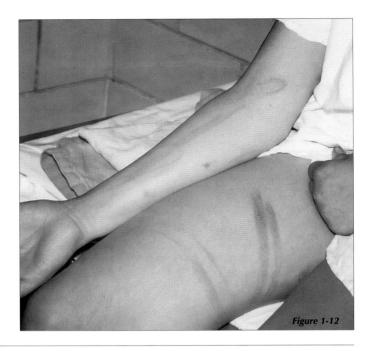

Figure 1-12

Figure 1-13. *This 14-month-old Southeast Asian boy was seen in the emergency room because he was having difficulty breathing. The mother said that the bruising to the back was due to her treating him for his illness with a "Chinese rub," a form of folk medicine. However, this is not what is typically seen with this practice. The bruising follows a bony pattern, lying over the ribs, sternum, and spine (**a** and **b**). On the child's back (**c**) there is a hint of that pattern.*

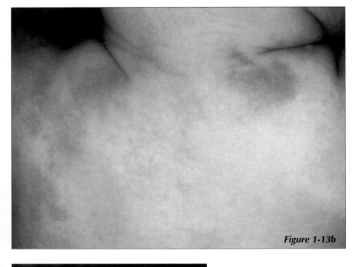

Figure 1-13b

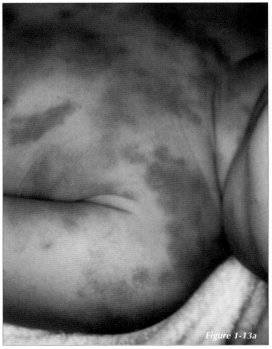

Figure 1-13a

Figure 1-13c

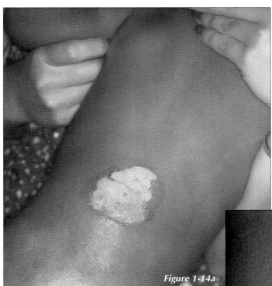

Figure 1-14a

Figure 1-14. *This 19-month-old boy was taken to the hospital by his grandmother. She noted the contact burn to his back **(a)**, which was healed over **(b)**. The child was in the care of his father, who was an alcoholic. He had given no explanation for the burn. The burn was reported as reason to suspect child abuse—there was no explanation for its cause, a third party sought medical attention, and the injury was old. The child's condition was also being followed in the lead clinic.*

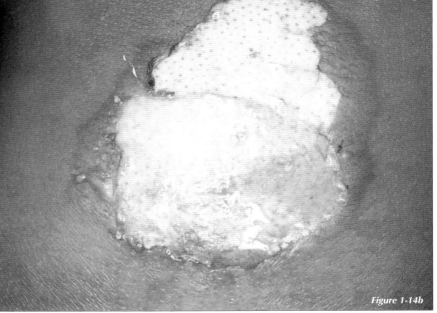

Figure 1-14b

Figure 1-15. *Eye injury to a 15-year-old boy beaten with a stick. The imprint of the instrument is central, with ecchymosis extending beyond the area of impact.*

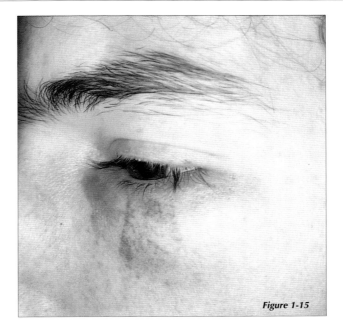

Figure 1-15

19

Figure 1-16. *This 22-month-old boy fell from a second-story window, supposedly landing in a wheelbarrow before striking the ground. There were no witnesses. All but one of the injuries were fresh. There was a large ecchymosis of the forehead, a swollen upper lip, and multiple abrasions of the neck, right shoulder and arm, left chin, and left thorax (**a** to **e**). An older appearing abrasion on the right elbow had been covered with a bandage (**f**). After their investigation, the police determined that the cause of the injury was consistent with the explanation and was accidental, due to a lack of supervision.*

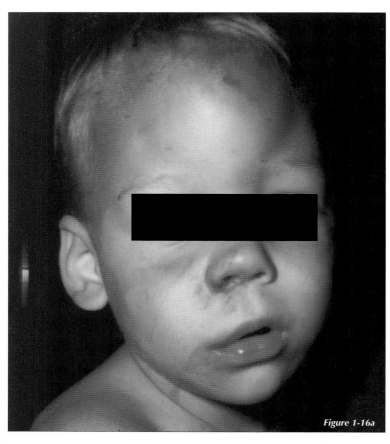

Figure 1-16a

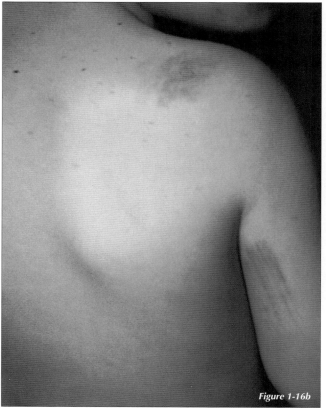

Figure 1-16b

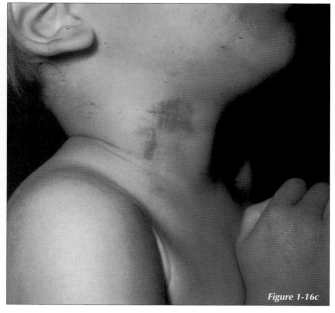

Figure 1-16c

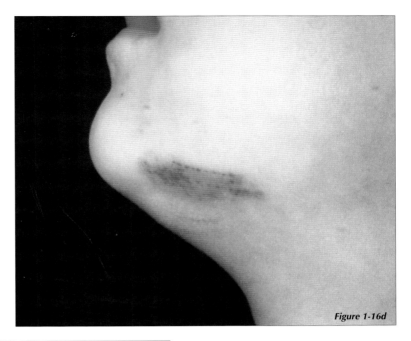

Figure 1-16d

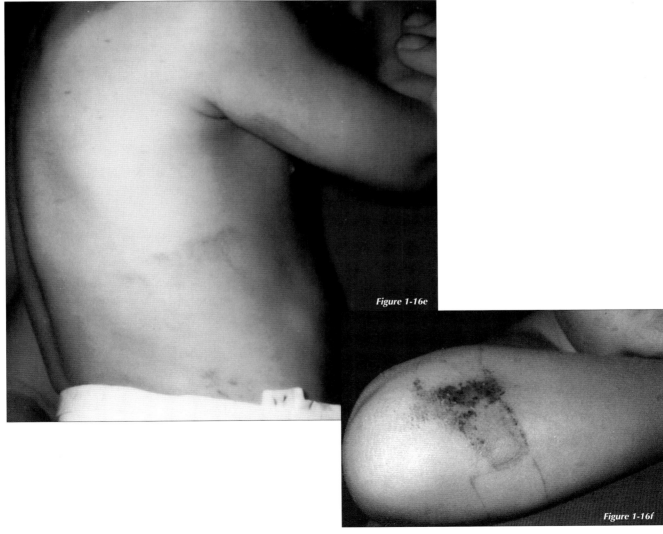

Figure 1-16e

Figure 1-16f

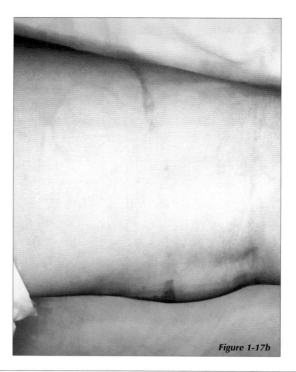

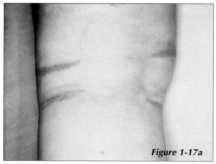

Figure 1-17. *This 7-month-old boy was taken to the emergency room by his babysitter. He had an upper respiratory infection and the sitter was concerned that the child had been abused because of the linear bruises on his legs (**a** and **b**). The hotline was called to report suspected abuse, but it was determined that the injuries were caused by tight elastic in his socks.*

Figure 1-17a

Figure 1-17b

Figure 1-18. *This 4-year-old girl was brought to the emergency room by her father and his girlfriend, who said she was found unconscious after falling down the stairs. (**a**) The child was severely malnourished. Her hair was patchy and thin. When the caretakers were asked how the child had lost so much hair, they said that she had a metabolic disease. She had numerous bruises, (**b** to **e**) which were not fresh, on multiple surface areas. She had a subdural hematoma from blunt trauma to the head, retinal hemorrhages, a splenic hematoma, a liver laceration and a contusion of the duodenum. She was also anemic. She died shortly after admission. The girlfriend was convicted of homicide.*

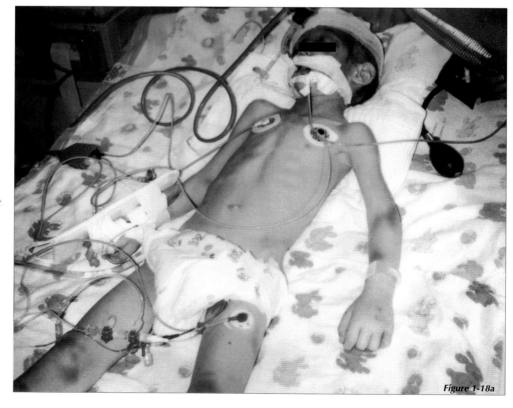

Figure 1-18a

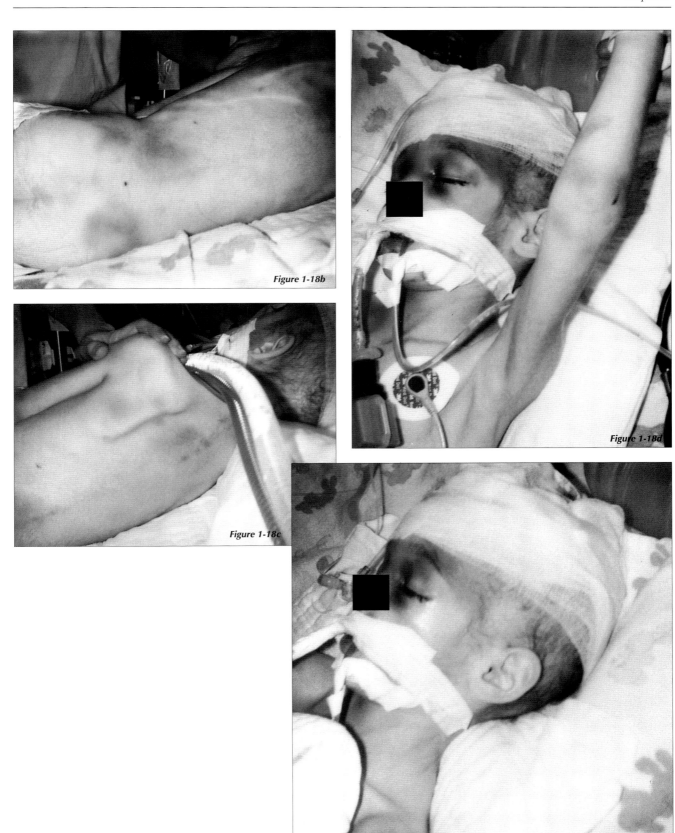

Figure 1-18b

Figure 1-18c

Figure 1-18d

Figure 1-18e

Figure 1-19. Dog bites on an 8-year-old boy. Note the prominent canine teeth marks.

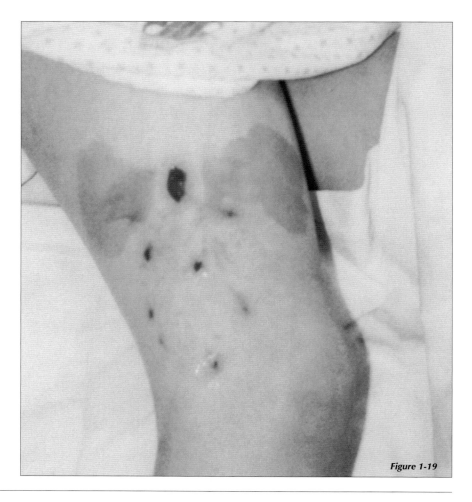

Figure 1-19

Figure 1-20. The injuries on this 8-month-old boy consisted of multiple coalesced, short, linear lesions principally on the dorsum of both hands (*a* to *d*). The caregiver said that he saw a rat coming out of the child's room and thought that was probably how the injuries occurred. When challenged, saying that these did not appear to be rat bites, the caregiver said that they had a puppy in the house, that the child liked to play with the puppy, and that the injuries were most likely caused by the puppy scratching the child. The injuries were believed by the healthcare workers to be secondary to disciplining the child with a hairbrush or similar instrument.

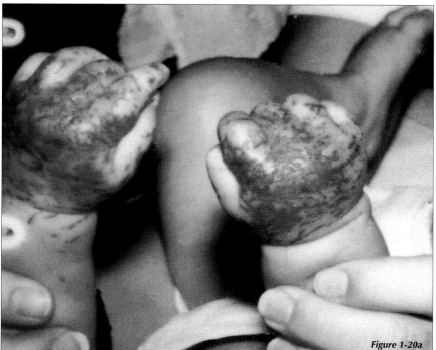

Figure 1-20a

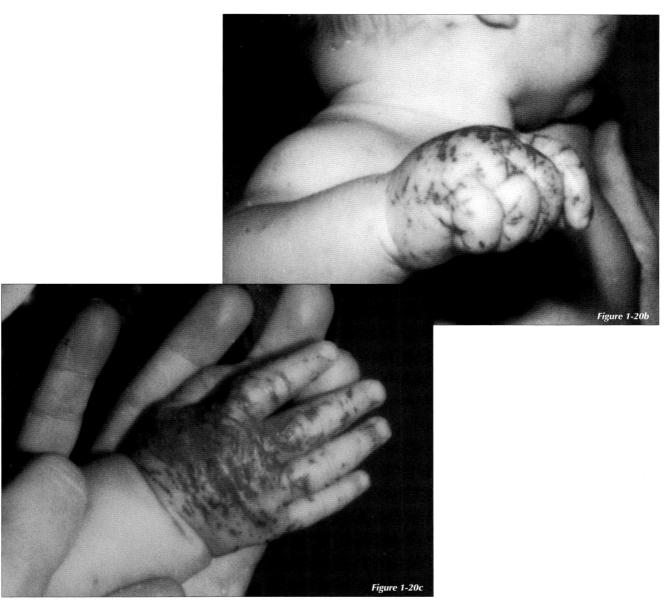

Figure 1-20b

Figure 1-20c

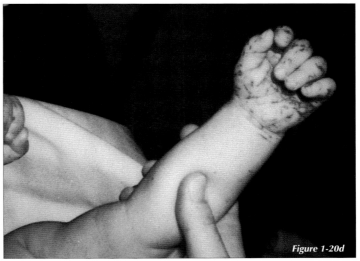

Figure 1-20d

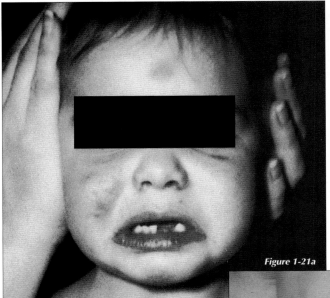

Figure 1-21. This 2-year-old boy presented with facial bruising (**a**), a large ecchymotic area on the abdomen (**b**), and an avulsed tooth (**c**). When confronted, the child's father admitted to losing patience with the child and beating him.

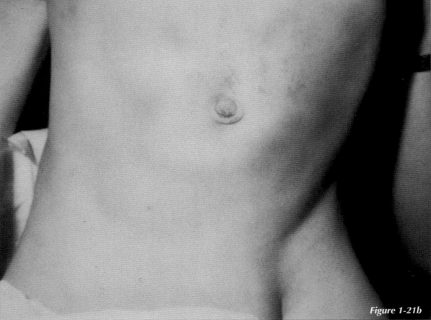

Figure 1-21a

Figure 1-21b

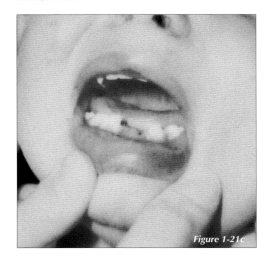

Figure 1-21c

Figure 1-22. *This exhibit was used in a criminal trial to demonstrate a human bite on the back of a 9-month-old boy. A forensic dentist was able to match the bite injury with the bite of the mother's boyfriend.*

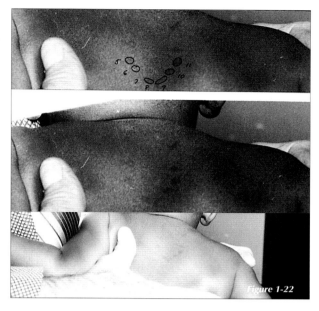

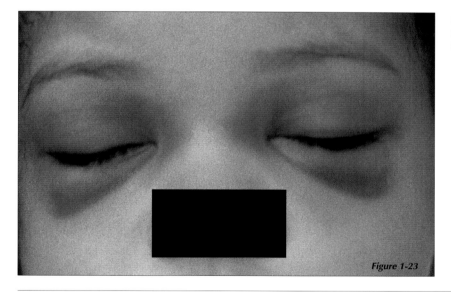

Figure 1-23. *This 2-year-old girl with bilateral black eyes supposedly walked into a door. Her nose was not broken.*

Figure 1-24. *Bruising of the buttocks. The lesion in the upper right area of the buttocks is a nevus and not related to the abuse.*

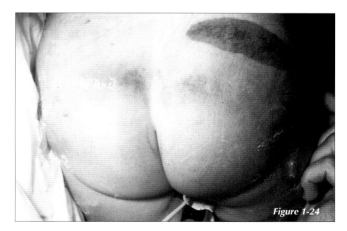

Figure 1-25. *Multiple bruises on a 3-year-old boy sustained in a "fall." These injuries involve the lateral face (**a**) and the genital area (**b** to **d**) and are abuse.*

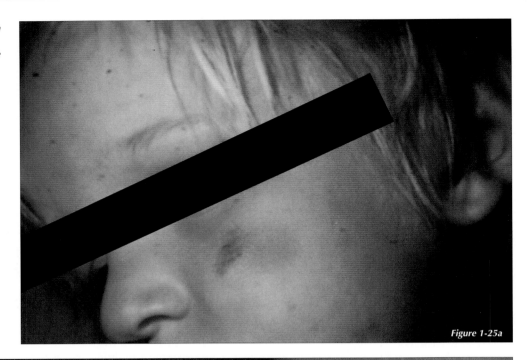

Figure 1-25a

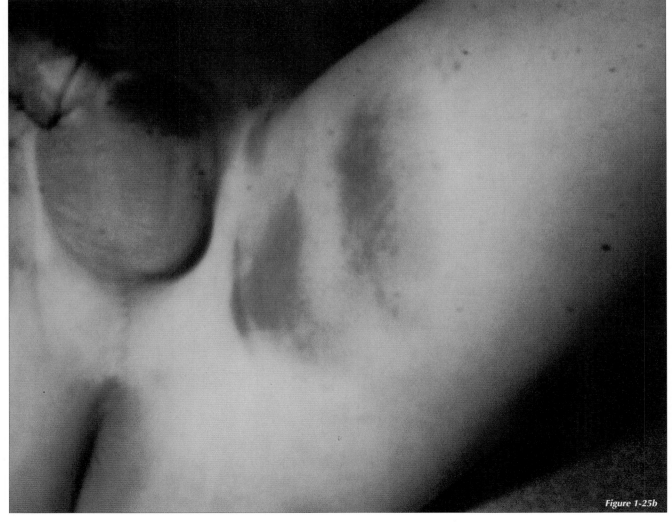

Figure 1-25b

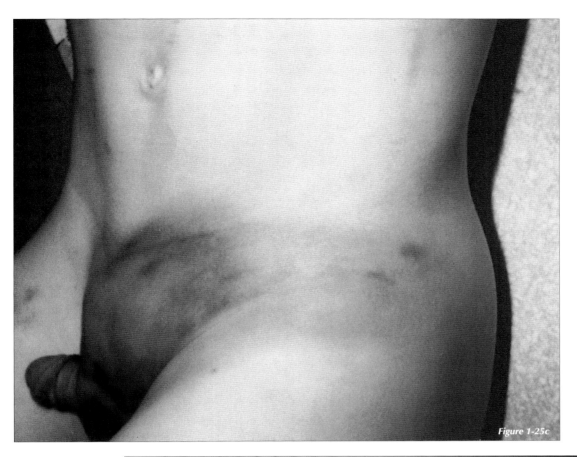

Figure 1-25c

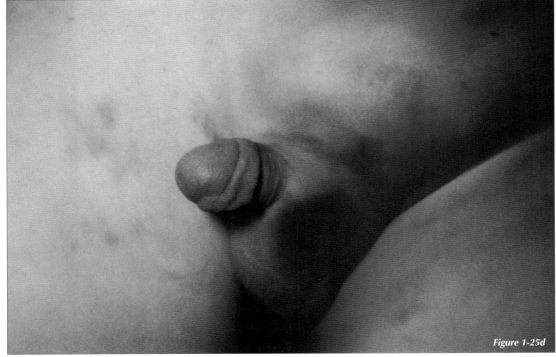

Figure 1-25d

Figure 1-26. *This 24-month-old girl was brought in by the police. Her mother had left her in the care of a 4-year-old sibling while she ran to answer a phone call next door. The 4-year-old ran after the mother, leaving the child unattended. Supposedly the 2-year-old child tried to follow them. A neighbor found the child naked in the middle of the yard, sitting in a dog run. The dog was a puppy. The neighbor said that the dog was to the side, away from the child, at the time. The mother stated that the child's injuries were inflicted by the dog. None of the injuries were bites, and none resembled dog scratches (**a** through **e**). The dog was chained. None of the injuries appeared to be made by a chain. The child also had an anal tear and several puncture wounds of the perianal area (**g**). Vaginal examination showed an imperforate hymen (under low power in **h**). Note that it appears to be fresher than the other wounds, which are in the process of healing. The arrow in **i** shows an anal puncture wound. The ecchymotic areas of the back (**b**) were parallel to one another. The abrasions on the back and chest (**b** and **c**) were all singular and linear. The child had lateral facial bruising and ecchymoses (**a**). The caregiver was reported for abuse. Neither the history nor the extent of the injury matched the injuries. The means of the injuries was not determined. **F** is shown for comparison, illustrating a 3-year-old child who was bitten numerous times by a dog.*

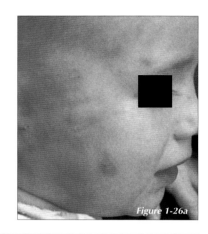

Figure 1-26a

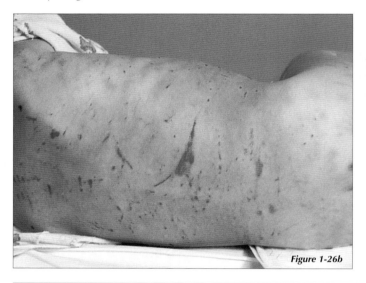

Figure 1-26b

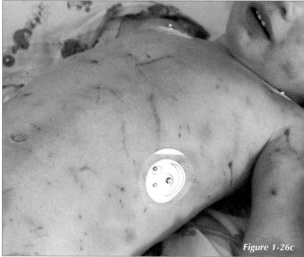

Figure 1-26c

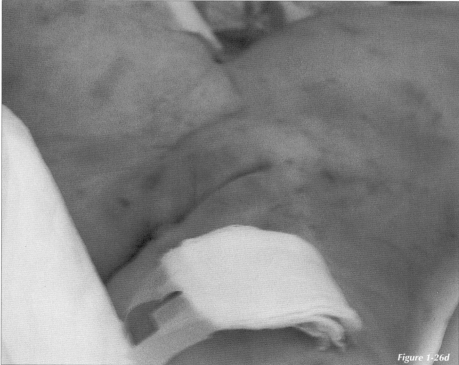

Figure 1-26d

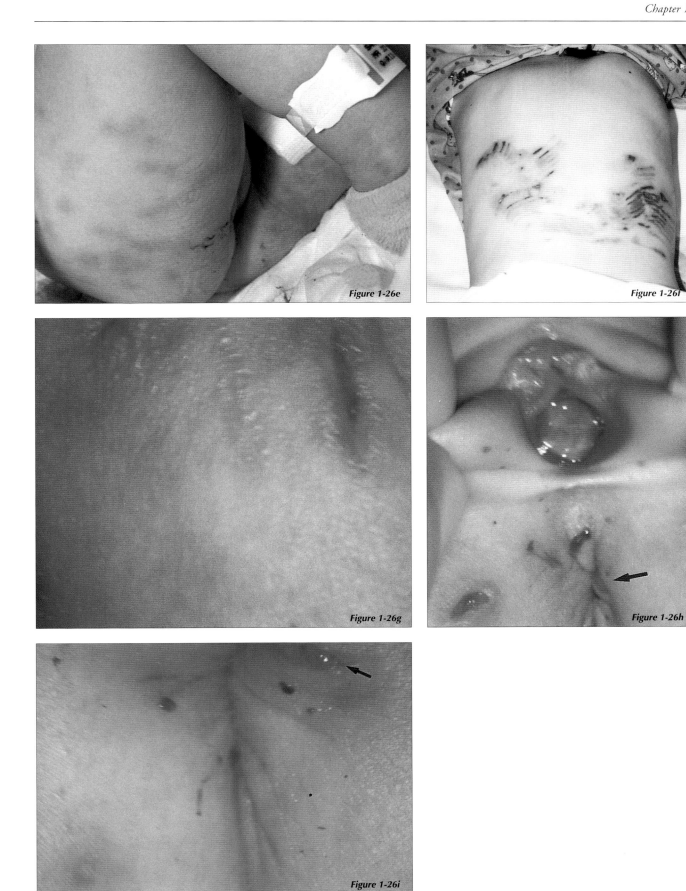

Figure 1-26e

Figure 1-26f

Figure 1-26g

Figure 1-26h

Figure 1-26i

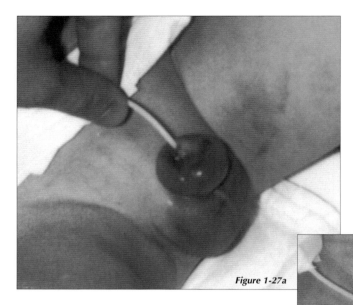

Figure 1-27. *This 25-month-old boy was in the care of his mother's boyfriend while his mother was asleep. The history was that the child had climbed up the back of a rocking chair that was propped against the wall. When told to get down, he quickly stepped down and the rocker lunged forward, throwing him over the arm of the rocker. He straddled the arm momentarily as he fell and struck his forehead on the floor. The glans and shaft of the penis were injured. The scrotum was ecchymotic but not swollen. The blood accumulation in the scrotum was probably drainage from the penile injury, as it followed fascial planes and settled in a more dependent area (**a** and **b**). After an investigation of the scene by a state child protection worker, the injury was determined to be consistent with an accidental straddle injury.*

Figure 1-27a

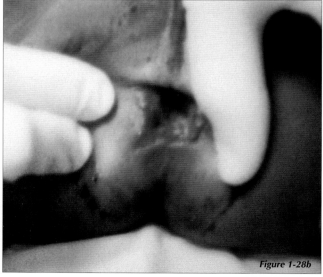

Figure 1-27b

Figure 1-28. *This 4-year-old boy was left in the care of his 16-year-old cousin while his father went to the store. When the father returned, the boy complained of anal pain. The father noted blood in the child's underwear and took him to the hospital. The boy was found to have a severe laceration of the anus extending into the rectum (**a** and **b**). He also had anal laxity and dilation. He initially said that he did not know how it happened but later described anal intercourse by the cousin. The cousin stated that the boy had fallen on an exercise bike.*

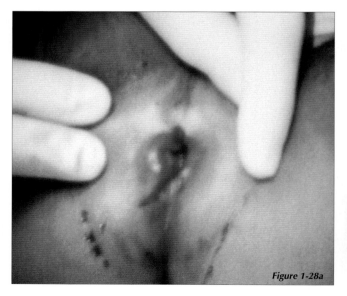

Figure 1-28a

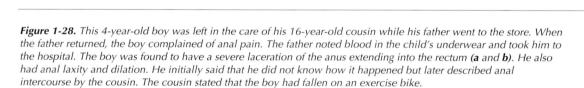

Figure 1-28b

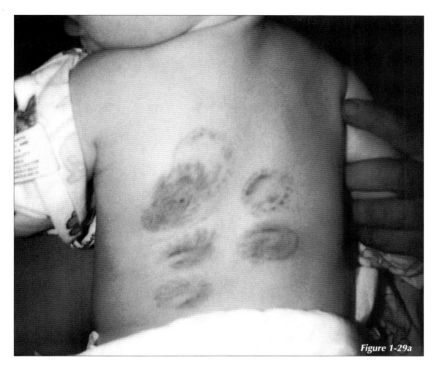

Figure 1-29. *Multiple bites on the back (**a**), chest (**b**), and side (**c**) of an 11-month-old girl. These were inflicted by a sibling. The case was reported for poor supervision.*

Figure 1-29a

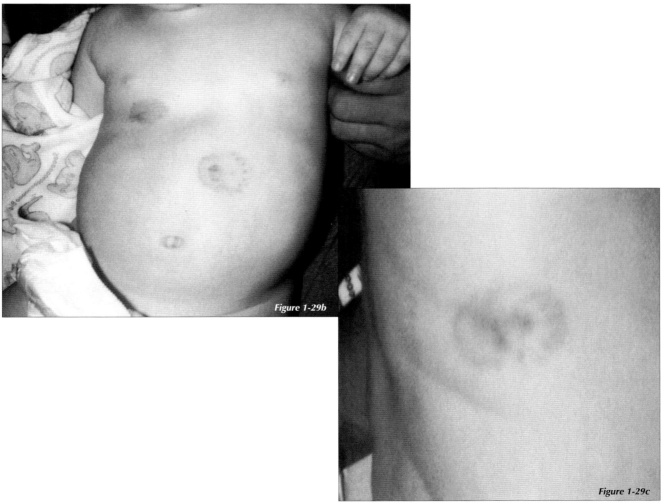

Figure 1-29b

Figure 1-29c

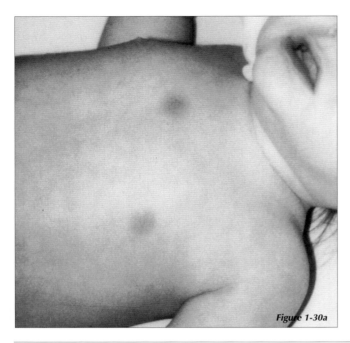

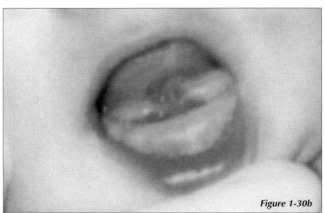

Figure 1-30. This 5-month-old infant was seen in acute care for a fever. She was found to have several small ecchymotic areas on the chest (a) and one on the hip. She also had a torn frenulum (b).

Figure 1-30a

Figure 1-30b

Figure 1-31. This 5-year-old exhibited bruising of the buttocks (a) and upper leg (b) following a spanking.

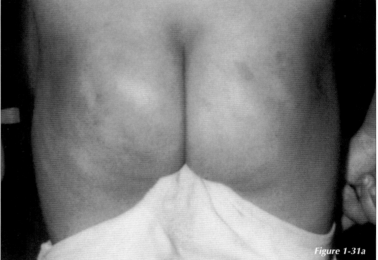

Figure 1-31a

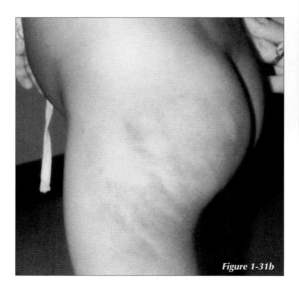

Figure 1-31b

Figure 1-32. This 4-year-old boy was seen in the emergency room following a near strangulation. He and his family were waiting in line at a restaurant. He was playing with a restraining rope when he was pushed into the rope by a sibling. The rope encircled his neck and burned him (*a through c*) but did not occlude the airway or blood supply. He was not unconscious. The event was witnessed by others. In intentional strangulation, the person generally loses consciousness and suffers facial petechiae.

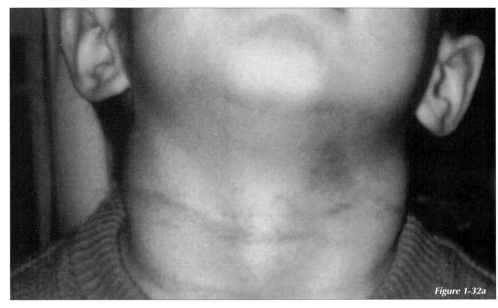

Figure 1-32a

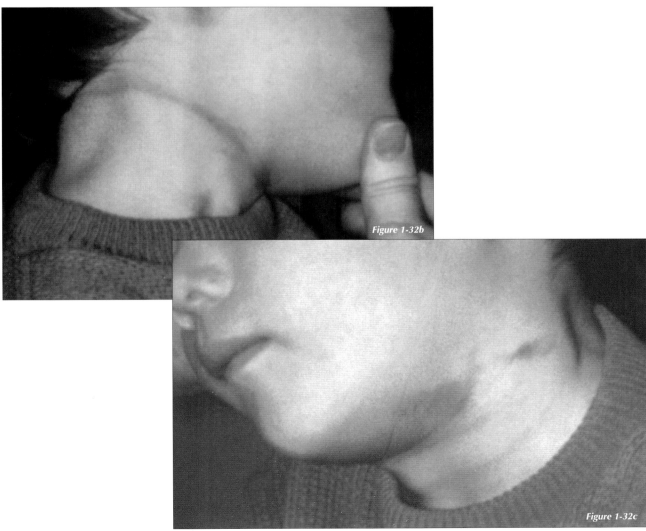

Figure 1-32b

Figure 1-32c

Figure 1-33. This 2-year-old boy was taken to the emergency room by his mother and her boyfriend. The mother said that the child had been vomiting for the past day, unable to hold any food or liquids down, and that he had a fever. The child had multiple bruises in various stages of healing (**a** through **d**) and on multiple surface areas, including the genitalia (**e**). When asked why the child had so many bruises, the mother said that he had been injured by their dog. The child had a post-traumatic pancreatic pseudocyst, requiring surgery, and a laceration of the pancreas. The child was well below the third percentile in height and weight. The child was in the care of his mother's boyfriend while the mother worked. It is important to note that although the child had a severe intra-abdominal injury there was no evidence of injury to the external abdominal wall.

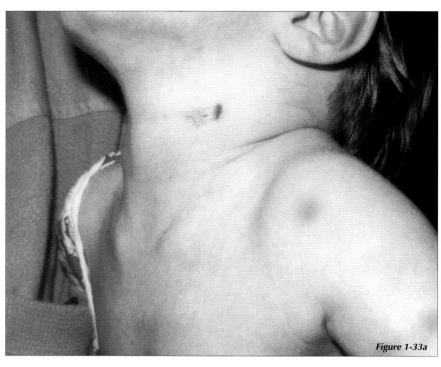

Figure 1-33a

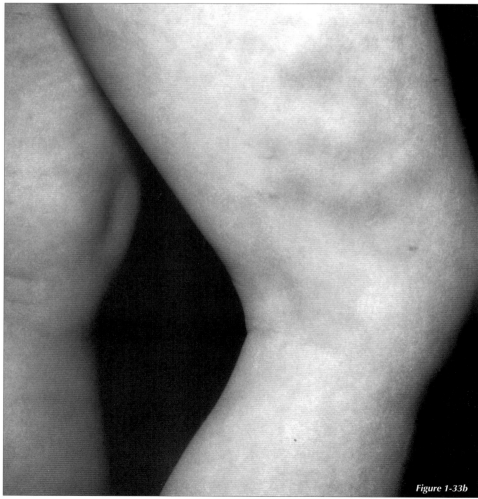

Figure 1-33b

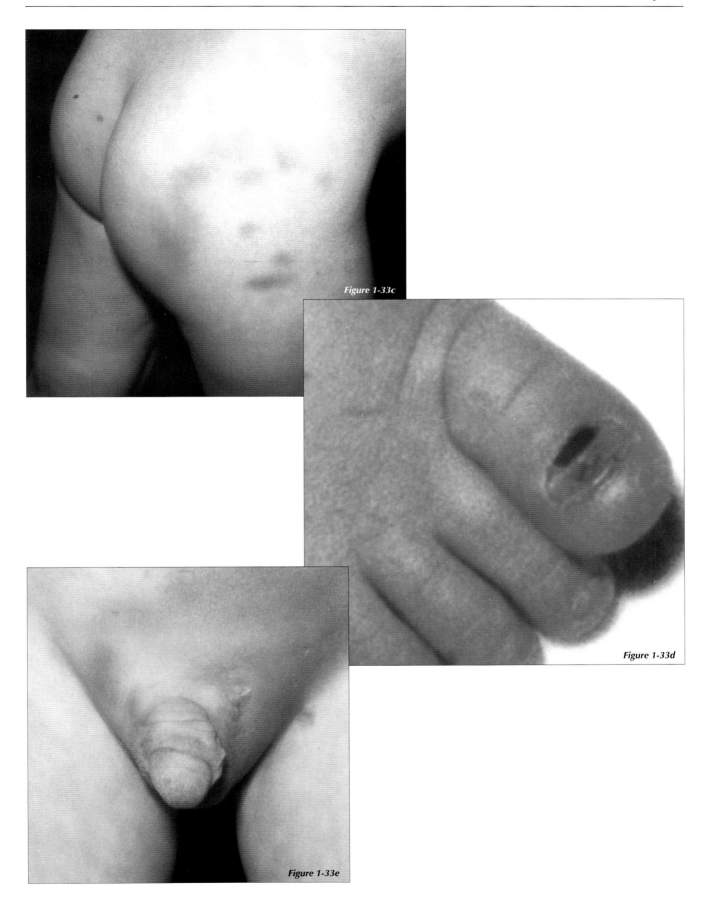

Figure 1-33c

Figure 1-33d

Figure 1-33e

Figure 1-34. This 15-year-old girl was beaten by her father. She had eye **(a)** and oral injuries **(b** and **c)**. The oral injuries are not noticeable when her mouth is closed.

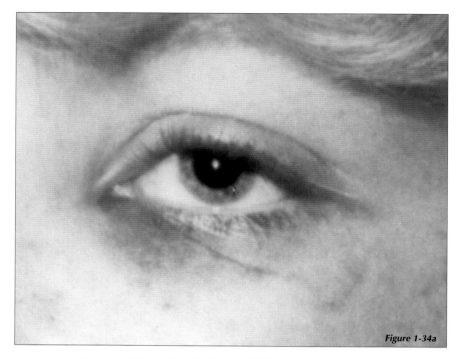

Figure 1-34a

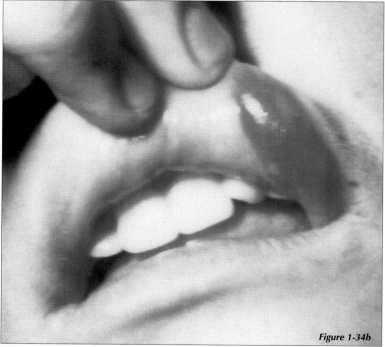

Figure 1-34b

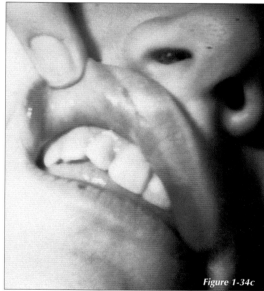

Figure 1-34c

Figure 1-35. **a**, *15-month-old with multiple bite marks to the back, abdomen, chest, and arm. Note in **b** the outer circle is the bite mark, the inner circle is the thrust mark, and the central ecchymotic area is the suck mark. The suck mark and/or the thrust mark are missing from some bites.*

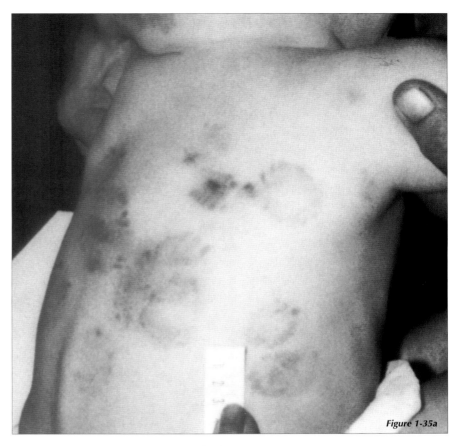

Figure 1-35a

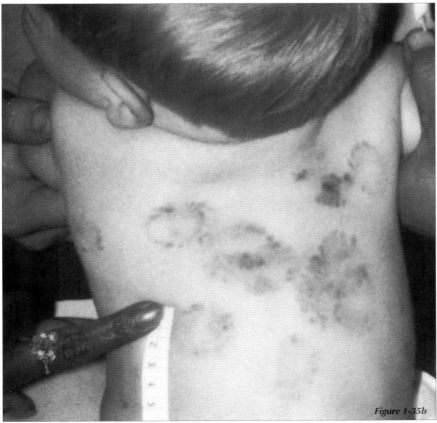

Figure 1-35b

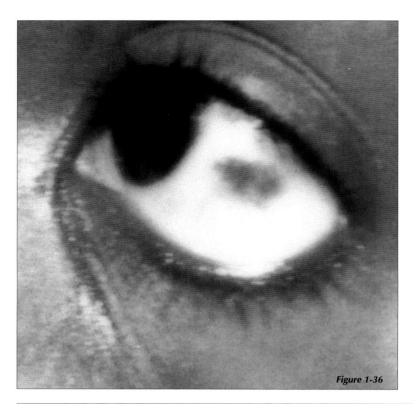

Figure 1-36. *This 5-year-old boy was seen in the emergency room for a conjunctival injury. He was intentionally struck in the eye by his mother's boyfriend. This should not be confused with the subconjunctival hemorrhage of suffocation. The latter differs in that it is thicker and more diffuse than this traumatic injury.*

Figure 1-36

Figure 1-37. *This 6-year-old boy was falsely believed to have been abused. He had bilateral epidemic keratoconjunctivitis, which is caused by several viruses (a and b), and bilateral flushing of the cheeks, which added to the impression of abuse.*

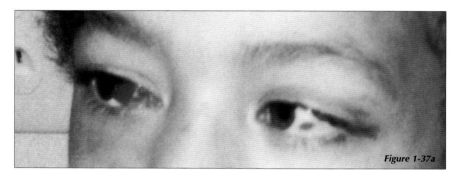

Figure 1-37a

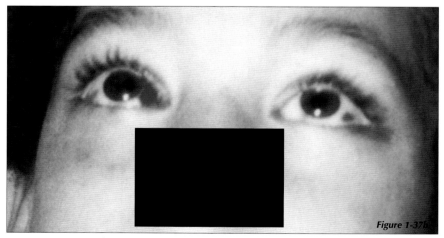

Figure 1-37b

Figure 1-38. *This 23-month-old boy had loop marks to his face (**a** and **b**) and an eye injury (**c**) as a result of a beating.*

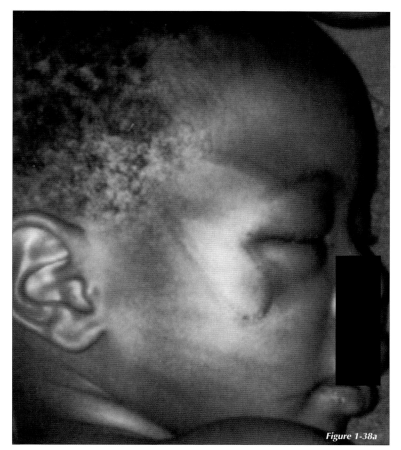

Figure 1-38a

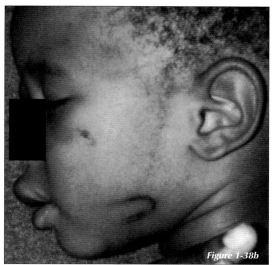

Figure 1-38b

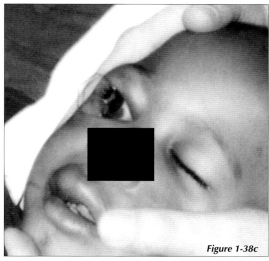

Figure 1-38c

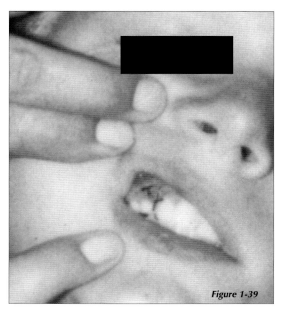

Figure 1-39

Figure 1-39. *An avulsed tooth in a 10-year-old boy with loop marks to his face and an eye injury as a result of a beating.*

Figure 1-40. This 3-year-old boy was first seen in a small community hospital emergency room with the history that he had a fever and had been vomiting for 2 days. Before coming to the hospital he had a convulsion. The child had a large hematoma of the left ear that supposedly occurred because he had been jumping on the bed and struck his ear against the bed post. He had bruises on his chin (**b**) and leg (**c**) and a torn frenulum (**a** and **b**). He had a skull fracture with a subdural hematoma, a lacerated liver and pancreas, a fractured humerus, and large patches of hair pulled out. In addition, he showed evidence of nutritional neglect.

The mother and her three children (the patient, a 4-year-old brother, and a 9-year-old sister) had been living and traveling across the country with a man and his 3-year-old son. The older sister related how the man had killed a younger brother and buried him somewhere in Oregon. Although the man severely abused the patient, his brother, and his sister, the man's own child was not physically abused.

After several days in the hospital the patient was recovering. Note the lid lag and flat affect (**d**) as well as the wasted extremities (**e**). (**f**) Recent injury to ear, caused by a blow to the side of the face. When the injury heals without medical intervention it leaves a distortion of the ear cartilage often called "cauliflower" ear.

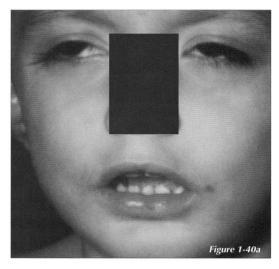

Figure 1-40a

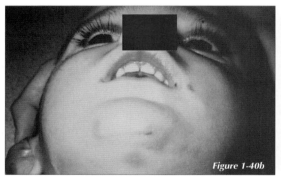

Figure 1-40b

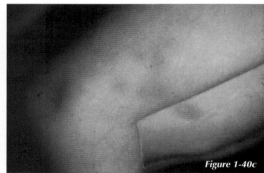

Figure 1-40c

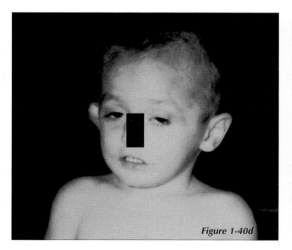

Figure 1-40d

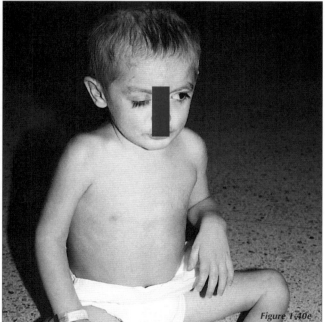

Figure 1-40e

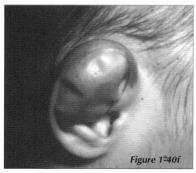

Figure 1-40f

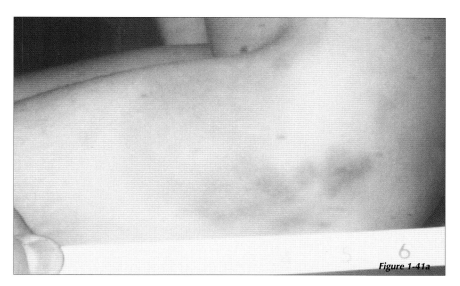

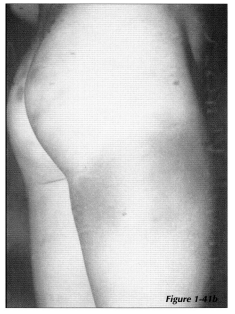

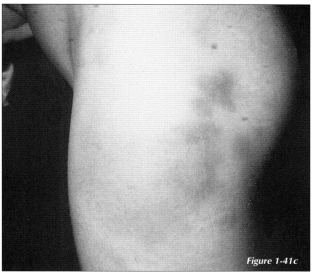

Figure 1-41. The 9-year-old sister of the patient in Figure 1-40 had multiple bruises in various stages of healing *(a* through *d)*. She had also been sexually abused.

Figure 1-41a

Figure 1-41b

Figure 1-41c

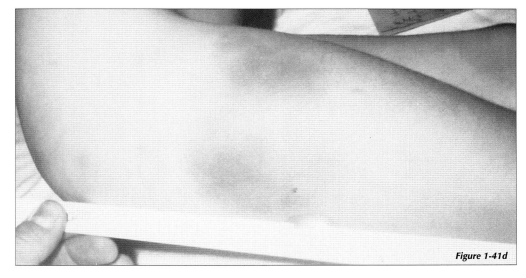

Figure 1-41d

Figure 1-42. *A 3-year-old who is recovering from a closed head injury caused by abuse. He previously had a hematoma of the right ear that had gone untreated and left a residual deformation of the cartilage (cauliflower ear, **a**). Compare with his normal left ear (**b**). This deformity can be congenital.*

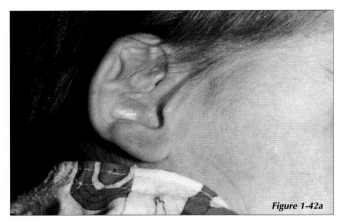

Figure 1-42a

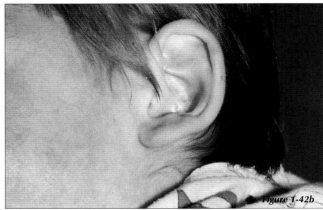

Figure 1-42b

Figure 1-43. *Scarred linear and loop marks in a 4-year-old boy.*

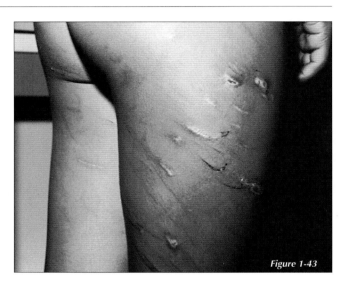

Figure 1-43

Figure 1-44. *This 6-year-old boy came to the emergency room with a history that he had accidentally injured his eye (**a**). An alert resident noted fresh loop marks on the child (**b**) and the child stated that his eye was struck while he was being whipped. He had a corneal abrasion.*

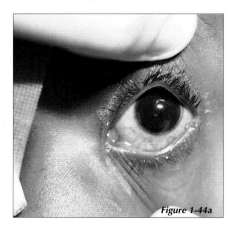

Figure 1-44a

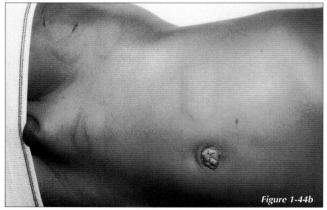

Figure 1-44b

Figure 1-45. *This 3-year-old girl supposedly fell down the stairs. She had fresh bruises, all of the same age, on every body surface (**a** through **c**). She had a closed head injury with a cerebral hemorrhage and blunt trauma to the abdomen. The 18-year-old mother was living with a 21-year-old man. When the history given was challenged, the mother admitted that she and her boyfriend "got stoned" and beat the child. Six weeks before this admission the child was seen in another hospital with similar but less serious injuries. The child was sent home with the understanding that the boyfriend would no longer have access to the child. The family was not monitored closely enough and the boyfriend returned. The child is presently in a rehabilitative hospital in a chronic vegetative state.*

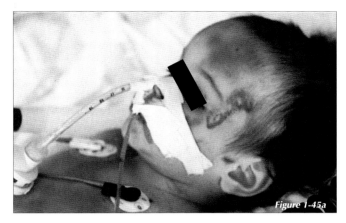

Figure 1-45a

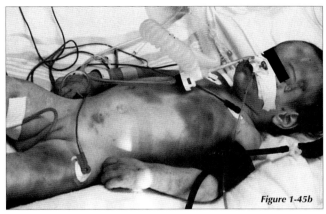

Figure 1-45b

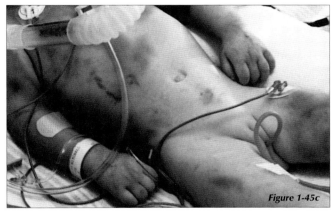

Figure 1-45c

Figure 1-46. *Pinch to the glans penis for wetting.*

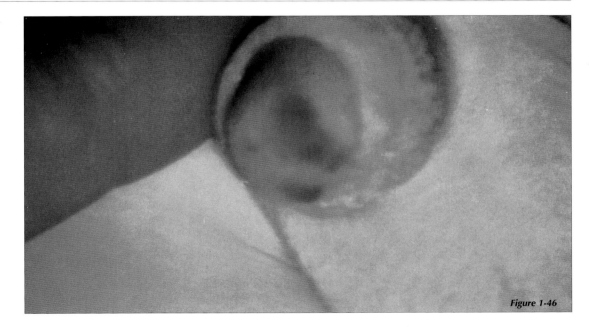

Figure 1-46

Figure 1-47. This 4-year-old girl was taken to the emergency room with swelling and ecchymosis of both hands (**a**). This is early Henoch-Schonlein purpura. Note the beginning of lesions on her lower legs. Within hours a more familiar pattern appeared on her buttocks and legs (**b**). Note the circumferential lesions of the lower extremities caused by pressure from the elastic of her socks (**c**).

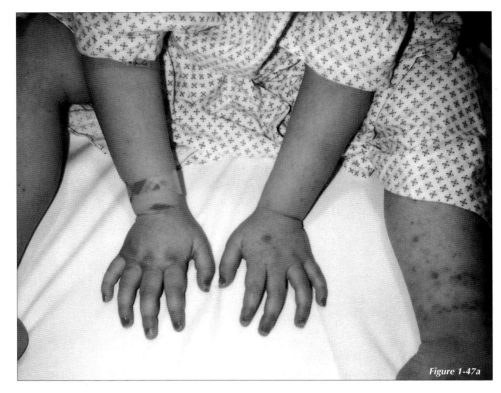

Figure 1-47a

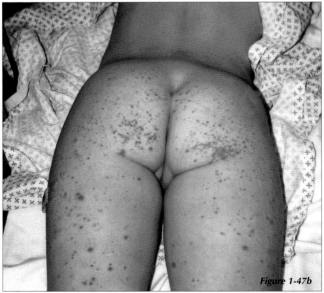

Figure 1-47b

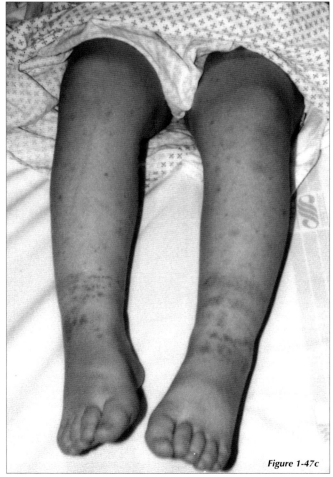

Figure 1-47c

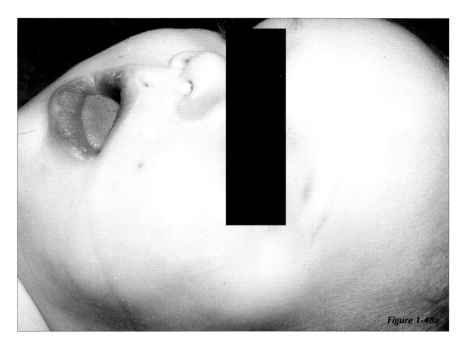

Figure 1-48a

Figure 1-48. a, This 5-month-old boy was seen in the emergency room with the history that he had accidentally aspirated pepper. He was dead on arrival. The caregiver stated that the pepper shaker was lying on the floor. The cap was apparently loose. The baby crawled over to the pepper shaker, grasped it, rolled over, the pepper fell onto his face, and he aspirated it. He stopped breathing. The actions described are beyond a 5-month-old child's developmental level. The mother later admitted that she was trying to break the child of sucking his thumb. In frustration she covered his mouth with a handful of pepper. The child had no external evidence of abuse. The pulmonary tree was loaded with pepper even to the alveoli (*b* to *d*). Note that there is no external evidence of trauma or pepper.

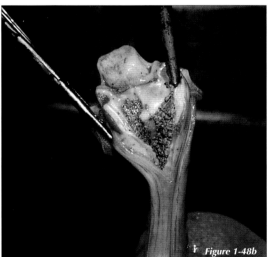

Figure 1-48b

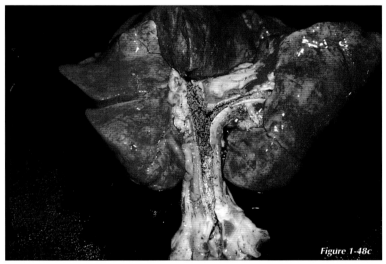

Figure 1-48c

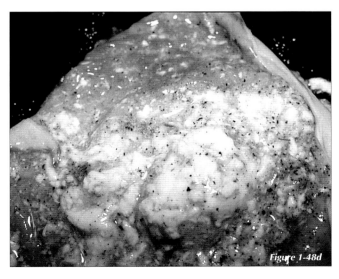

Figure 1-48d

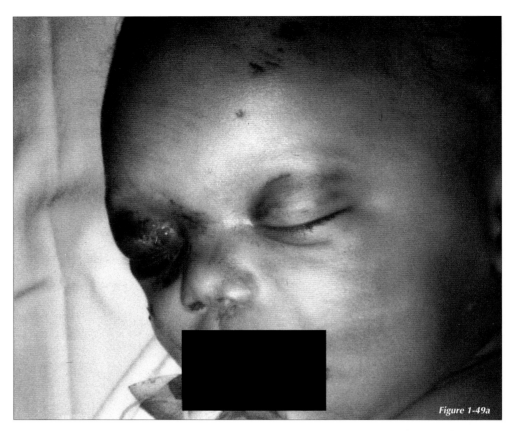

Figure 1-49. *This 5-month-old girl was beaten with a broom by her father in a domestic argument with her mother (a to d).*

Figure 1-49a

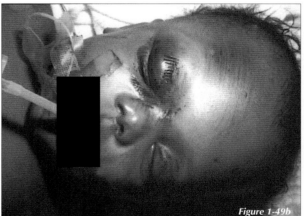

Figure 1-49b

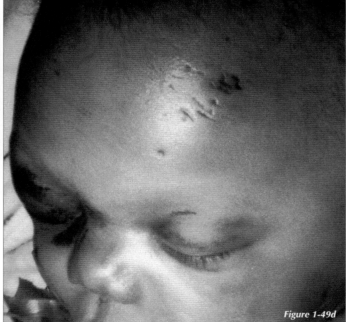

Figure 1-49d

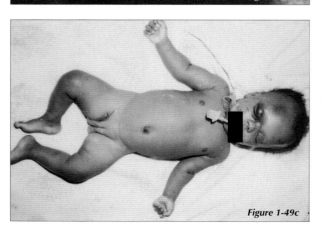

Figure 1-49c

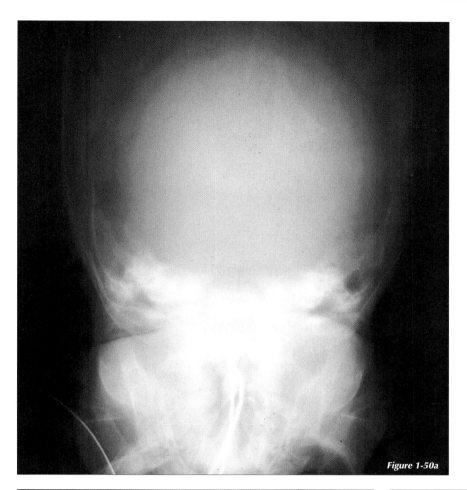

Figure 1-50a

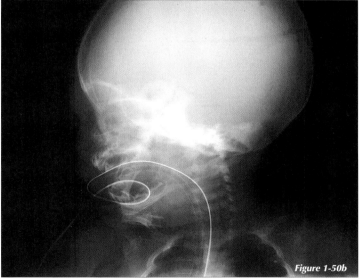

Figure 1-50b

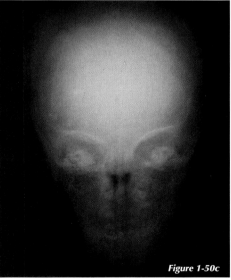

Figure 1-50c

Figure 1-50.
Radiographs
*(**a** to **c**) of the child*
in Figure 1-49. She
had multiple skull
fractures.

Figure 1-51.
Two children with Ehlers-Danlos syndrome. This condition has been mistaken for abuse. The skin is fragile, thin, and resembles cigarette paper in consistency. These children bruise easily and scar extensively. (Courtesy Dorothy K. Grange, M.D.)

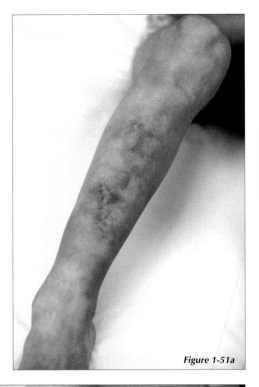

Figure 1-51a

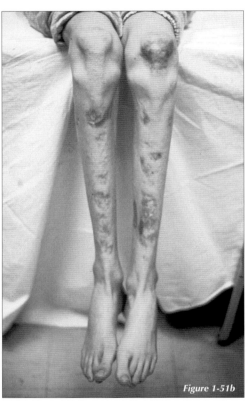

Figure 1-51b

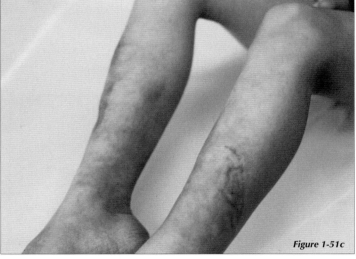

Figure 1-51c

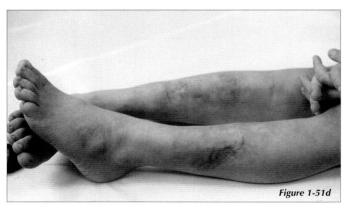

Figure 1-51d

Figure 1-52. *Child with burns to his face, back (**a** to **c**), and buttocks. He also had multiple cigarette burns, old (**d**) and new (**e**), two of which are shown here. He had choke marks to his neck (**f**). His mother was a former mental hospital patient who had been noncompliant with her antipsychotic medication regimen for several years. She had two other children who had been removed permanently a year earlier because of abuse. Although this child was 3 1/2 years old, the mother had successfully eluded state protective services all that time. He had no immunizations. (Courtesy James J. Williams, M.D.)*

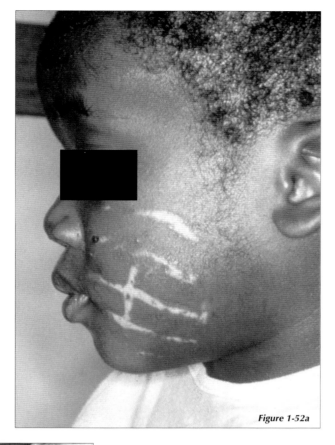

Figure 1-52a

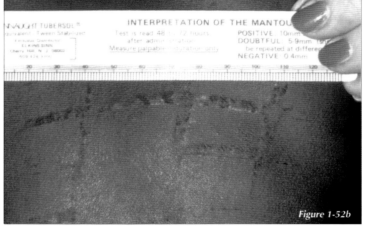

Figure 1-52b

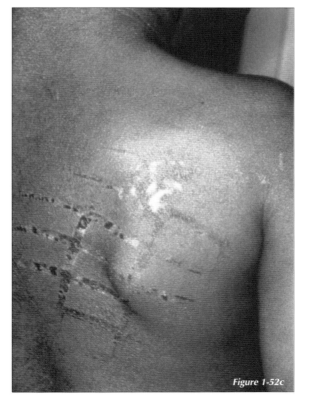

Figure 1-52c

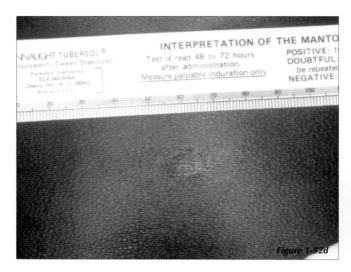

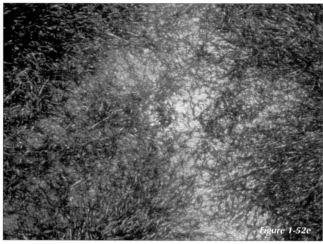

Figure 1-52e

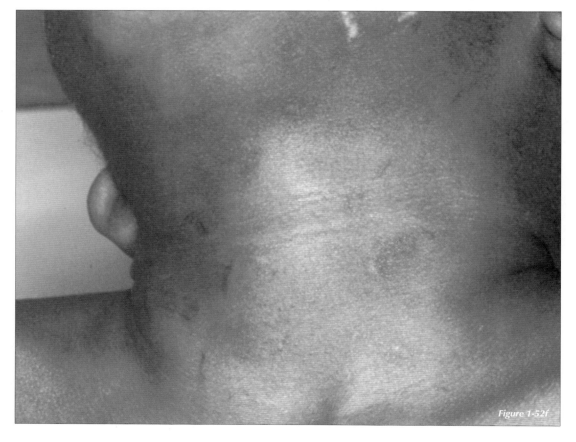

Figure 1-52f

Figure 1-53. *This 4-month-old girl was seen by social services and found to have linear bruising of her neck **(a).** The line of bruising was anterior and, with a sweep upward, ended at the posterior base of the ear **(b).** The mother's boyfriend admitted to picking her up by the back of her shirt and suspending her in the air until she stopped crying. (Courtesy Officer S. Krakowiecki and Investigator S. Blair.)*

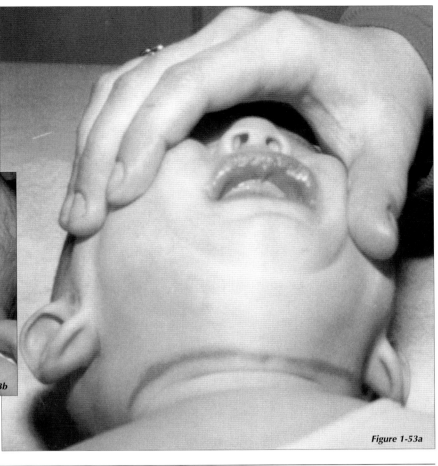

Figure 1-53a

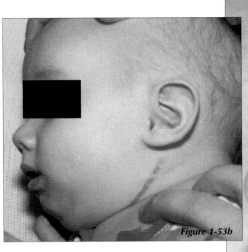

Figure 1-53b

Figure 1-54. *This 3-year-old boy had dried blood in his external ear canal. His eardrum had ruptured as the result of a slap to the side of the head.*

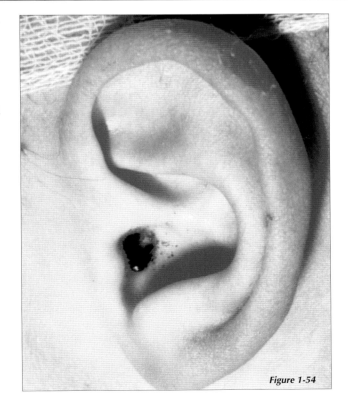

Figure 1-54

Figure 1-55. A 10-month-old boy who was taken to the emergency room by his parents because he was irritable. They noted bruising of his abdomen and chest **(a)** and abrasions to the side of his face **(b)**. He had been left in the care of an adolescent male. The injuries to his face were done by a pick comb **(c).** Liver enzyme levels were elevated as a result of blunt trauma to the abdomen.

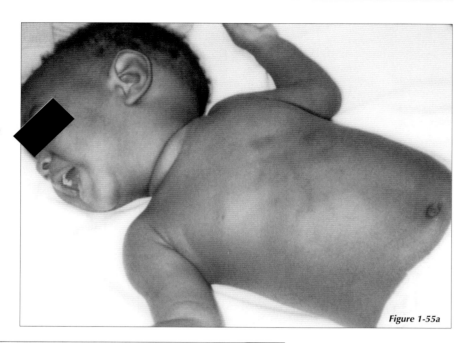

Figure 1-55a

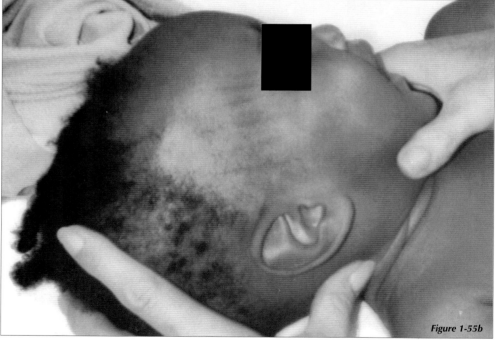

Figure 1-55b

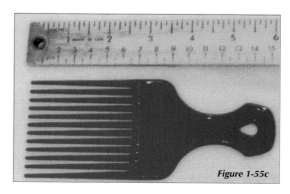

Figure 1-55c

Figure 1-56.
Housestaff believed this injury of the upper and lower lip to be abuse. It turned out to be a self-induced suck mark.

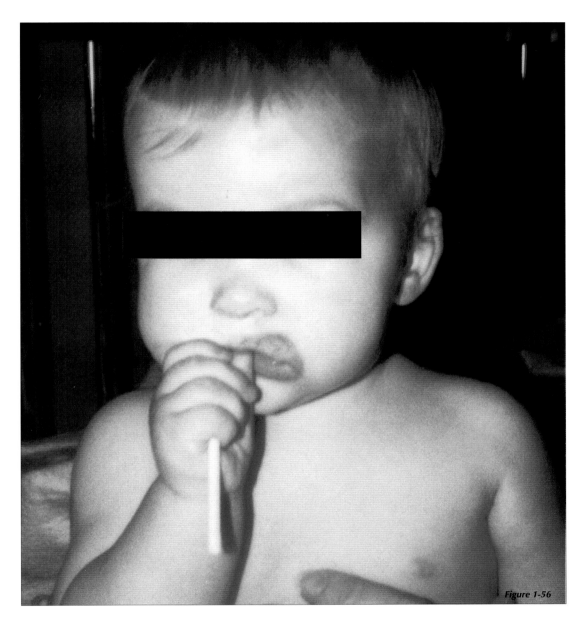

Figure 1-56

BURNS
PART 1

JAMES A. MONTELEONE, M.D.
ANTHONY J. SCALZO, M.D.

Children who are burned abusively are marked or branded with the outward manifestation of parental violence, emotional imbalance, impulsivity, educational and cultural deprivation, and poverty. Intentionally burning a child is a controlled, premeditated, or even sadistic action. In terms of severity among the various forms of abuse, burns rank first. They cause both physical and emotional trauma at the time of the incident, and often produce long-term physical and psychological scarring.

It has been estimated that burns are the third most common form of childhood accidental death in the United States, causing more than 1300 deaths each year. The numbers of burns not brought to medical attention and those that go unreported as abuse are probably significant. In general, the victim of abusive burning is young, 3 to 4 years of age at most. The abuser who burns typically is educationally or culturally deprived, single or divorced, unemployed, abuses women also, and may be isolated, suspicious, rigid, dependent, and immature.

The six categories of burn injury are flame, scald, contact (with a hot object), electrical, chemical, and ultraviolet radiation (sunburn). Abusive burns generally cluster in the scald and contact categories, although there are rare reports of the others. Children's skin is much thinner than adult skin, so serious burning occurs more rapidly and at lower temperatures.

Medical treatment of the injury must be the first priority in burn patients. Once these needs are met, efforts are directed toward obtaining a careful history outlining the time, nature, extent, and location where the burn occurred. All cases in which abuse by burning is suspected must be investigated thoroughly. Again, the evaluator's focus is on whether the injury could have occurred as the caregiver described and whether the child is developmentally capable of performing the actions reported.

When a child presents with a burn and one or more of the following factors are found, the evaluator should consider abuse:

1. Multiple hematomas or scars in various stages of healing

2. Concurrent injuries or evidence of neglect such as malnutrition and failure to thrive (especially suspicious are bone injuries such as old rib fractures and distal tibial, metaphyseal, or spiral fractures)

3. History of multiple prior hospitalizations for "accidental" trauma

4. An inexplicable delay between time of injury and first attempt to obtain medical attention (In some cases, if the parent has medical training, such as an R.N. or M.D., the delay may be because the parents tried initially to care for the burn on their own.)

5. Burns appearing older than the alleged day of the accident, similarly indicating ambivalence about seeking care and possibly risking exposure of the abuse

6. An account of the incident not comparable with age and ability of the child (An example is that of an infant who "crawled into the hot bathtub" when the infant is only a few months old and developmentally incapable of doing so.)

7. The responsible adults allege that there were no witnesses to the "accident" and the child was merely discovered to be burned, thus hoping to discourage further inquiry

8. Relatives other than the parents bring the injured child to the hospital or a nonrelated adult brings the child (unless there is a good explanation for the parents' absence, such as when a child is being cared for by a babysitter while the parents are out of town)

9. The burn is attributed to action of a sibling or other child (Although this is often an explanation for abusive burns, it should be noted that siblings can be abusive.)

10. The injured child is excessively withdrawn, submissive, or overly polite, or does not cry during painful procedures

11. There are scalds of the hands or feet, often symmetrical, appearing to be full thickness in depth, suggesting that the extremities were forcibly immersed and held in hot liquid

12. There are isolated burns of the buttocks or perineum and genitalia or the characteristic doughnut-shaped burn of the buttocks, which in children can hardly ever be produced by accidental means

13. The responsible adults give different stories as to the cause of the burn or change their stories when questioned

The burns presented in this chapter illustrate the patterns found in abusive versus accidental burns. The inability to match the caregivers' descriptions to the patterns observed revealed that the majority of these were abusive injuries. The young ages of the victims are typical of the findings with abusive burns.

Figure 2-1. *An intentional steam iron burn of a 6-year-old boy. Note how clear the pattern is and the visibility of the steam jet holes.*

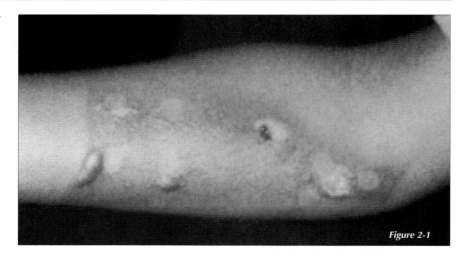

Figure 2-1

Figure 2-2. This child was first seen when he was 26 months old. While in the care of a 14-year-old babysitter he supposedly burned his right hand on a space heater (*a*). It was determined to be an accidental injury. Four months later he again appeared in the emergency room and the parent reported that she had given him a bath the evening before. She did not see the burns until the following day when she noted that the skin on his buttocks was coming off (*b* to *d*). He had a large ecchymotic area on the lower back and a smaller one on the left thigh. These were confluent linear marks. The burning was a part of discipline.

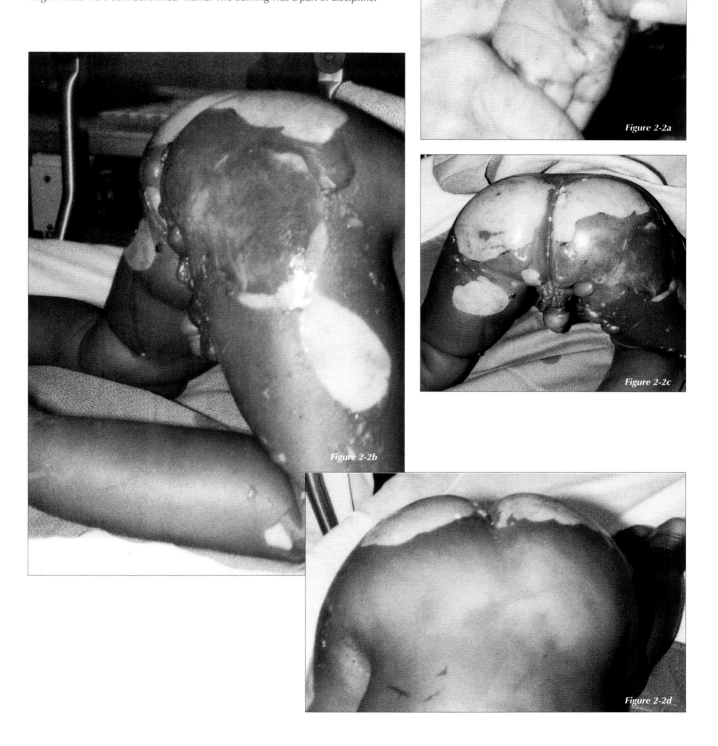

Figure 2-2a

Figure 2-2c

Figure 2-2b

Figure 2-2d

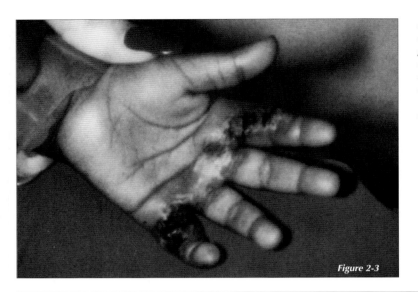

Figure 2-3. This 11-month-old girl was taken to the emergency room with a second-degree burn of the left palm and a linear burn at the base of the fingers. She had no other injuries. The wound is fresh. The child supposedly sustained the injury when she grasped a hot curling iron sitting on the table, which is consistent with the injury. There were no indicators suggesting abuse, so the injury was determined to be accidental.

Figure 2-4. This 8-month-old girl was seen in the emergency room with a second-degree burn of her right cheek. She received the burn from a curling iron. Two older siblings were using the iron at the time, when one of them suddenly turned with the hot curling iron in her hand. She did not realize that the girl was in the second person's lap. The curling iron momentarily touched the child's cheek. The wound is fresh, and the child has no other injuries. The family had no previous reports of abuse, and the wound was consistent with the history. It was determined to be accidental.

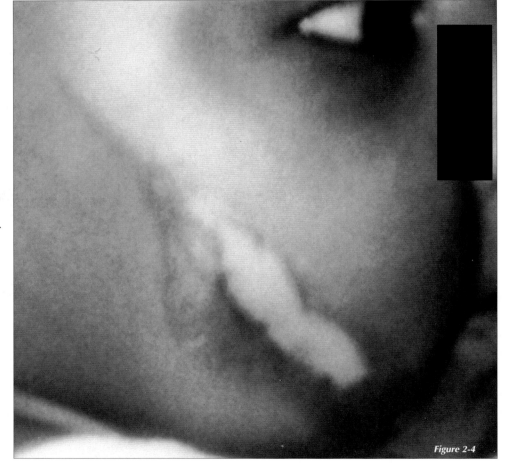

Figure 2-5. This 12-month-old girl was seen in the emergency room with a history of having been burned while sitting in her mother's lap. The mother was holding a hot liquid when the child suddenly moved, causing her to spill the liquid on the child's foot. This was the only area affected. The dorsum and sole of the right foot were burned and the distal foot and area across the instep spared (**a** to **c**). The pattern is irregular at the ankle (**d**) and consistent with a flow of liquid. The point of impact was on the instep. The child raised her foot at impact and the liquid flowed behind and up the ankle. She was wearing a sandal, which accounts for the spared areas.

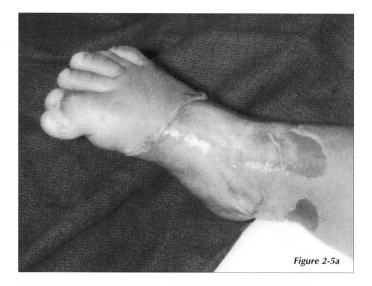

Figure 2-5a

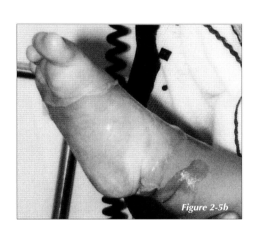

Figure 2-5b

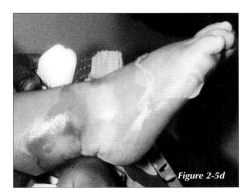

Figure 2-5d

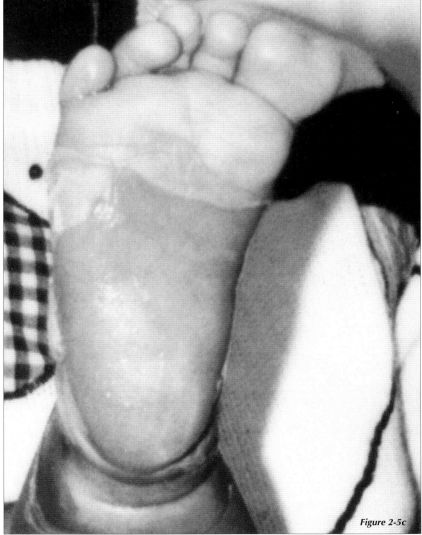

Figure 2-5c

Figure 2-6. *A chemical burn in a 3-year-old girl (**a** and **b**). The child supposedly sat on a bench on which a leaky battery had previously been placed. An investigation supported the explanation.*

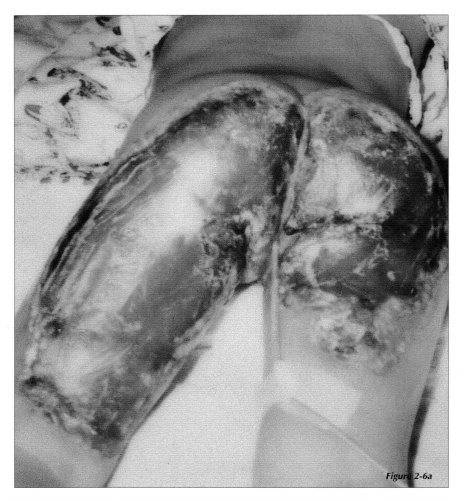

Figure 2-6a

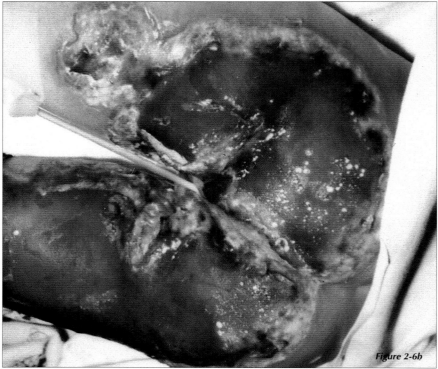

Figure 2-6b

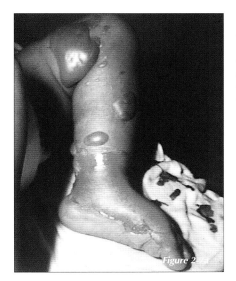

Figure 2-7. *The history given for this burn was that the caregiver had run hot water in the bathtub to wash clothes. She left the tub unattended. When she returned she found the 17-month-old standing in the tub. The history does not fit the injuries. There are two levels of burned areas, and each foot has a different degree of burn (**a** to **c**). Note the stocking-glove pattern on both feet. The left foot has third-degree burns, the level of burn is well above the ankle, and the bottom of the foot is spared. The right foot has second-degree burns, and the burn level is below the ankle. Note splash burns to the upper left leg and right arm (**d** and **e**). This was probably an immersion burn. The left leg was forcibly held in the water, which would explain the sparing of the sole of that foot. The right foot was free and spent less time in the hot water; it was the source of the splash burns.*

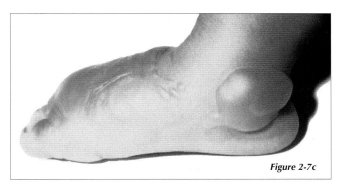

Figure 2-7c

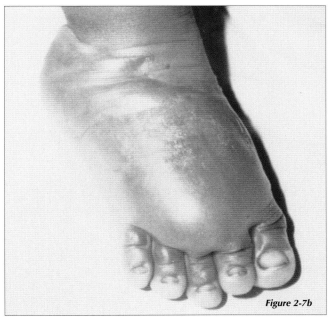

Figure 2-7b

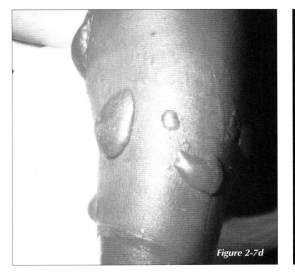

Figure 2-7d

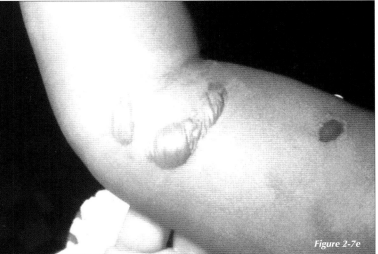

Figure 2-7e

Figure 2-8. *Multiple scarred cigarette burns in a 4-year-old girl who stated that her stepmother would discipline her with a lit cigarette (**b** to **f**). A fresh burn is under the bandage (**a**).*

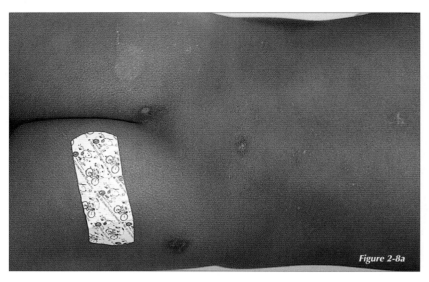

Figure 2-8a

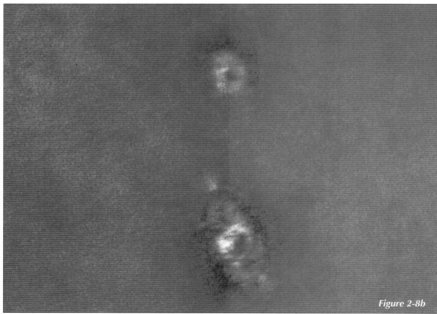

Figure 2-8b

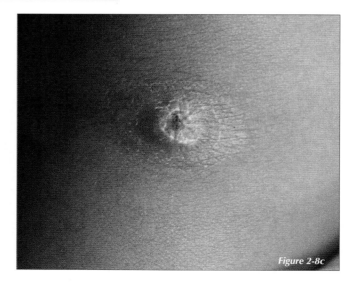

Figure 2-8c

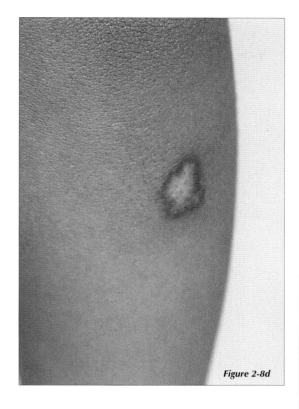

Figure 2-8d

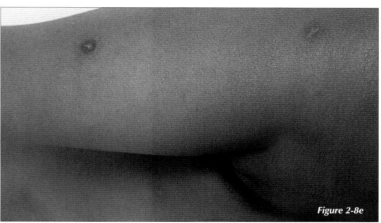

Figure 2-8e

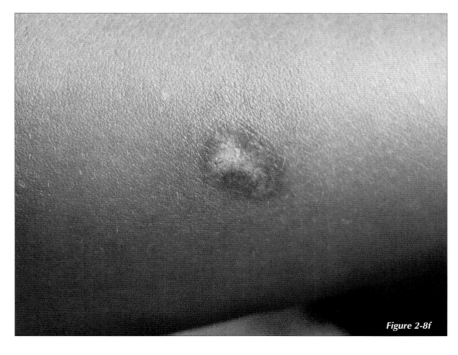

Figure 2-8f

Figure 2-9. Doughnut-shaped burn (see Figure 2-22).

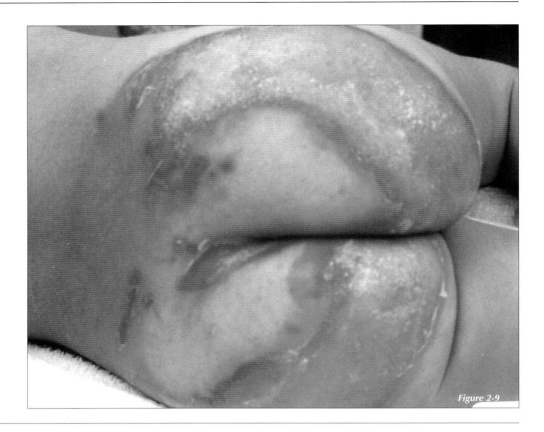

Figure 2-9

Figure 2-10. Pattern burn to buttocks from the top of a space heater.

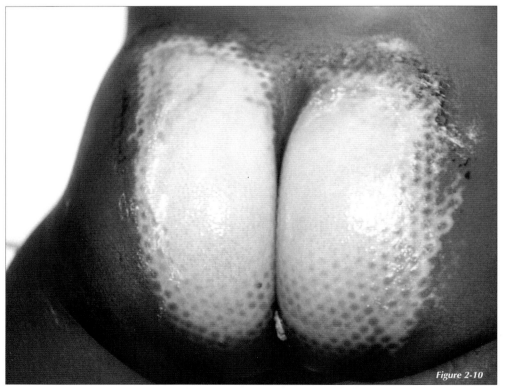

Figure 2-10

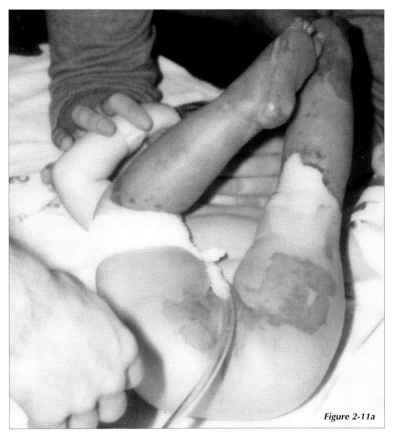

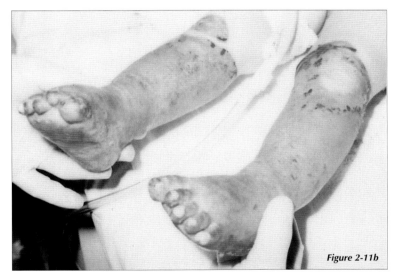

Figure 2-11. *This 20-month-old girl was in the care of her mother's paramour. He stated that while she was sitting in the bathtub, she accidentally turned on the hot water tap. She was supposedly sitting in about 4 inches of bath water at the time. He had left the room momentarily, but, when he heard her cry, he pulled her out of the water. The history is not consistent with the injuries. **A** through **c** clearly show that this is an immersion burn. Note the stocking-glove sign at the knees and the spared area in the popliteal area of the left leg. Her leg was flexed at the time of the injury or was protected by his hand as he dipped her.*

Figure 2-11a

Figure 2-11b

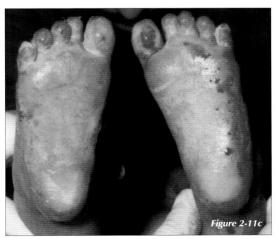

Figure 2-11c

Figure 2-12. *Intentional immersion burns in an 18-month-old boy (**a**). Note how both palms are affected (**b** and **c**). The history given was that he had accidentally turned on the hot water tap in the bathroom sink.*

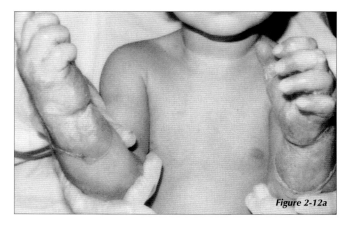

Figure 2-12a

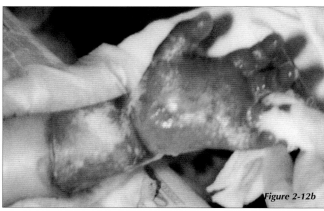

Figure 2-12b

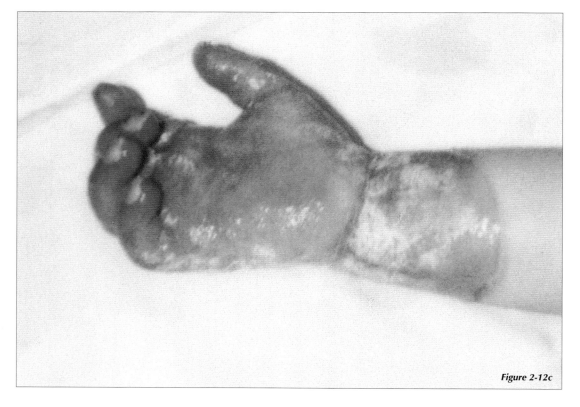

Figure 2-12c

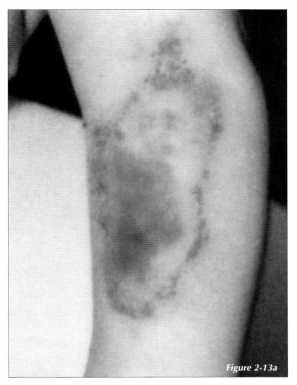

Figure 2-13a

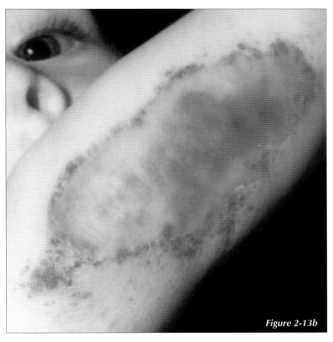

Figure 2-13. *This accidental contact burn was sustained when the child fell against a space heater (**a** and **b**). The history was consistent with the injury, and the child was otherwise in good health with no further injuries. The family was not known to state protective services. There was some concern because there was a delay in seeking help. The caregiver stated that she had hesitated to come for treatment because she did not think the injury was serious enough to require medical help.*

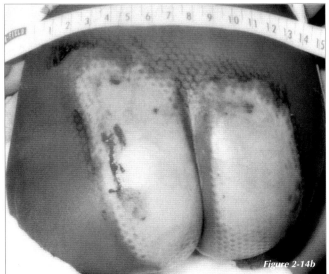

Figure 2-13b

Figure 2-14. *This 15-month-old girl was allegedly burned after climbing onto a space heater and sitting on it; however, the burn is not on the sitting part of the buttocks (**a**). The pattern on the burn is the same as the top of the heater (**b**) and could only have been made by contact with the top of the heater. The child had no other injuries, and if she had climbed onto the hot space heater she would have also burned her hands and legs.*

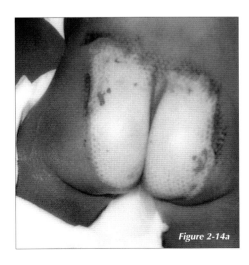

Figure 2-14a

Figure 2-14b

Figure 2-15. This 30-month-old boy suffered scald burns to the face (**a**), buttocks (**b**), left shoulder (**c**), and behind each ear (**d** and **e**). The child's mother said that she had left him in the care of relatives with whom she shared a house. When she returned home they told her the child had been burned. No one witnessed the burn. They found the child crying outside the bathroom and assumed that he had burned himself. The child was extremely dirty with embedded dirt and feces in the soles of his feet (**f**). The house was overcrowded and the children living there were poorly supervised. The child was unable to speak and could not relate what had happened to him. The injuries were considered abuse.

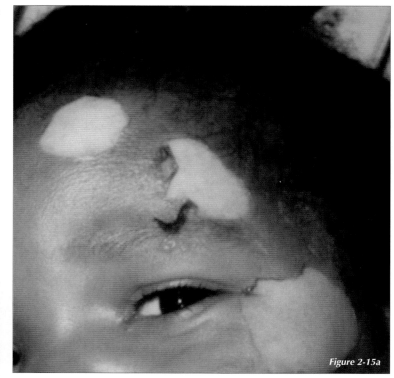

Figure 2-15a

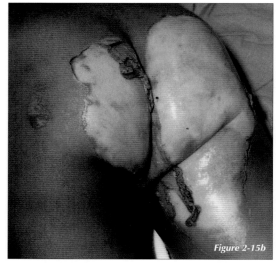

Figure 2-15b

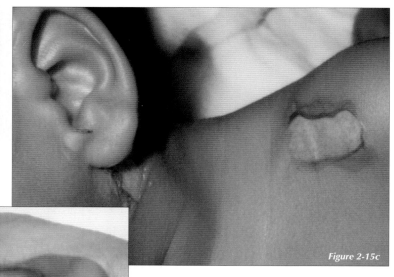

Figure 2-15c

Figure 2-15d

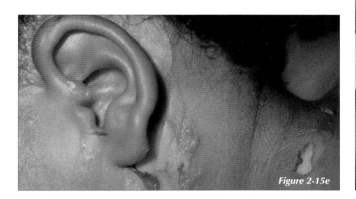

Figure 2-15e

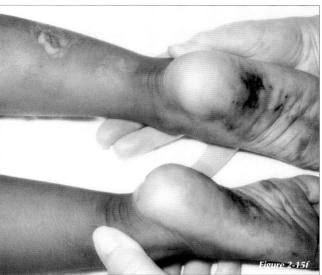

Figure 2-15f

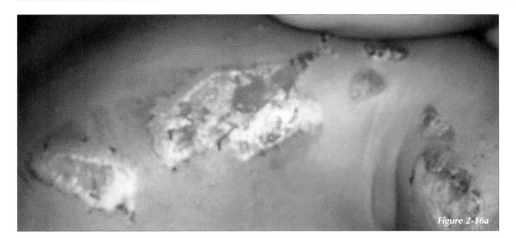

Figure 2-16a

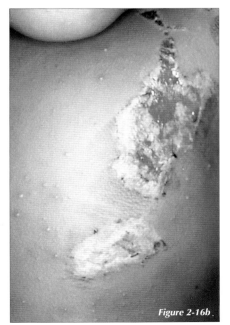

Figure 2-16b

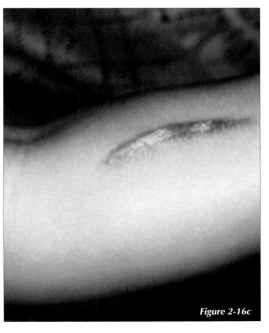

Figure 2-16c

Figure 2-16. *This 13-month-old boy was taken to the emergency room by his mother. She stated that he had been in the care of a 16-year-old cousin while she went to the grocery store. When she returned, the babysitter told her that he had been burned by a curling iron. She had placed the curling iron in the kitchen but did not see how the burn took place. She heard him crying and assumed that he had taken the curling iron off the table and burned himself. The child had second-degree burns of the left lateral chest and left upper arm (**a** and **b**). When the arm was flexed, the two areas were contiguous. The child had been seen in the emergency room just a week earlier with a curling iron burn of his left forearm (**c**). The incident was reported as suspicious of abuse because it fulfilled several of Stone's criteria.*

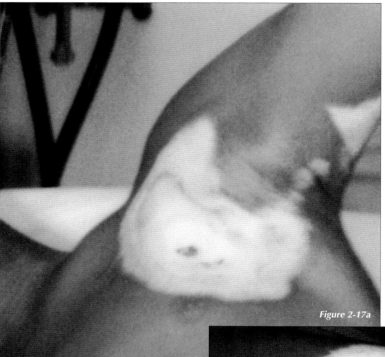

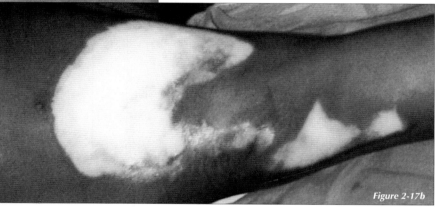

Figure 2-17. This 9-year-old boy was taken to the emergency room with a second- and third-degree burn of the upper anterior arm and chest (**a** and **b**). The boy initially stated that it was the result of having put his finger in to an electrical socket. This was challenged because the injury was not an electrical burn. There was no evidence of an exit burn or an injury of the finger. Because of the inconsistency, he was reported to state protective services. He finally stated that he had received the burn after he caught his arm in a wringer washer (**c** and **d**). The apparatus had sprung; the lower roller, which was active, continued to turn and he was unable to free his arm. When asked why he had lied initially, he said that if his grandmother had found out that he was playing with the machine, he would have been in trouble. A torn shirt was recovered to substantiate the history.

Figure 2-17a

Figure 2-17b

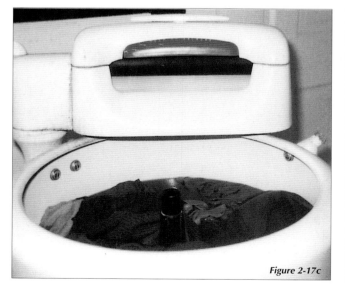

Figure 2-17c

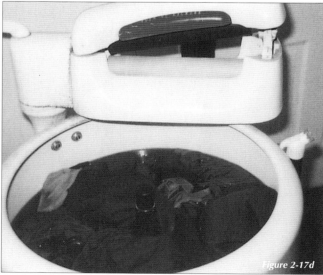

Figure 2-17d

Figure 2-18. *This 18-month-old girl was taken to the emergency room with the history that she had pulled hot liquid off a table onto her face. She had second-degree burns of her face with a burn over the bridge of the nose, above her lip, and the sides of her mouth. The chin was spared. She had burns on the inside of her lips and on her tongue. This is a child who was forced to drink hot liquid. In addition, she was found to have a healing fracture of the left radius and ulna.*

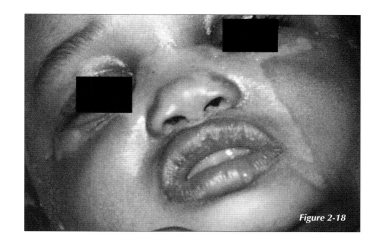

Figure 2-18

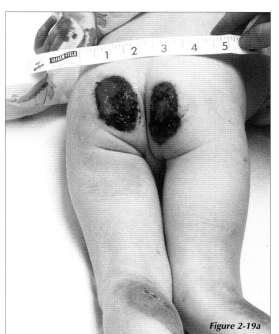

Figure 2-19a

Figure 2-19. *(a) Bilateral buttocks and posterior calf burns in a 23-month-old boy brought to medical attention 2 1/2 weeks after injury. The child was reportedly riding a tricycle that was caught between a wall and a heater (b). It is difficult to imagine how this happened or how it could have resulted in accidental burn of this degree and multiple locations. The measured temperatures at the bottom of the unit (in the range of the child) would require 20 minutes to sustain a burn of this magnitude. The stove top found in the home (c) was suspected by child care professionals as the source of the buttocks burns. The stove shown (d) has a partially open right side oven door. This was probably the source of burns to the posterior legs, which would have been at the correct height if the child was placed on the stove top.*

Figure 2-19c

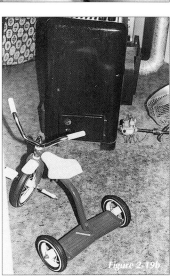

Figure 2-19b

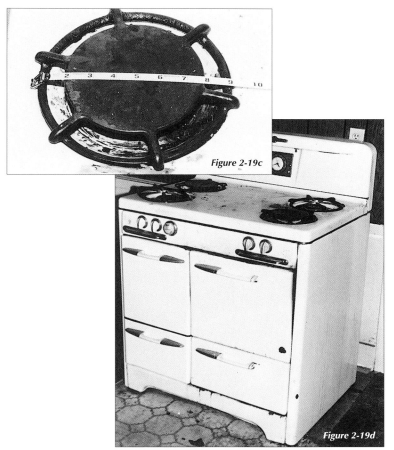

Figure 2-19d

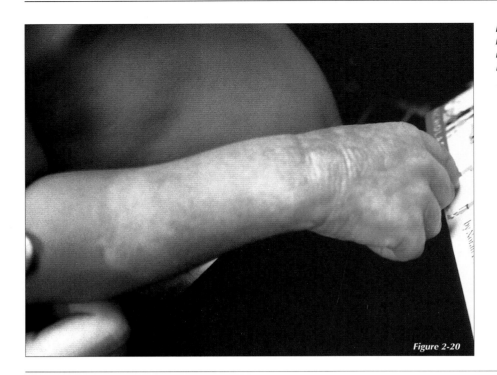

Figure 2-20. *This is a healed immersion burn, stocking-glove pattern, in a 20-month-old boy. The caregiver stated that it was a splash burn.*

Figure 2-20

Figure 2-21. *Scald burn of a 1-year-old child showing spared skin in the inguinal area due to flexion of the hip when the burn occurred.*

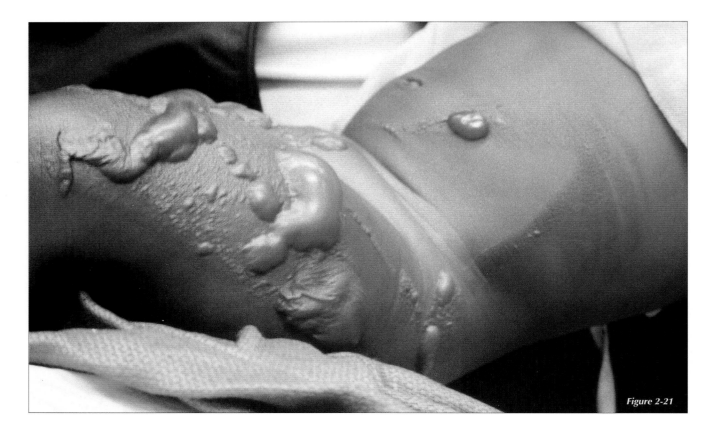

Figure 2-21

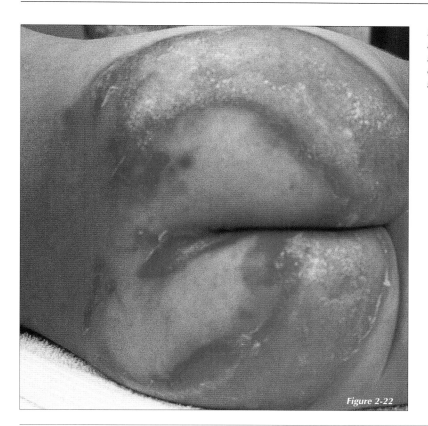

Figure 2-22. Doughnut-shaped burn of the buttocks in a 3 1/2-year-old girl. Note the central area of spared skin. The child was forcibly held against the relatively cooler bottom of a sink while hot water burned the area surrounding the center.

Figure 2-23. Healed abusive burn to the buttocks.

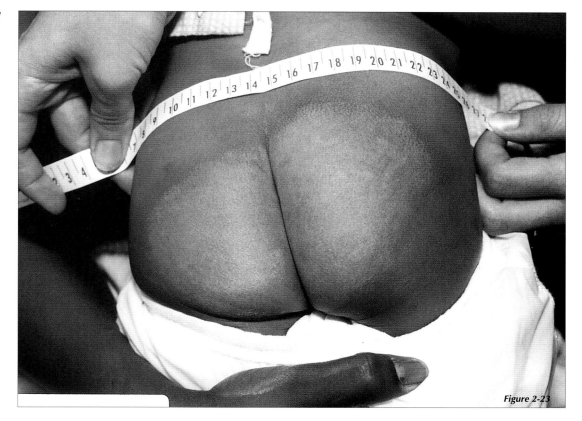

Figure 2-24. *This 28-month-old boy supposedly sat on a curling iron (**a** and **b**). The injury is not on the sitting part of the buttocks and is suspicious for abuse.*

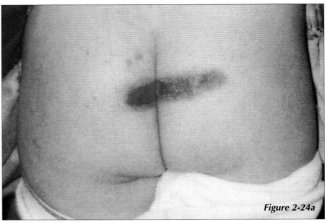

Figure 2-24a

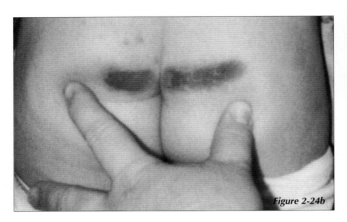

Figure 2-24b

Figure 2-25. *This 10-month-old boy was in the care of his mother's paramour. The caregiver said that the child accidentally sat on a furnace grid. The grid pattern was present. The case was reported to state child protective services because of a delay in seeking medical assistance, the age of the child, and the location of the injury. It was determined to be accidental.*

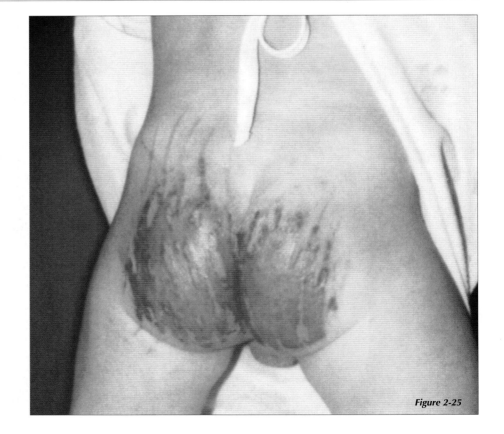

Figure 2-25

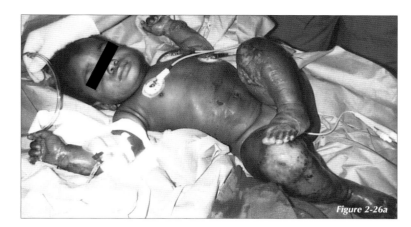

Figure 2-26a

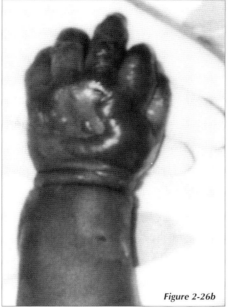

Figure 2-26. This 5-month-old girl had second-degree burns to the hands (**b** and **c**), legs (**a**, **d**, and **e**), and feet (**f**). The history was that the child's older sibling, a 4-year-old girl, drew the bath water and then placed the child in the tub. An investigation of the home determined the injury was accidental. A case was opened for poor supervision.

Figure 2-26b

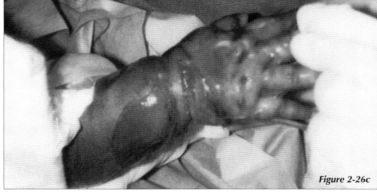

Figure 2-26c

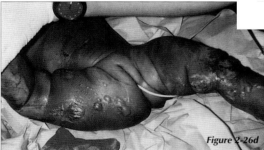

Figure 2-26d

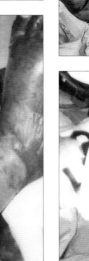

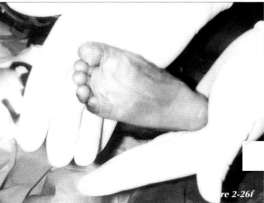

re 2-26f

Figure 2-26e

Figure 2-27. *This 2-year-old girl was seen in the emergency room for respiratory distress. While there, the staff noted two healed burns to the right shoulder (**a**), one healed burn to the right forearm (**b**), and a more recent burn to the left lower leg (**c**). They were said to be accidental curling iron burns. The child had a past history of premature birth and a long stay in the intensive care nursery. At 1 year of age she was admitted with a drug ingestion. This injury was reported as abuse.*

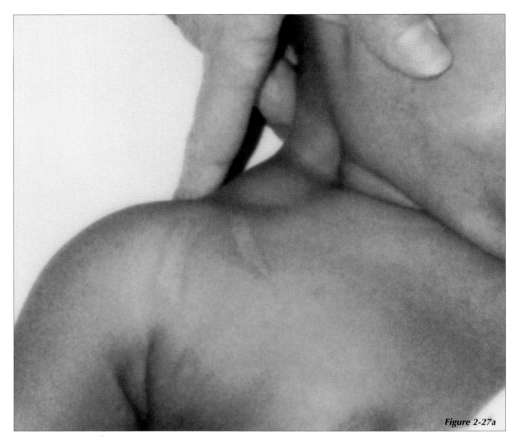

Figure 2-27a

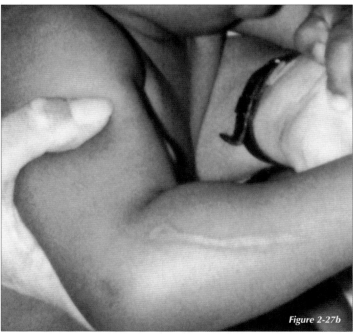

Figure 2-27b

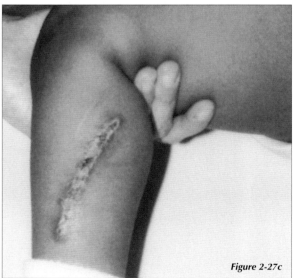

Figure 2-27c

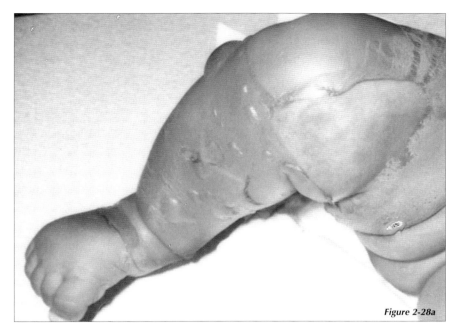

Figure 2-28a

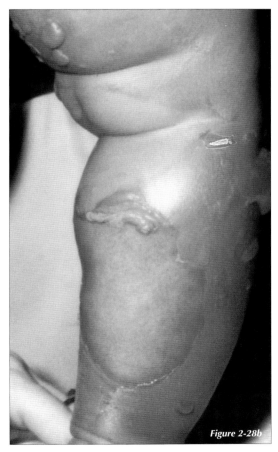

Figure 2-28b

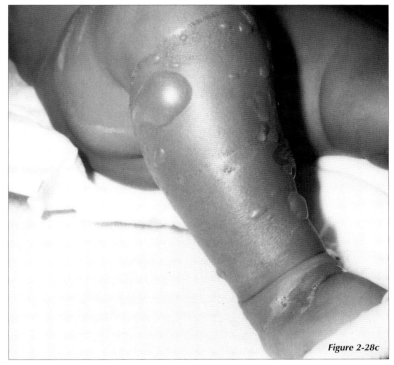

Figure 2-28c

Figure 2-28. *This 7-month-old girl was supposedly left in the bathtub by the mother while the water was running. When the mother returned, she found that the child had been burned. Only the right leg was involved, but the burn extended to the mid-thigh (**a** and **b**). The knee of that leg was spared, as was the popliteal area. The leg must have been flexed with the knee above the water. The distal end of the right foot was also spared and thus must have been above the water. Note the stocking-glove line just below the knee (**c**). The injuries are inconsistent with the history and most likely resulted from the child having been dipped in the hot water.*

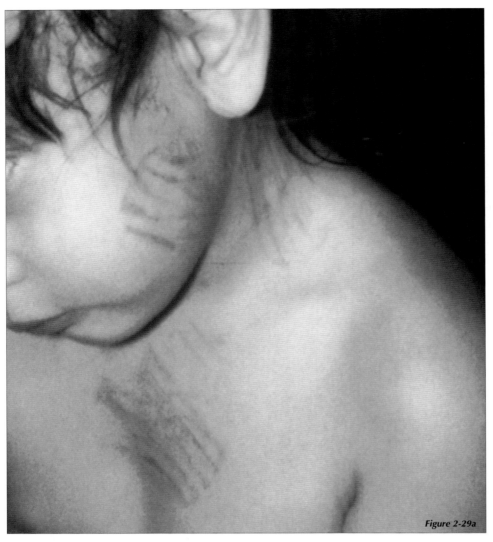

Figure 2-29. *This 30-month-old girl was taken to the emergency room by her foster mother, who was concerned because after every visitation the child had with her biological mother she returned with injuries. The biological mother said that the child was clumsy. On this particular visit, the child had multiple pattern burns on her face (**a**), chest (**b**), and arms (**c**), which the biological mother said were caused by a blow dryer. She said the child caused the burns by moving too much. In addition, the child had a conjunctival injury (**d**), bruising on the upper back (**e**), and a healed circular burn to the buttocks (**f**).*

Figure 2-29a

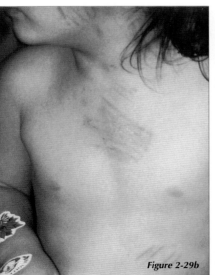

Figure 2-29b

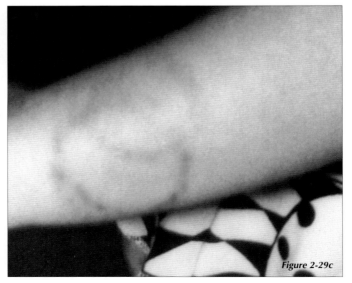

Figure 2-29c

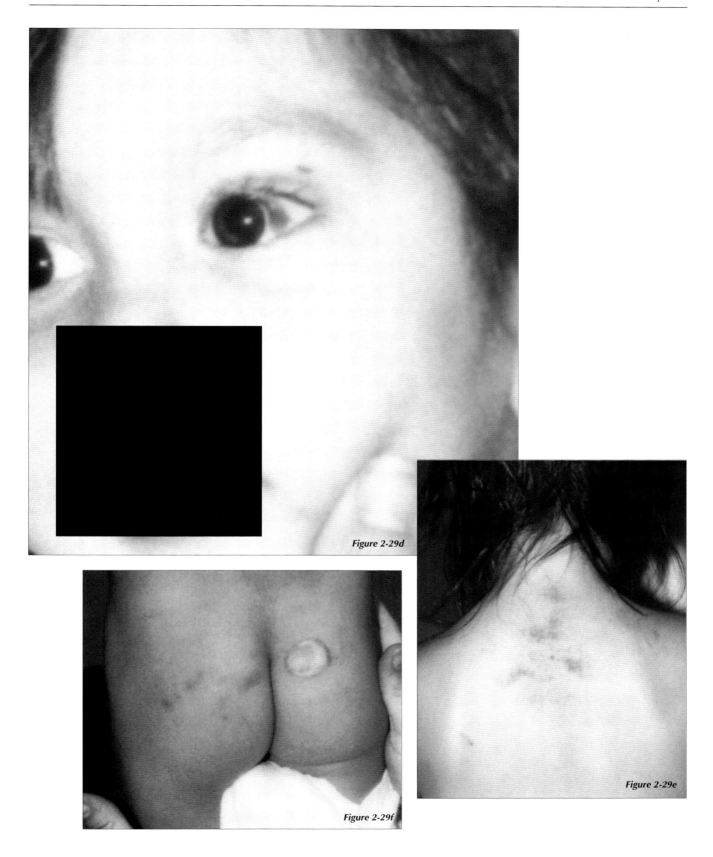

Figure 2-29d

Figure 2-29e

Figure 2-29f

Figure 2-30. This 33-month-old girl was taken to the emergency room by her mother and the mother's paramour. They said that they noted the burns to the child's back after returning from a trip. The child was in the backseat of the car. They said that she was restless but did not give any other reason to suspect that she was injured. They had no idea how the injury had occurred. They suggested that it might have been sunburn or caused when the sun heated the back of the car seat. The child had second-degree burns of the back to the gluteal crease on her left side, including the left buttock (**a**). The burns extended laterally on the torso to midchest on her right and higher on her left (**b** and **c**). Her left arm was almost completely involved, sparing only her hand to the wrist and her shoulder on that side (**d**). Her right arm had a small area of burn medially and at the elbow (**e**). The burn involves multiple surface areas and the pattern is not consistent with a sunburn, since there are no clothing lines. She was said to have been wearing a bathing suit. It is not a contact burn. The host surface would have had to have been contoured. This is an immersion burn and involves hot liquid. It was reported as abuse. The child was placed in foster care for 6 months, then returned to her mother and her husband. One month later she returned with another, similar burn. Again the caregivers denied abuse and had no idea how she was burned.

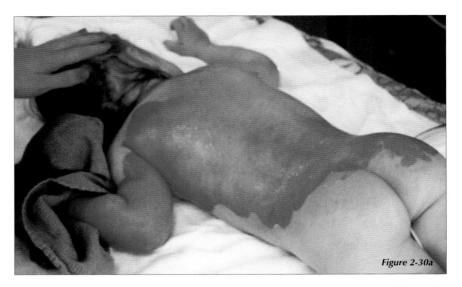

Figure 2-30a

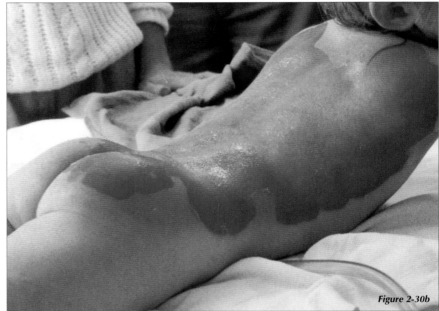

Figure 2-30b

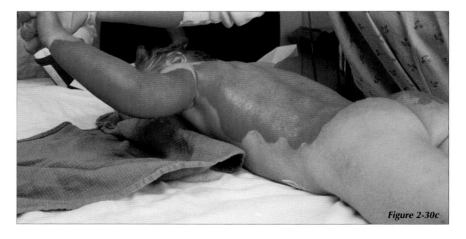

Figure 2-30c

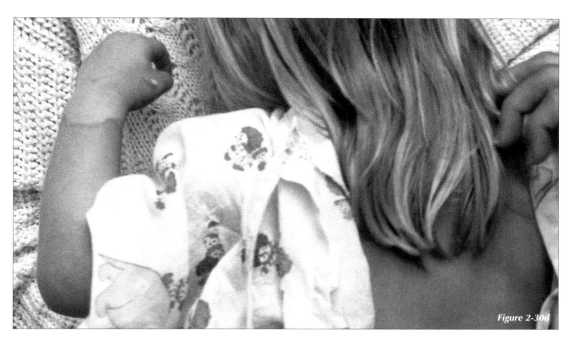

Figure 2-30d

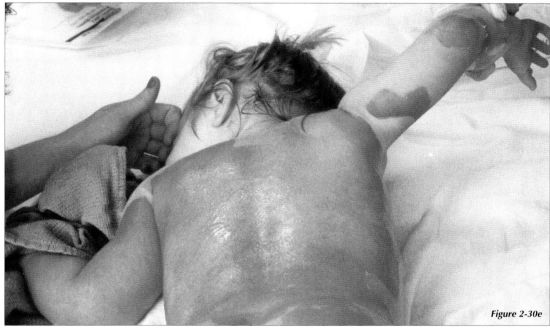

Figure 2-30e

Figure 2-31. *This 4-year-old boy was taken to the emergency room by his parents for a burn to the dorsum of his right foot (a). The burn was said to be accidental. The child supposedly had accidentally placed his foot on the top of a space heater. Abuse was suspected because the injury appeared older than the parents had indicated, the injury was in an unusual location, and the child had healed loop marks on his back (b) and a well-healed burn scar to his chest (c).*

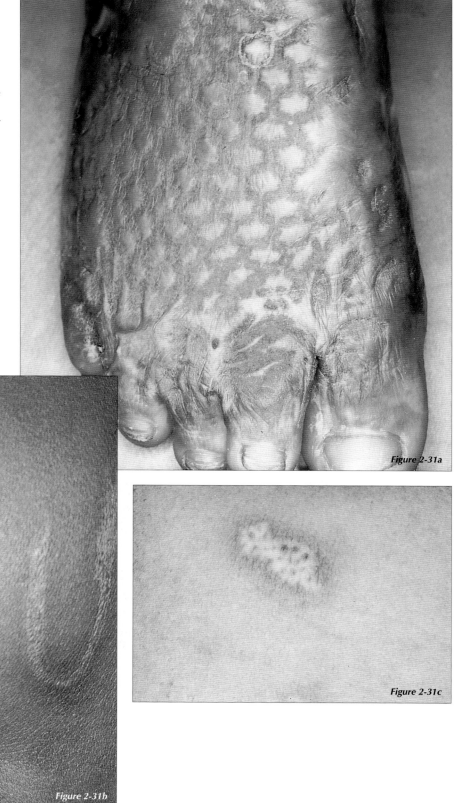

Figure 2-31a

Figure 2-31b

Figure 2-31c

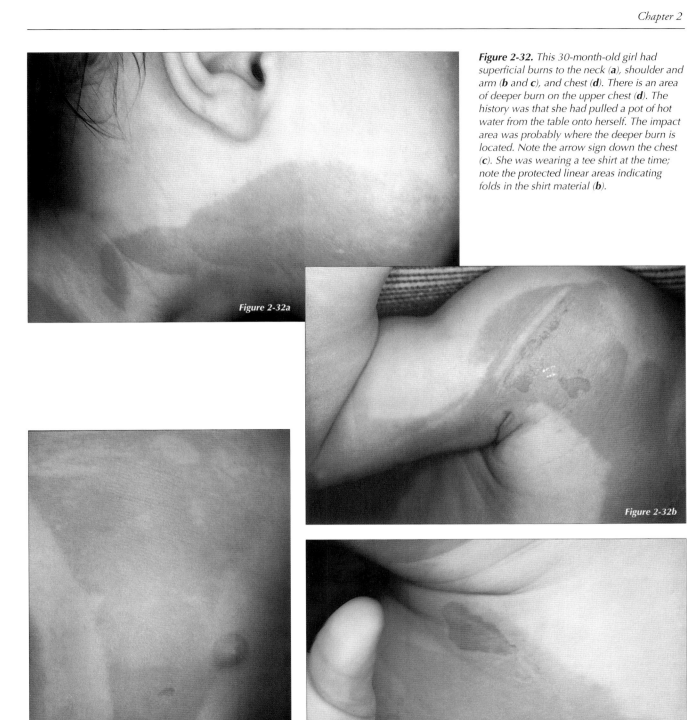

Figure 2-32. This 30-month-old girl had superficial burns to the neck (**a**), shoulder and arm (**b** and **c**), and chest (**d**). There is an area of deeper burn on the upper chest (**d**). The history was that she had pulled a pot of hot water from the table onto herself. The impact area was probably where the deeper burn is located. Note the arrow sign down the chest (**c**). She was wearing a tee shirt at the time; note the protected linear areas indicating folds in the shirt material (**b**).

Figure 2-32a

Figure 2-32b

Figure 2-32c

Figure 2-32d

Figure 2-33. This child was brought in by the mother for burns she noted on the child's genitalia after a visitation with her estranged husband. The mother could not explain the burns to the genital area. Although all of the injuries were of the same age, the emergency room staff felt that each injury represented a separate incident. The injuries were limited to the scrotum and glans penis (**a** to **d**). The instrument was believed to be a curling iron. The injuries were probably the result of discipline for soiling. The father denied injuring the child. The mother had recently been released from a psychiatric hospital.

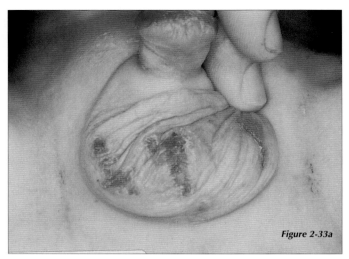

Figure 2-33a

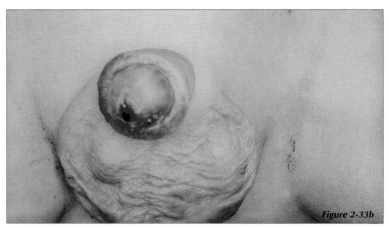

Figure 2-33b

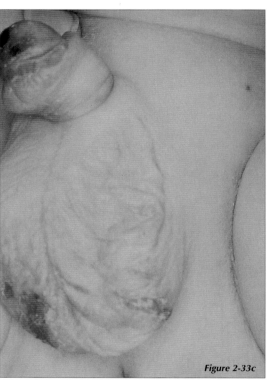

Figure 2-33c

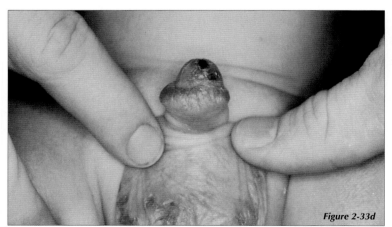

Figure 2-33d

Figure 2-34. *Cigarette burns, recent (**a**) and healing (**b**).*

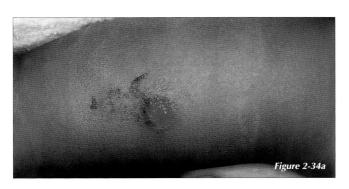

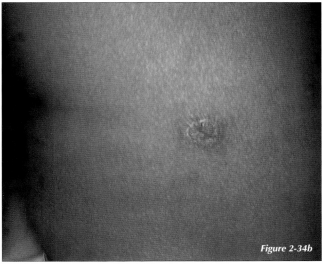

Figure 2-34a

Figure 2-34b

Figure 2-35. *This 4-year old child had first- and second-degree burns of the legs (**a**) and buttocks (**b**) and was said to have "jumped" into the tub of hot water without checking the temperature. Although the child had stocking-glove burns of the legs, the injury was thought to be consistent with the history. Note the irregular border of the burn and the angulation. The child was said to have emotional problems, and her intent was questioned.*

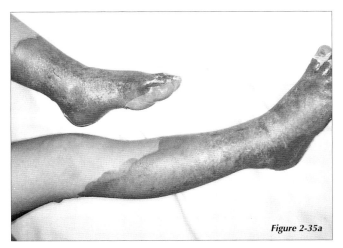

Figure 2-35a

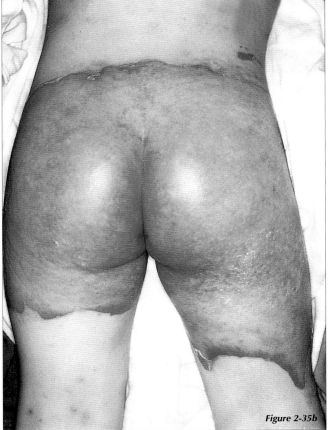

Figure 2-35b

Figure 2-36. *Two-year-old boy with a deep burn to the dorsum of the left hand. The history given was that the child accidentally placed his hand under the hot water tap. Because of the severity of the burn and the location, as well as the delay in seeking medical help, it was reported as suspected child abuse. An investigation by police corroborated the story, finding that the hot water heater was set at high and that the hot water temperature could have caused this degree of burn in a short time. Note the arrow signs down the fingers.*

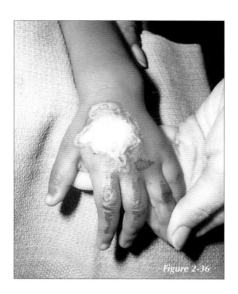

Figure 2-37. *This 3-year-old child supposedly fell against the radiator in the bathroom. Three things suggested abuse: there was a delay in seeking help; the injury involved three surface areas, including both the buttocks and the back of the hand (a to c); and the injury was blamed on a sibling.*

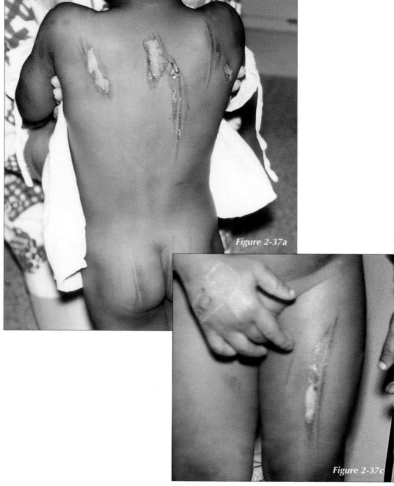

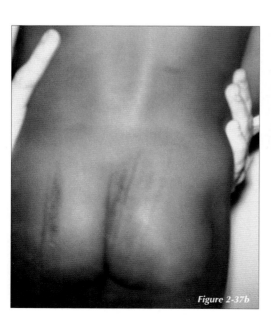

Figure 2-38. This 5-year-old boy "ran into his mother while she was carrying a pot of hot water." It was a suspicious burn because three surface areas were involved. There was an arrow sign to the back (*b*), but none on the thigh (*c*). The scalp was spared. The boy was steadfast in his insistence that it was accidental. It was postulated that the child struck the pot of hot water with his head, at the left forehead area (*a*). Liquid splashed down the front to a flexed leg. The remainder of the liquid spilled down his left neck and back area.

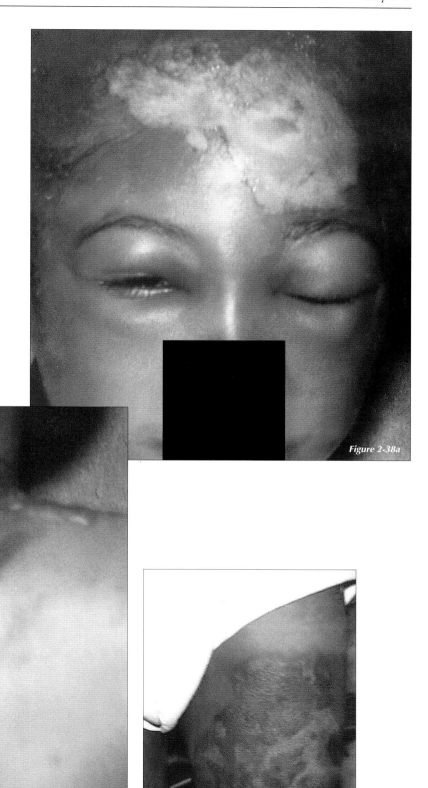

Figure 2-38a

Figure 2-38b

Figure 2-38c

Figure 2-39. This 22-month-old boy was brought in by ambulance with convulsions. The child was found to be hypoglycemic and had an elevated ethanol level. The mother stated that her boyfriend had given the boy alcohol. In addition, the child was found to have a healed contact burn to the left forearm (**c**), a flow burn to the back of his right hand (**a** and **b**). The mother "did not know" how the child had been burned.

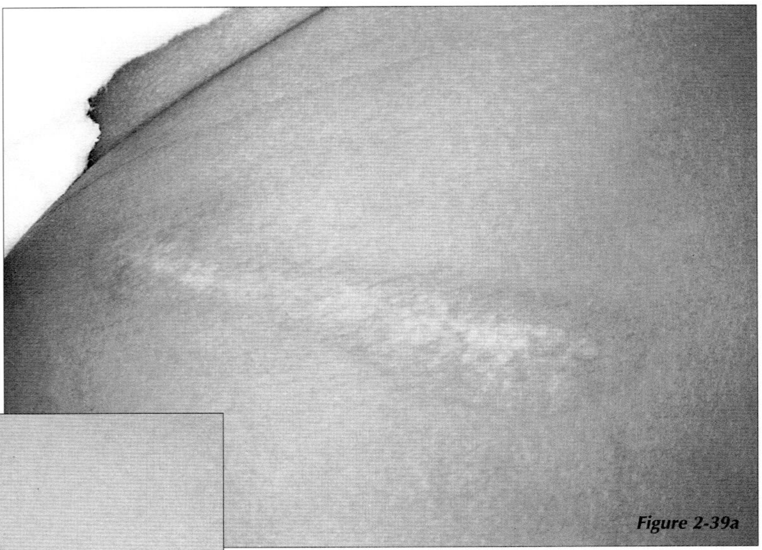

Figure 2-39a

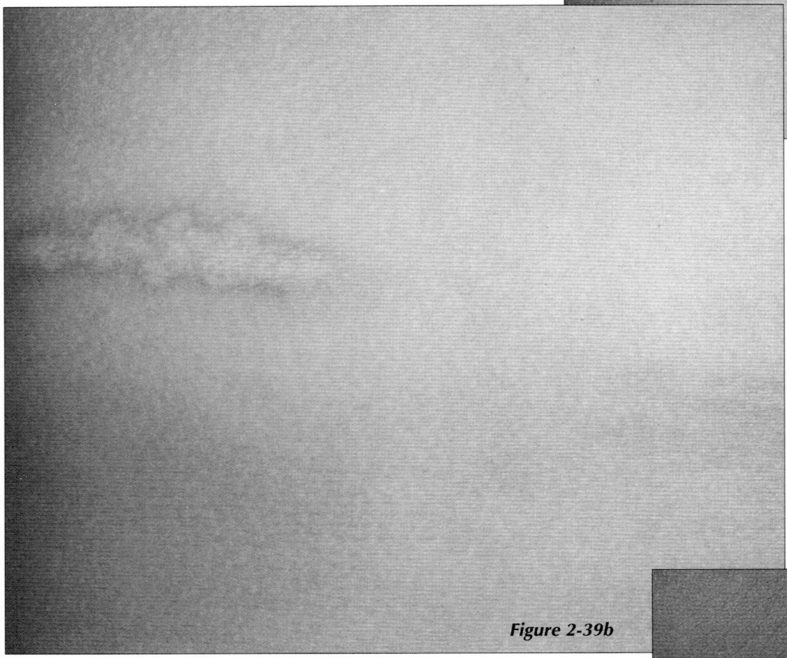

Figure 2-39b

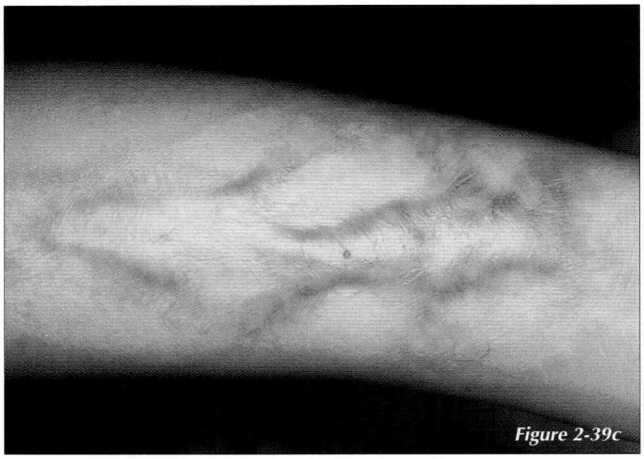

Figure 2-39c

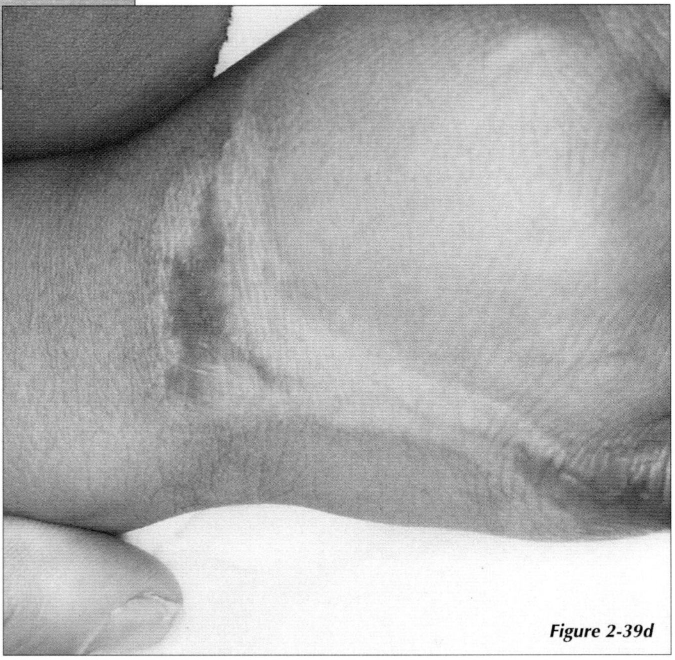

Figure 2-39d

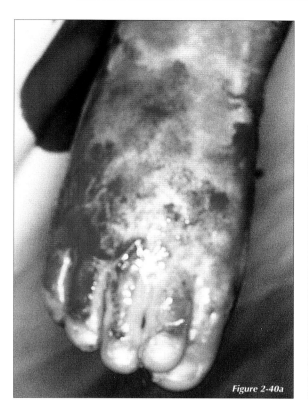

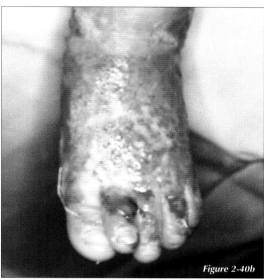

Figure 2-40. *This 18-month-old boy was "taking a bath and while the mother was not looking, he accidentally turned on the hot water tap." Both feet had second- and third-degree burns and a stocking-glove line above the ankle (**a** and **b**). No other areas were burned. This is abuse. The history does not fit the findings because the child would have had to have been standing in the tub to sustain these injuries. Had he been sitting or standing in water and turned on the hot water, the cooler water of the tub would have dissipated the heat.*

Figure 2-40a

Figure 2-40b

Figure 2-41. *This 3-year-old girl was taken to the emergency room for second- and third-degree burns of the hands (**a** and **b**). She supposedly accidentally stuck her hands in running hot water. The child stated that "mommy was mad at me and put my hands in the water." Compare this injury with the immersion injury. There is no stocking-glove sign. The palms are relatively spared. In addition to the child's history, a measurement of the water temperature by the investigator confirmed that the water temperature was not hot enough to give an instant burn.*

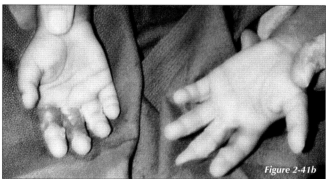

Figure 2-41b

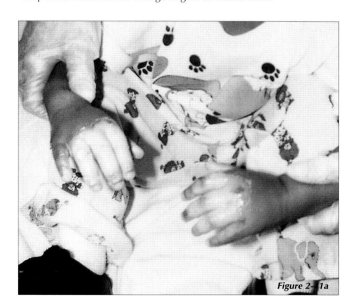

Figure 2-41a

Figure 2-42. *Intentional curling iron burns on a 6-year-old boy inflicted by his stepmother (**a**, **b**, **c**, and **e**). Note the shape of the burn to the neck (**d**). This wound was the most recent. Its configuration was caused by the child flexing his neck on the iron. When he was 2, he was abused by his biological mother, who burned his buttocks and injured his penis.*

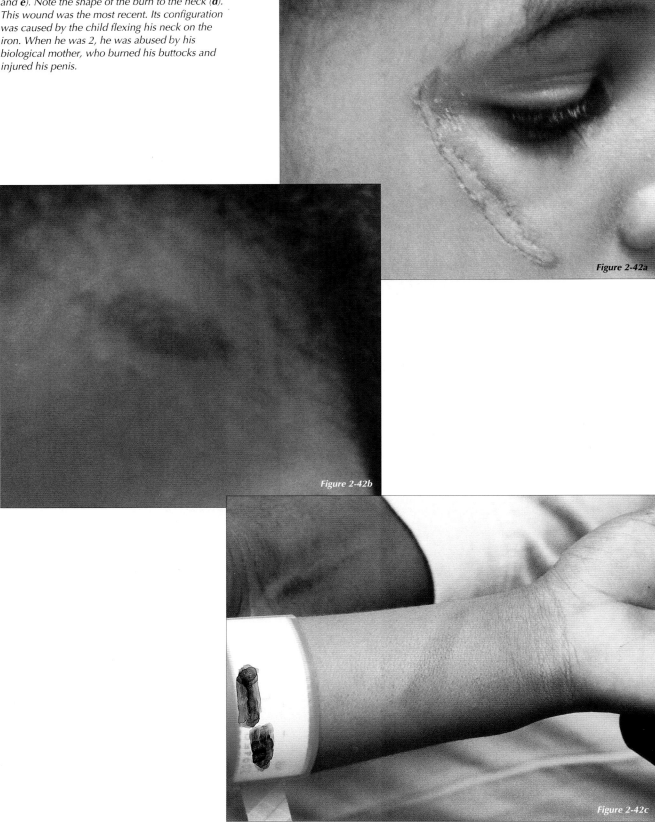

Figure 2-42a

Figure 2-42b

Figure 2-42c

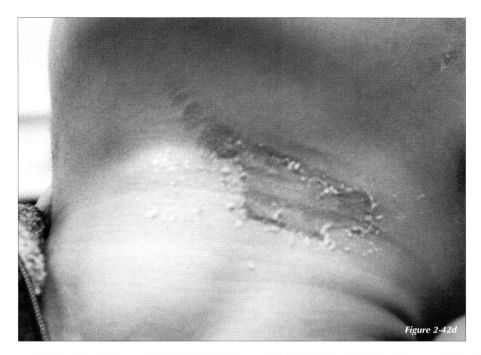

Figure 2-42d

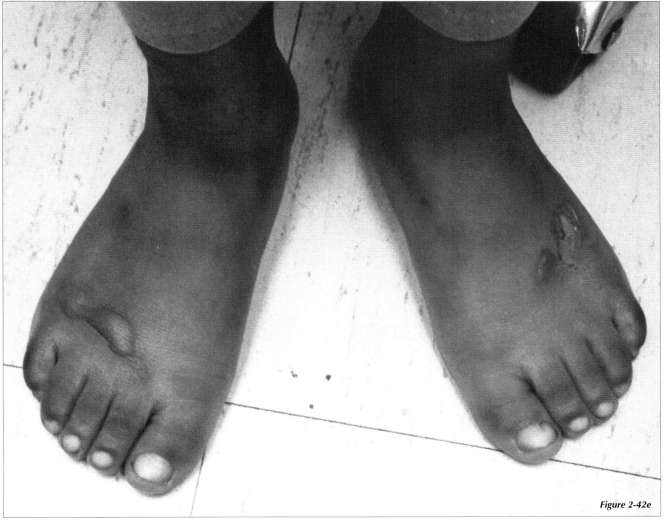

Figure 2-42e

Figure 2-43. *This 15-month-old girl was in the care of a babysitter. The sitter said she spilled hot grease and the "hot grease got under her Pampers." She had second-degree burns to the diaper area (a and b) and a circular burn to her right arm (c). The injuries are not consistent with the history. There was no diaper line burn, which would be expected for grease to fall cleanly into the diaper area without first touching the abdomen. The diaper would limit the flow of liquid. In addition, there was no grease-soaked diaper. This is most likely a water scald burn.*

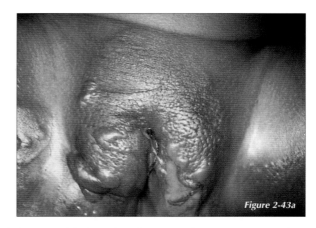

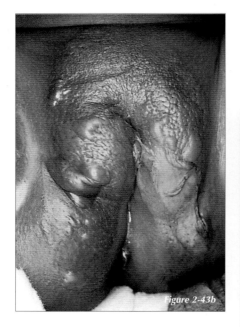

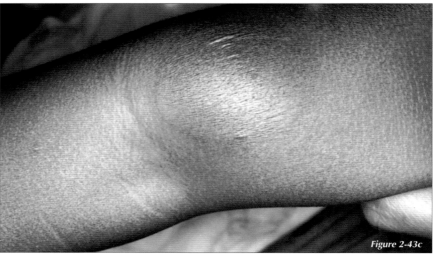

Figure 2-44. *This 16-month-old boy was burned by a curling iron sitting on a counter. He grabbed it with his hand (a). He released it and it fell, striking his left upper arm (b). Note the hand injury and the glancing burn injury to his arm. This is consistent with the history. The child had a previous admission to the hospital for a Pine Sol ingestion.*

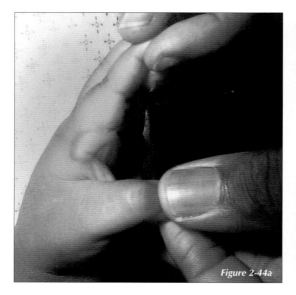

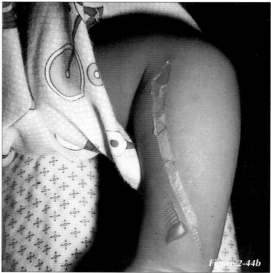

Figure 2-45. This is a pattern burn to the dorsum of the right hand and lower arm. The child is a 3-month-old girl. She supposedly accidentally touched the space heater. The pattern matches the grids of a space heater. The child was healthy, and there were no other injuries. The case was reported to child protection personnel so that they could inspect the home and make sure that there were no safety hazards.

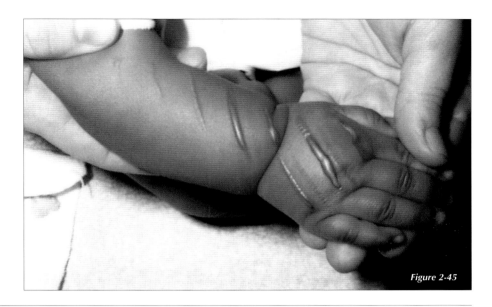

Figure 2-45

Figure 2-46. This 5-year-old boy fell onto a space heater (*a*) while his mother was chasing him around the house to whip him with an extension cord. There is a loop mark on his right upper back (*b*).

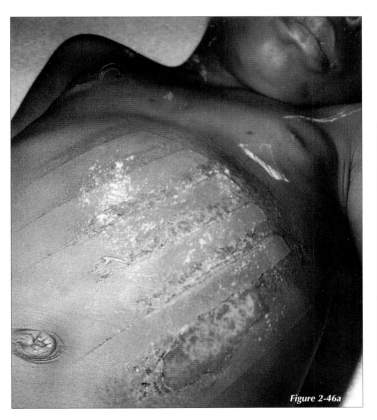

Figure 2-46a

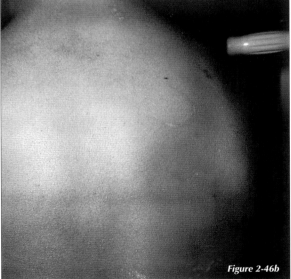

Figure 2-46b

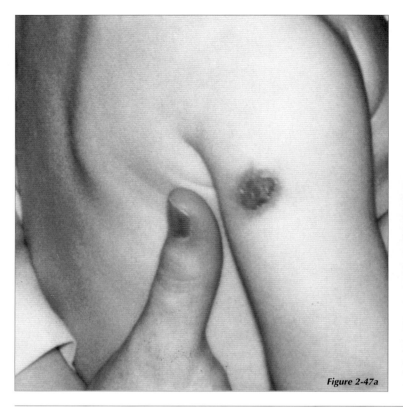

Figure 2-47. This 9-month-old girl had two circular healing burns, of different ages, to the back of the right upper arm (**a**) and the dorsum of the left hand (**b**). No history was given to explain the injuries. The caregivers stated that they might have been caused by popping grease or a cigarette ash. The poor history, the age of the wounds, and the patient's age made this case suspicious of abuse.

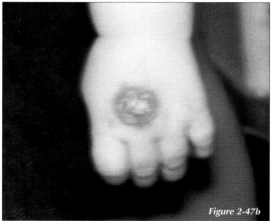

Figure 2-47a

Figure 2-47b

Figure 2-48. This 17-month-old girl was seen in the emergency room with swollen feet. She had mild first-degree burns of the feet. The child was in the care of her mother's boyfriend, who said that she received the mild burn when he "gave her a bath after she soiled herself." She had an ecchymotic area behind her ear (**a**) and a deep healing injury to her right foot (**b**). The case was reported to the hotline as suspected abuse.

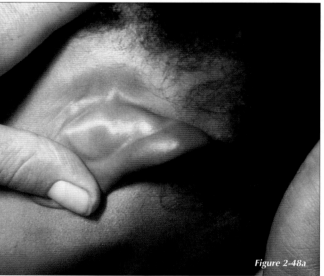

Figure 2-48a

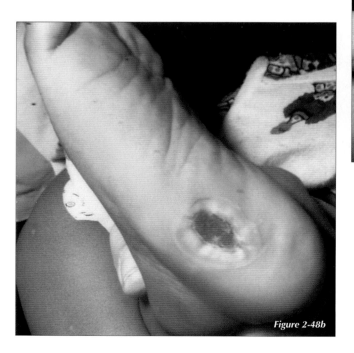

Figure 2-48b

Figure 2-49. *This 6-month-old boy was branded by his mother's boyfriend with a square-shaped object, which was not found. The object seems to have been carefully applied on the left shoulder with minimal overlapping to form a larger burn pattern. (Courtesy James J. Williams, M.D.)*

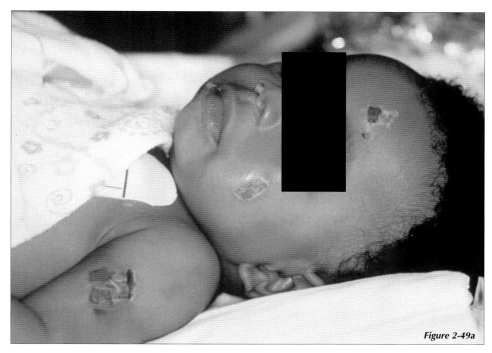

Figure 2-49a

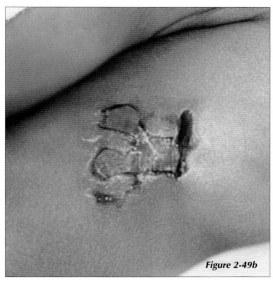

Figure 2-49b

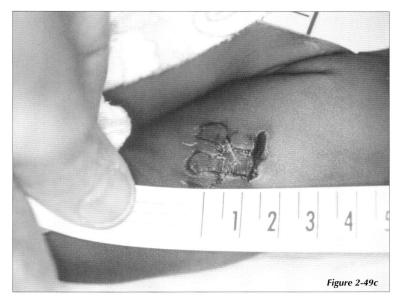

Figure 2-49c

Figure 2-50. Fourteen-year-old boy who was seen in the emergency room and found to have this burn scar. He said it was a gang initiation brand. It was done with a heated coat hanger, bent into this "J" shape.

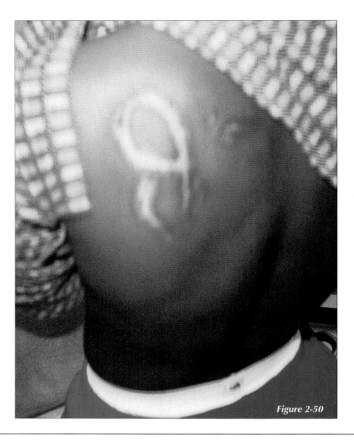

Figure 2-51. This 18-month-old boy had several characteristic healed burn lesions on his face (shown here), abdomen, and thighs. The mother's boyfriend would touch him with the heated end of a cigarette lighter when he cried. Note the pattern of the burn.

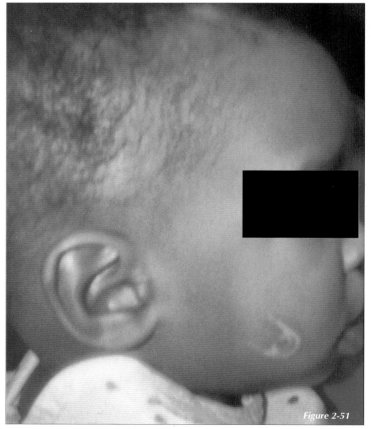

Burns
Part 2

Christian Paletta, M.D.

Figure 2-52. This 18-month-old boy has second- and third-degree immersion burns to both lower extremities. This child was originally admitted to another hospital and was transferred with the diagnosis of "scalded skin syndrome" believed to be secondary to an infectious process. This appeared more like an intentional immersion burn, showing a combination of thermal and chemical burn characteristics. Body x-rays revealed a healing tibial plateau fracture. Because of progressive swelling, a compartment syndrome developed in the affected leg and required a fasciotomy. It was later determined that this child was one of several being cared for by a particular caregiver. He had soiled his diaper and she had run out of diapers into which to change him. Therefore she dipped him in a mixture of hot water, ammonia, and Pine Sol to both cleanse him and punish him for soiling his diapers.

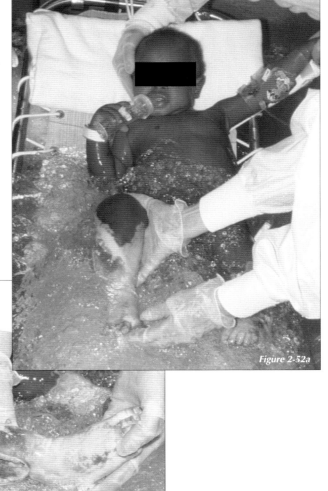

Figure 2-52a

Figure 2-52b

Figure 2-53. *A 9-month-old girl with circumferential second- and third-degree burns of the left hand. While in the babysitter's arms, the child placed her hand in boiling water on the stove. After an investigation, the injury was determined to be accidental. Escharotomies were required for all of the fingers because of ischemia. A split-thickness skin graft was needed because of the depth of the burn.*

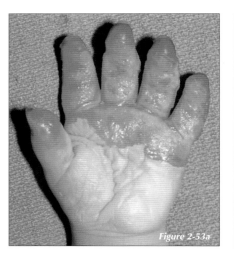

Figure 2-53a

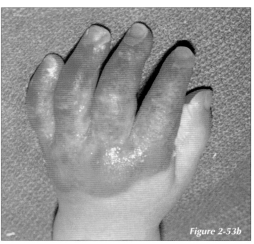

Figure 2-53b

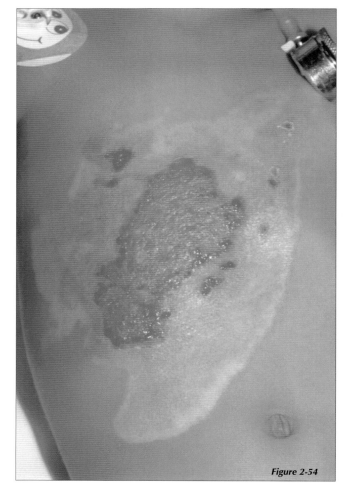

Figure 2-54

Figure 2-54. *This 2-year-old child had first-, second-, and third-degree burns of the anterior abdominal wall skin. The cause of the burn was never determined. Skin grafting was required for the central portion of the burned area. After discharge, the child was lost to follow-up. It was later learned that the child died at age 3 of "natural causes." A funeral director informed police about many bruises on the child's body. A more thorough autopsy revealed a total of 88 blunt wounds and a bite mark, all of which had been inflicted within 36 hours before the child's death. The direct cause of death was found to be peritonitis from a ruptured small intestine. The child's stepfather was later convicted of murder. The stepfather quoted the Bible on disciplining children: "The Bible tells us to take up a rod and beat your child to deliver his soul from hell."*

Figure 2-55. *This 18-month-old sustained second- and third-degree burns of both legs from hot water immersion (**a** and **b**). She was noted to be malnourished and required nutritional support before skin grafting could be done. Investigation by social services determined that the burns were most likely accidental. She was readmitted 6 months later with a large third-degree burn on her back (**c**). Her mother and stepfather stated that she was asleep in the back seat of their car when battery acid spilled onto her back. According to their account of the burn, she did not awaken when she was burned. They noted the burn after they arrived home and were getting her ready for bed. After a thorough investigation, it was determined that the burns were inflicted by her stepfather. She was then placed in foster care and has subsequently been adopted.*

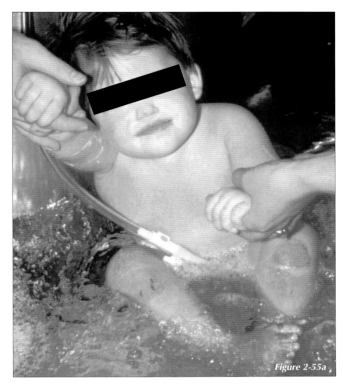

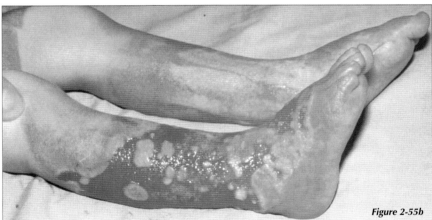

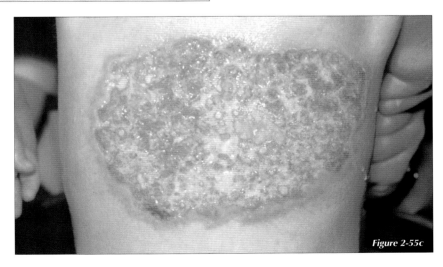

Figure 2-56. This 3-year-old boy had a second- and third-degree burn on the dorsum of the left wrist. The injury was made with a hot iron, inflicted as a form of discipline.

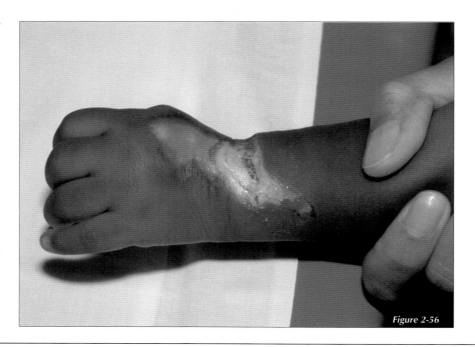

Figure 2-56

Figure 2-57. This 12-month-old girl has second-degree burns to both hands and wrists following immersion in hot water in her bathtub. While suspicious of abuse, it was determined that the injury was accidental. The mother was filling the tub and left the girl alone in the room. When she returned, she found the child standing next to the tub with both hands suspended in the hot water. It was reported to the hotline. There was a witness to the event.

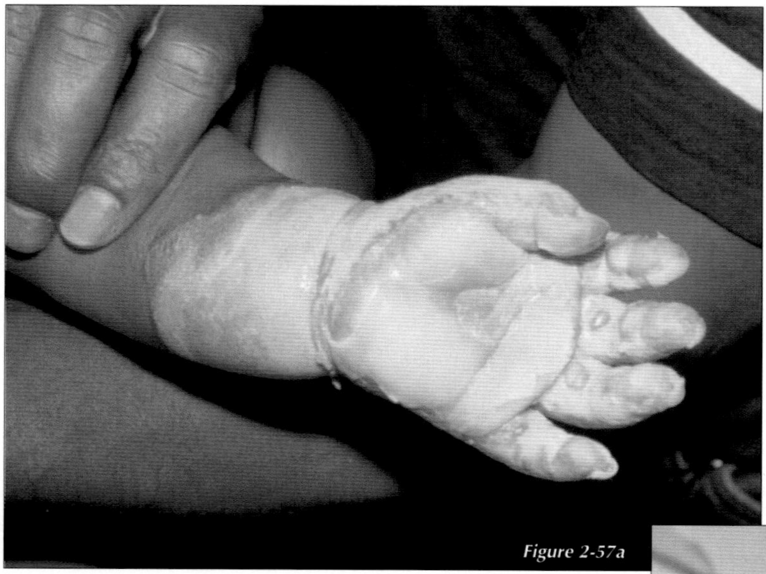

Figure 2-57a

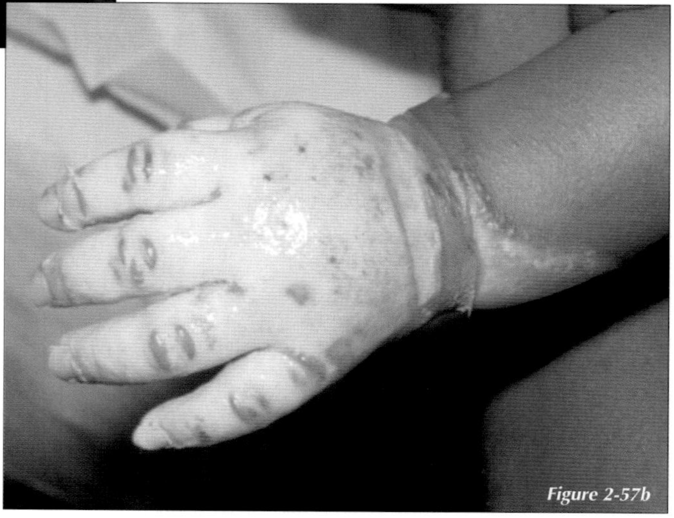

Figure 2-57b

Figure 2-58. This 3-year-old girl has an oral commissure burn. This occurred when she bit down on an electrical cord. This is a fairly common childhood burn and is rarely the result of abuse.

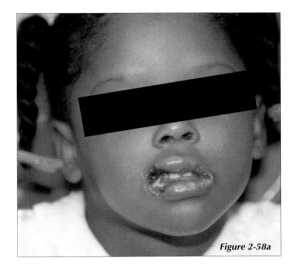

Figure 2-58a

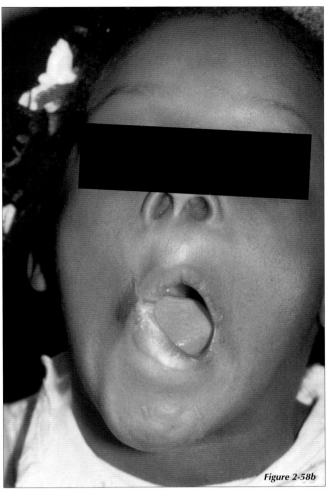

Figure 2-58b

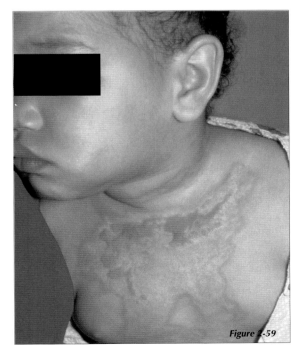

Figure 2-59

Figure 2-59. Fourteen-month-old girl who sustained a second-degree burn of the upper chest when she spilled boiling water from the microwave oven. She was wearing a shirt at the time, as seen from the upper edge of the burn. The material held the liquid and distorted the arrow sign. Upper trunk and shoulder-upper arm burns such as this are usually accidental.

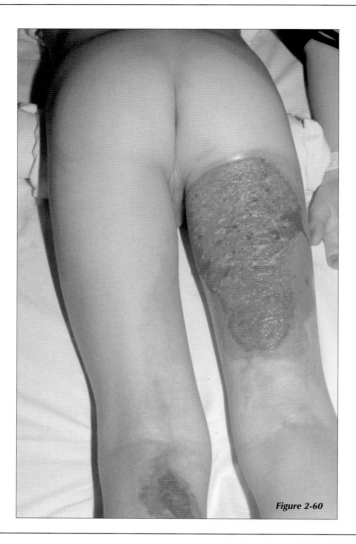

Figure 2-60. *A 10-year-old boy with a third-degree burn to his right posterior thigh. The burn was caused by an ignited lighter, which set his clothes aflame. While they may involve neglect, flame burns are rarely a direct result of abuse.*

Figure 2-60

Figure 2-61. *This 4-year-old has a second-degree burn to the right foot. This was caused by stepping barefoot onto hot coals in a campground. While burns to the lower extremities are often a warning sign for child abuse, isolated plantar burns, such as this, are most commonly accidental.*

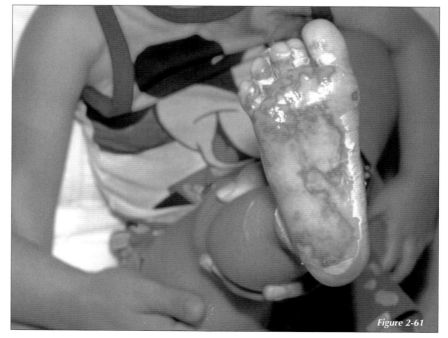

Figure 2-61

Urologic and Genital Lesions

George F. Steinhardt, M.D.

The finding of injuries in the genital areas is frequently indicative of abuse, particularly sexual abuse. However, in this chapter we present a number of cases in which the lesions were mistaken for abuse, yet represent nonabusive situations. It is important to clearly diagnose inflicted versus nonabusive injuries. Errors in diagnosis can be both catastrophic and costly for the child and family. If inflicted injury is not recognized, the child is left in the care of persons who may injury him or her again. If the diagnosis of inflicted injury is incorrect, parents are wrongfully accused and investigated and the child and parents may be separated.

Conditions that produce lesions in the urologic or genital area and can be mistaken for abuse include the following:

1. Henoch-Schonlein purpura

2. Poison ivy

3. Hair injury

4. Paraphimosis

5. Edema from idiopathic causes

6. Genital warts

The following cases illustrate both these nonabuse situations and the effects of abusive behavior.

Figure 3-1. *Genital warts in a 10-month-old boy. The child's mother had a history of genital warts. There was no other physical evidence of abuse, and the case was not reported to child protective services.*

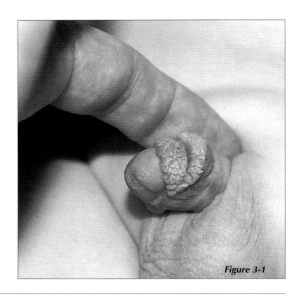

Figure 3-1

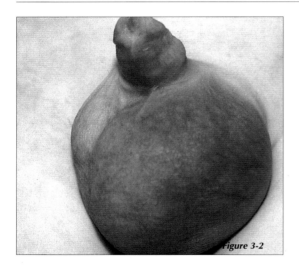

Figure 3-2

Figure 3-2. *Genital lesions that can be mistaken for abuse—scrotal swelling and ecchymosis due to Henoch-Schonlein purpura.*

Figure 3-3. *Genital lesions that can be mistaken for abuse—penile edema due to poison ivy (see also Chapter 4, Dermatology).*

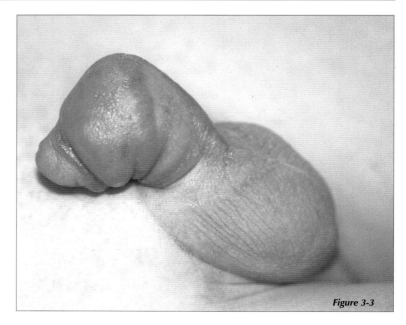

Figure 3-3

Figure 3-4. *Genital lesions that can be mistaken for abuse—hair injury. This erythematous and edematous penis (**a**) was produced by a hair wrapped around the glans (**b**).*

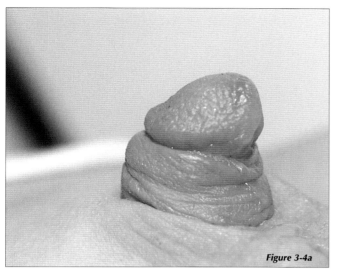

Figure 3-4a

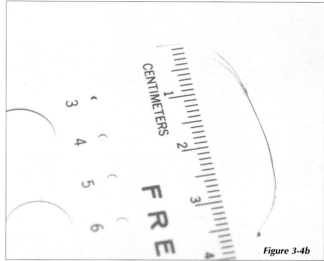

Figure 3-4b

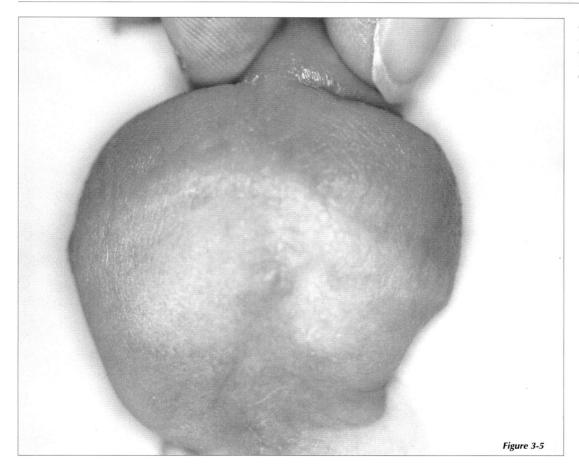

Figure 3-5

Figure 3-5. *Genital lesions that can be mistaken for abuse— idiopathic scrotal edema.*

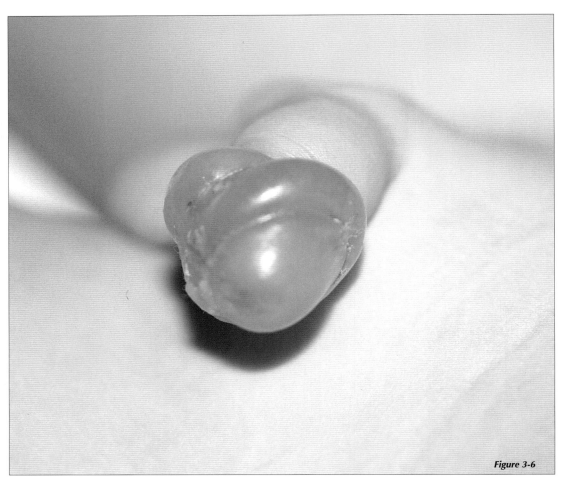

Figure 3-6. Genital lesions that can be mistaken for abuse— paraphimosis.

Figure 3-6

Figure 3-7. Genital lesions that are abusive. This 5-year-old retarded child had penile narrowing below the glans (**a** and **b**) believed to be due to a stricture. The caregiver was trying to control the boy's bed-wetting.

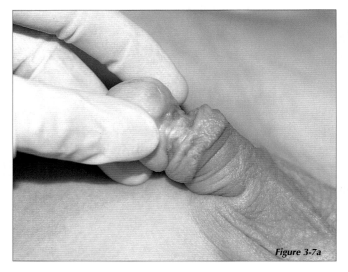

Figure 3-7a

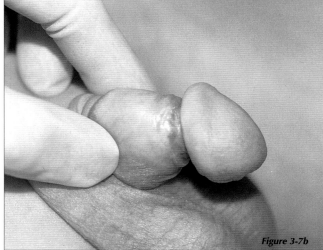

Figure 3-7b

Figure 3-8. Genital lesions that are abusive. Severe penile injury due to a stricture used by the caregiver to control bed-wetting.

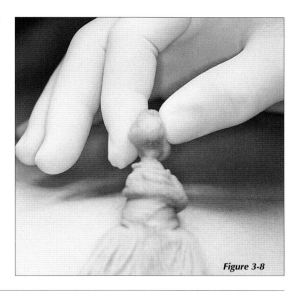

Figure 3-9. Scald burn of the penis. No history was given, and the case was reported as suspected abuse.

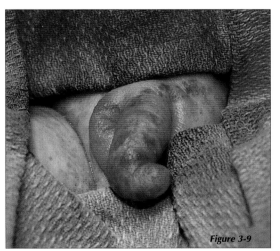

Figure 3-10. Flame burn of the penis that was believed to be caused by a cigarette lighter (*a* and *b*).

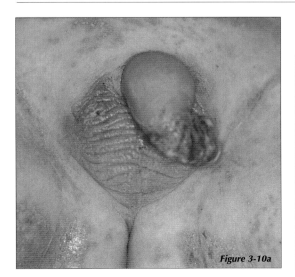

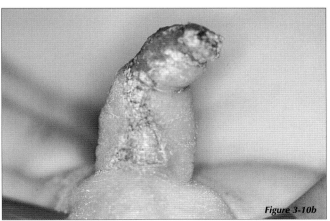

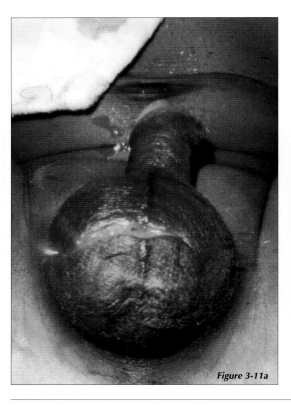

Figure 3-11. *This 38-month-old boy was seen in the emergency room with a deep laceration of the scrotum* **(a)***. The wound was infected and several days old when first seen* **(b)***. The history given was that the child was struck with a hammer by a playmate. Because of the delay in seeking help, the area of the injury, and the difficulty in fitting the injury to the history (one would expect a crushing injury with a hammer), the case was reported as suspected abuse. The child would only say, "Mommy hurt me."*

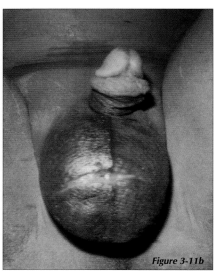

Figure 3-11a

Figure 3-11b

Figure 3-12. *This 30-month-old boy was taken to the emergency room by his mother. The end of the glans penis was cleanly amputated* **(a)***. There was no evidence of crushing injury. His mother stated that he was alone in the kitchen. She heard him cry out and run to her. She noted that he was bleeding from his penis and assumed that he slammed the kitchen cabinet door on himself. There were two older siblings in the home, but the mother stated that they were not in the kitchen at the time. The end of the glans was recovered at the home and grafted back on* **(b)***. The police investigated the scene and felt that the door was too dull to create such a clean amputation. After several days in the hospital, the child stated that "Sissy cut me."*

Figure 3-12a

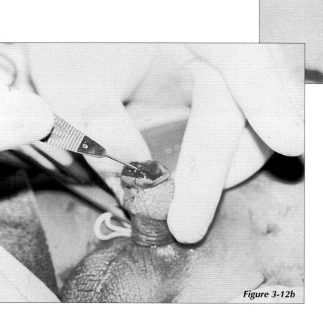

Figure 3-12b

DERMATOLOGY

ELAINE C. SIEGFRIED, M.D.

This chapter provides examples of cutaneous manifestations of abuse as well as conditions that mimic abuse. History, physical examination, and directed laboratory evaluation, including skin biopsy, can often, but not always, establish a diagnosis or provide evidence to support allegations of abuse.

Figure 4-1. *Genital psoriasis has sharp, symmetrical borders and distribution. Genital involvement is characteristic of "inverse" psoriasis.*

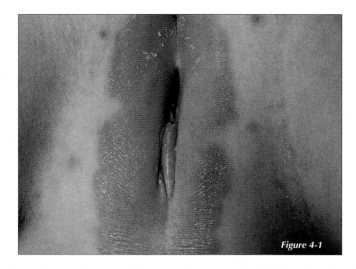

Figure 4-2. *Lichen sclerosis et atrophicus is characterized by atrophy with "cigarette paper" wrinkling and purpura with figure-of-eight vulvar and perianal involvement. Hypopigmentation may be striking in dark-skinned persons. Pruritus and burning are common symptoms. Skin biopsy may be necessary to distinguish this condition from recurrent trauma.*

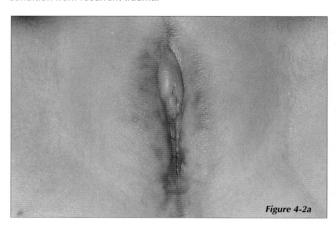

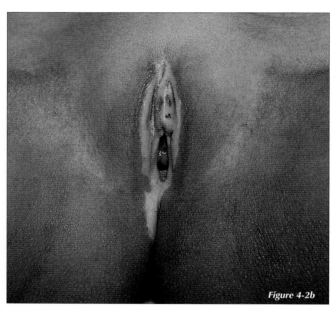

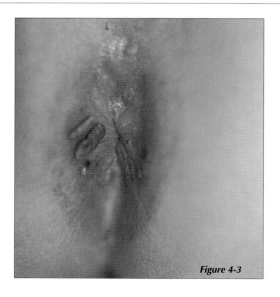

Figure 4-3. *This 9-year-old boy presented with pigmented condyloma. Biopsy revealed the features of bowenoid papulosis and HPV-16, the subtype most often associated with carcinoma. Screening culture was also positive for Chlamydia, additional supportive evidence of sexual abuse, although the patient never disclosed any history of this.*

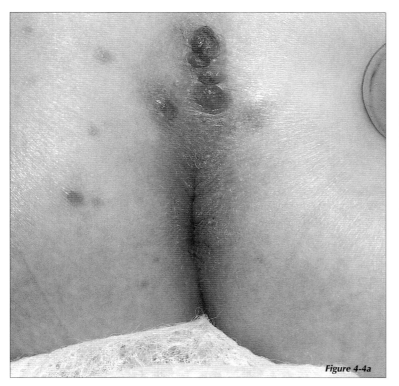

Figure 4-4a

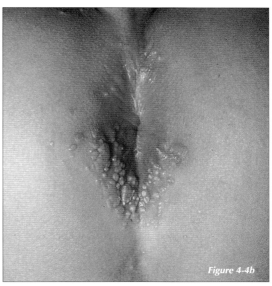

Figure 4-4b

Figure 4-4. *These are examples of perianal molluscum contagiosum in two children (a and b). In this area, lesions are often grouped (or agminate) and may not appear as typical dome-shaped papules with central umbilication. Perianal molluscum is often acquired innocently.*

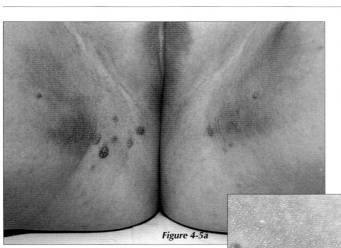

Figure 4-5a

Figure 4-5. *This 10-year-old girl presented with inguinal papules, assumed to be condyloma, and gave a credible history of ongoing sexual abuse by her father. The atypical lesions were proven by biopsy to be irritated molluscum contagiosum (a and b). The child had vaginal findings consistent with ongoing abuse. Despite no physical evidence of genital warts, a vaginal smear was positive for HPV-16.*

Figure 4-5b

113

Figure 4-6. *This 5-year-old with a history of "cold sores" developed vulvar pain and vesicles during hospitalization for meningococcal meningitis. A positive Tzanck smear and culture for HSV-2 verified the diagnosis of herpes genitalis. No history or other physical evidence of sexual abuse was elicited.*

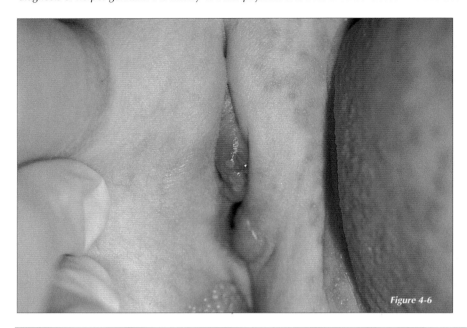

Figure 4-7. *This 12-month-old developmentally delayed boy was admitted to the hospital for "penile cellulitis." Skin examination supported the diagnosis of exogenous injury—specifically chemical or thermal burn. Note the sharp geometric border, with sparing of the inguinal fold.*

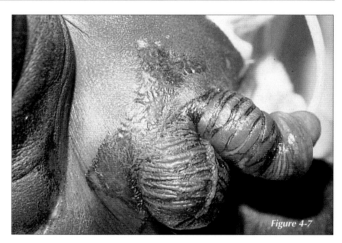

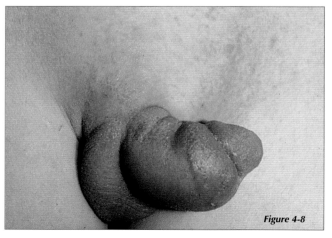

Figure 4-8. *Allergic contact dermatitis is often associated with marked edema at sites with thin skin, such as eyelids and genital areas. (See also Chapter 3.)*

Figure 4-9. *This 2-year-old boy presented with an 18-month history of perianal and anal condyloma, most likely acquired by vertical transmission and spread proximally by acetaminophen and suppositories.*

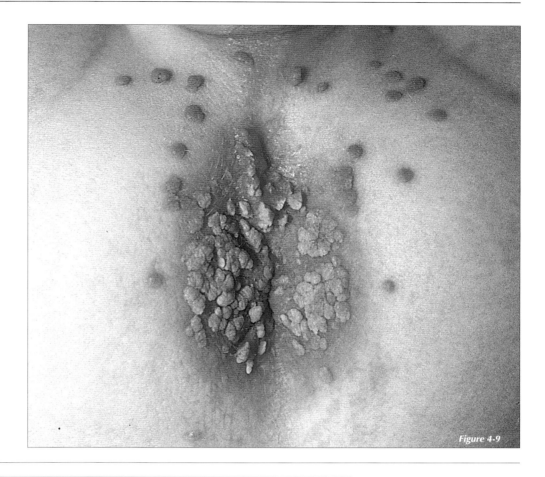

Figure 4-10. *This pigmented papule on a 5-year-old boy proved to be condyloma on skin biopsy. No history or other physical evidence of abuse was elicited.*

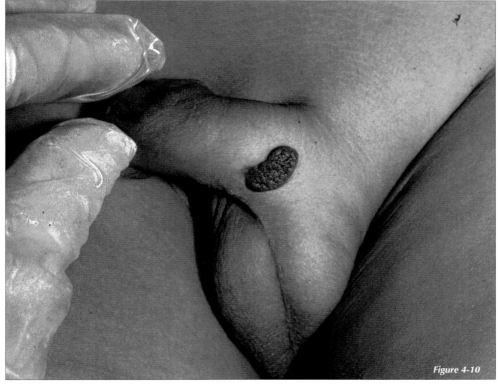

Figure 4-11. *This 15-year-old girl presented with vulvar burning and friable introital mucosa. Skin biopsy confirmed the diagnosis of pemphigus vulgaris. This disorder may occur in older children or adolescents and can present without the typical truncal blisters. Bullous pemphigoid is another immunobullous disease that causes vulvar erosions and occurs in young children. Vulvar bullous pemphigoid has been misdiagnosed as sexual abuse.*

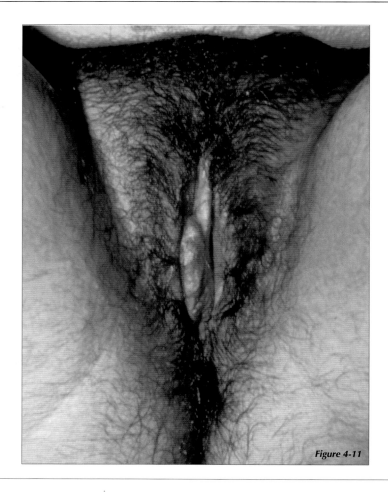

Figure 4-11

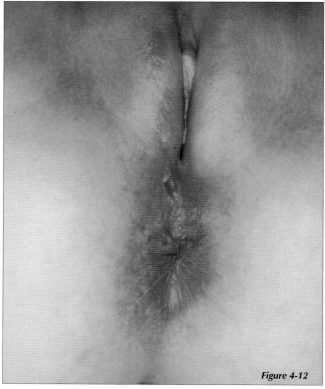

Figure 4-12

Figure 4-12. *This 4-year-old girl had a 2-year history of vulvar pain accompanied by a persistent unilateral linear plaque of skin thickening, redness, and erosions. Her history suggested a risk of sexual abuse by a previous caregiver. However, the clinical and histologic morphology of the lesion supported the diagnosis of inflammatory linear verrucous epidermal nevus (ILVEN).*

Figure 4-13. *This 2-year-old presented with a 2-month history of painful defecation and boggy perianal erythema. Cultures supported the diagnosis of perianal group A streptococcus dermatitis. The condition resolved after a course of erythromycin and topical mupirocin ointment.*

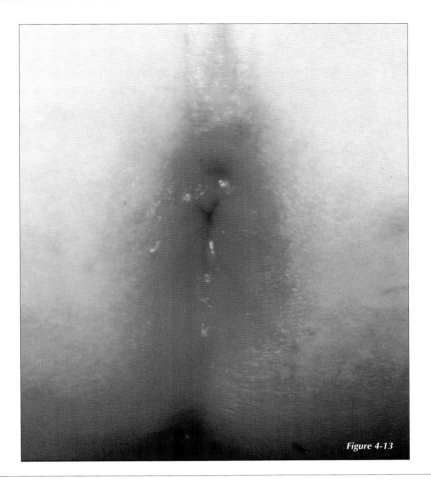

Figure 4-13

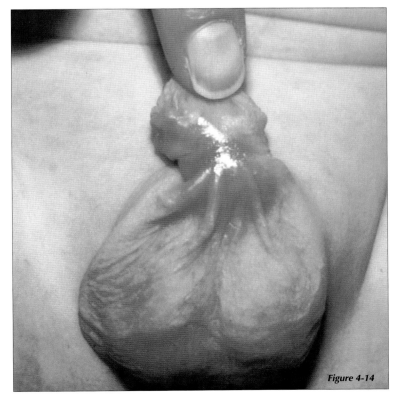

Figure 4-14

Figure 4-14. *This 1-year-old presented with a 4-month history of persistent tender penile erythema and fissuring, with occasional blisters, unresponsive to a variety of topical medications. Skin cultures supported the diagnosis of bullous impetigo caused by Staphylococcus aureus. The condition cleared after a 5-day course of mupirocin.*

Figure 4-15. *This 12-year-old institutionalized child presented with recurrent linear lesions on his extremities. Close inspection revealed incomplete blanching and intact overlying skin, diagnostic features of purpura. The linear configuration is very suggestive of pinch marks produced by an overly tight, prolonged grasp.*

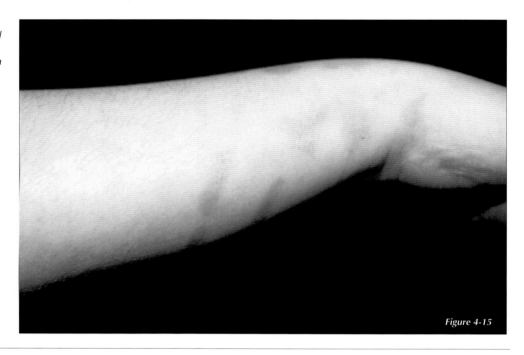

Figure 4-15

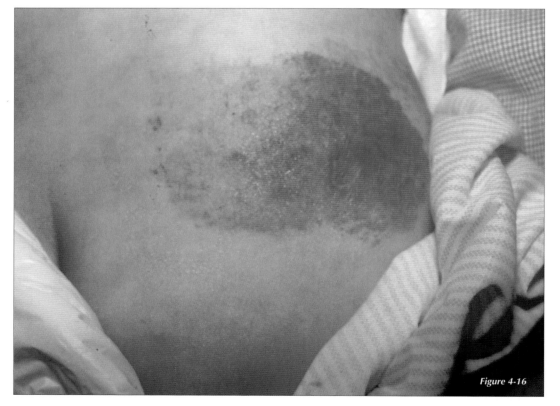

Figure 4-16

Figure 4-16. *This 1-year-old presented with an acute ulceration occurring within a hemangioma that had been present since 1 month of age. The lesion had shown no signs of rapid proliferation for 6 months. Skin biopsy of the ulcer showed superficial epidermal necrosis, suggestive of a burn.*

Figure 4-17. *This 2-month-old presented with a rapidly enlarging infantile hemangioma with typical ulceration within a skinfold.*

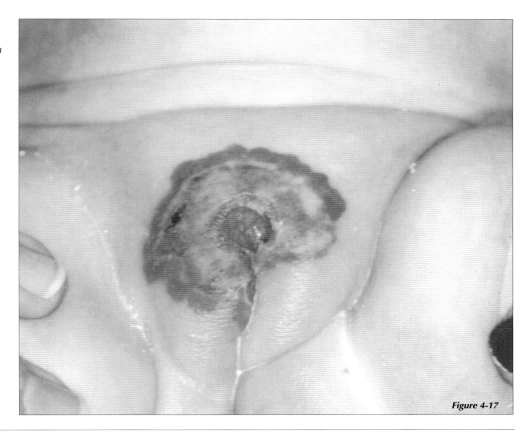

Figure 4-17

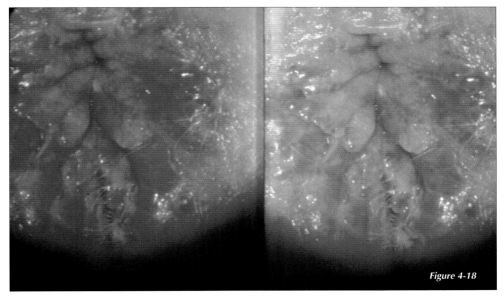

Figure 4-18

Figure 4-18. *This is a 2-year-old boy with a 6-month history of perianal lesions presumed to be condyloma. He was worked up for sexual abuse and finally scheduled for CO_2 laser ablation under general anesthesia. At that time, the lesions were noted to be friable and a biopsy was taken, confirming the diagnosis of Langerhan's cell histiocytosis. (Courtesy Duane Whitaker, M.D., University of Iowa.)*

Dental Injuries

Lynn Douglas Mouden, D.D.S., M.P.H., F.I.C.D., F.A.C.D.

Falls are the causative factor in many dental injuries in children. Frequently the injury will occur when the child falls against an unyielding surface. Avulsions and torn frenulum are the most common results of these injuries.

In abusive injury to the mouth area, the adult generally strikes the child forcefully, or the child may fall when trying to escape the adult's attack. The cases presented in this chapter show the results in abuse situations. Avulsions and torn frenulum usually occur, as shown here.

Figure 5-1. *Displaced upper primary left cuspid with the root forced labially through the cortical palate.*

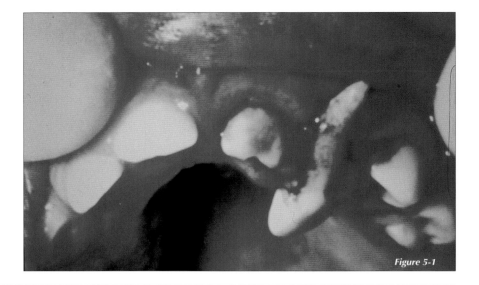

Figure 5-2. *Avulsed permanent central incisor in a 14-year-old boy who was abused over several years with repeated beatings to the head and neck areas.*

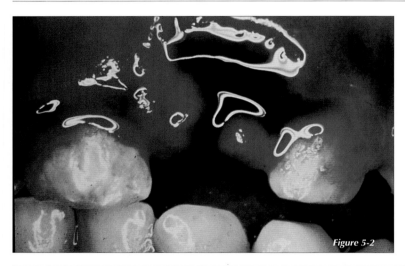

Figure 5-3. *Torn frenulum in a 5-month-old child who was force-fed due to a reluctance to take spoon feeding. The injury was done with a plastic "infant spoon."*

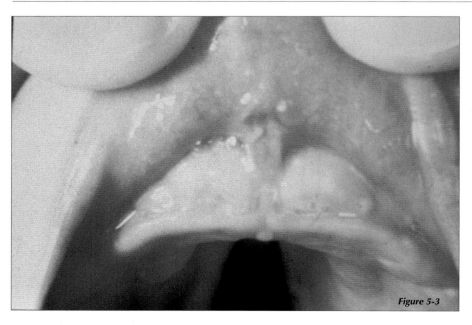

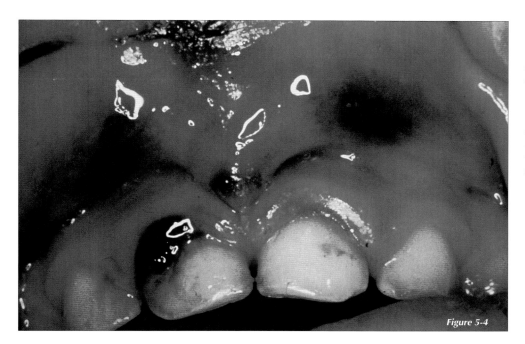

Figure 5-4. Torn frenulum, lacerated lip, and subluxated central incisor in an 8-year-old struck with an open-handed slap. The injuries include an upper lip lacerated by the upper incisors, ecchymosis of the upper lip and vestibule, and subluxation of the permanent right central incisor, as evidenced by bleeding of the periodontal ligament.

Figure 5-5. Severely torn frenulum in a child who fell against a stationary object during a beating by the parent. The incident resulted in severe laceration of the labial frenulum.

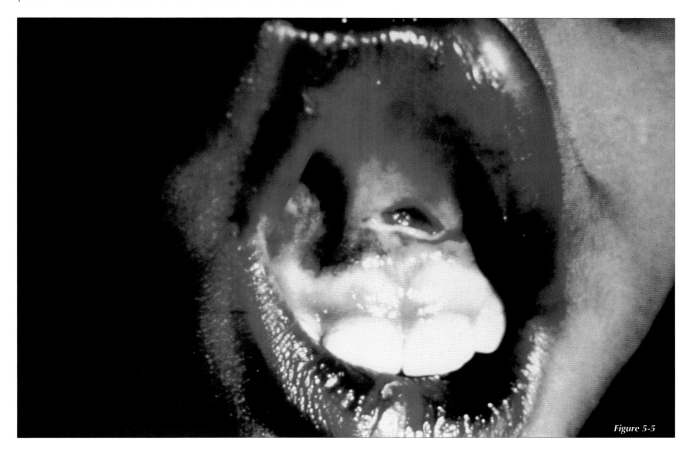

OPHTHALMOLOGY

OSCAR A. CRUZ, M.D.

The presenting signs of child abuse involve the eyes in less than 10% of cases. Ocular sequelae of abuse can include edema, amblyopia, retinal hemorrhages, or even sexually transmitted infection.

The entity most often associated with ophthalmic manifestations of child abuse is shaken infant syndrome. Retinal hemorrhages result from the shaking and can be subretinal, intra-retinal, predominantly in the bipolar layer, or in the nerve fiber layer. As the severity of the hemorrhages increases, there is a corresponding increase in acute neurologic damage.

Ocular injuries that are not associated with abuse include periorbital edema and subconjunctival hemorrhage, injury occurring during the birth process, and injury sustained when cardiopulmonary resuscitation is administered. Retinal hemorrhage may be produced by these latter two processes and must be differentiated from that produced by abusive behavior. The evaluator must look at the patterns of injury and the circumstances (age of the child, presence of medical risk factors, concomitant injuries) to make an accurate determination of causation.

Figure 6-1. This 7-month-old infant presented with lethargy and failure to thrive. The retinal hemorrhages seen in each eye (**a** and **b**) were the only physical findings of shaken infant syndrome. These are the typical white-centered hemorrhages most often seen with severe injury.

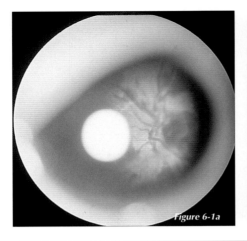

Figure 6-1a

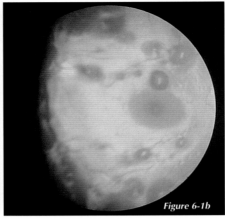

Figure 6-1b

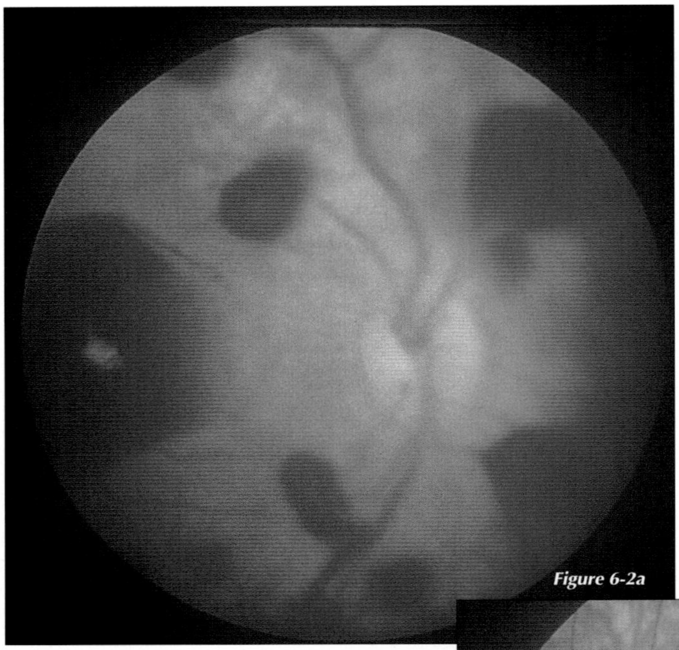

Figure 6-2. a, Retinal hemorrhages, including macular hemorrhage, in a 10-month-old child. **b,** Same child 7 years later with severe optic nerve atrophy secondary to the nerve fiber layer destruction associated with retinal hemorrhages.

Figure 6-2a

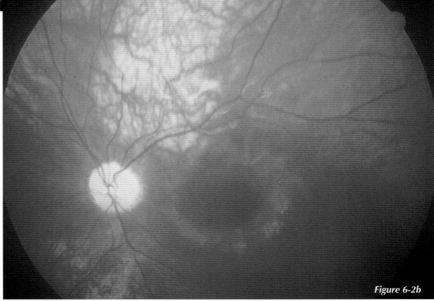

Figure 6-2b

Figure 6-3. *Papilledema secondary to cerebral anoxia in a 5-month-old child who had died of suffocation.*

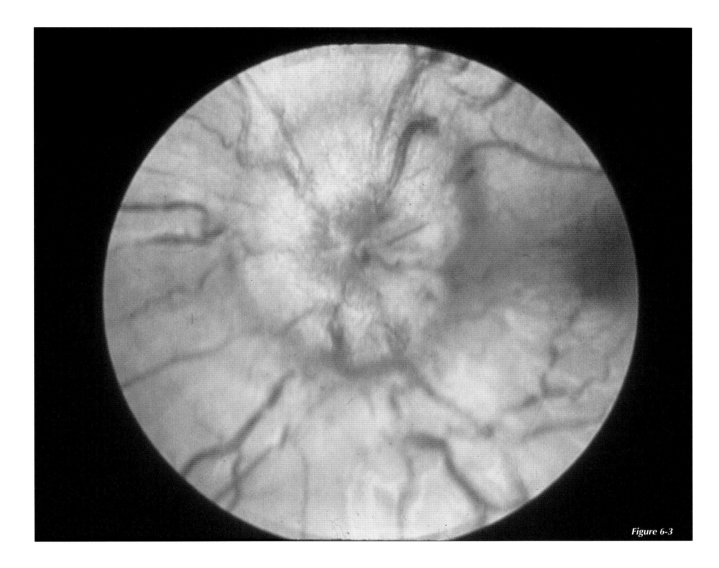

Figure 6-3

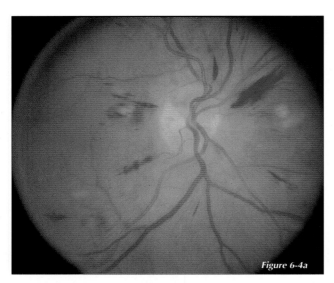

Figure 6-4a

Figure 6-4. *Varying degrees of retinal hemorrhages (a to d) in shaken infant syndrome. (Courtesy E. Dodson.)*

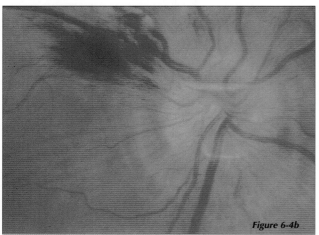

Figure 6-4b

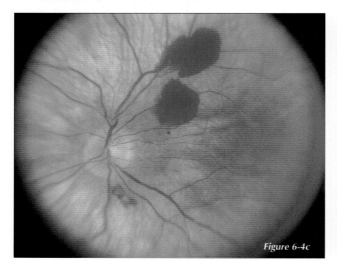

Figure 6-4c

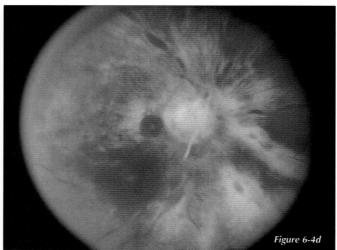

Figure 6-4d

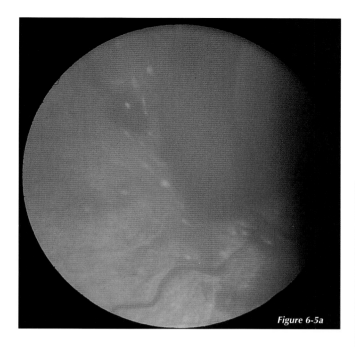

Figure 6-5. Two large retinal hemorrhages (**a** and **b**) with shaken infant syndrome.

Figure 6-5a

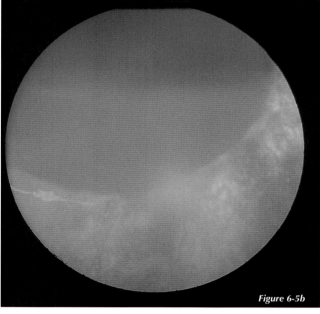

Figure 6-5b

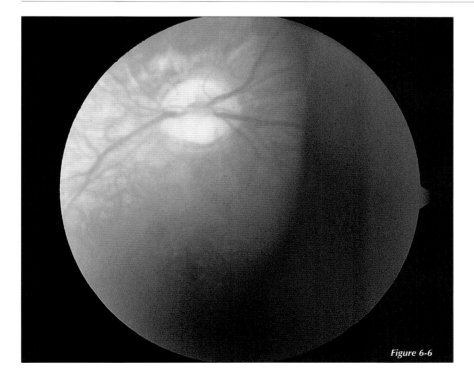

Figure 6-6. Pale optic nerve, a residual effect of retinal hemorrhages, in an abused child with shaken infant syndrome.

Figure 6-6

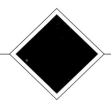

PART TWO

Radiologic Investigations

RADIOLOGY OF CHILD ABUSE

ARMAND E. BRODEUR, M.D.

Radiology serves a threefold role in child abuse cases:

1. Identifying traumatic injury
2. Recognizing abusive origin
3. Employing the optimal imaging modality to document findings

The radiologist is able to identify the type, extent, and age of the child's injury and distinguish between accidental and inflicted trauma.

The radiologist can employ a variety of imaging modalities, including X-ray films, nuclear medicine techniques, computerized tomography, magnetic resonance imaging, and ultrasound. These offer advantages or disadvantages that differ with type of injury, placement of injury, and age of the child.

The ability to determine the age of an injury can be critical to the radiologic diagnosis of child abuse. Differentiating between abuse and accident depends as much on when the injury occurred as on what the injury is and how it occurred. Dating injuries can illuminate discrepancies between the radiologic findings and the history provided, with incongruities often indicative of abuse. The presence of old and new fractures, suggesting that abuse took place over a period of time, is a strong indicator of nonaccidental injury in children. Multiple injuries in various stages of healing is pathognomonic for child abuse.

For a detailed description of abusive injuries and the types of surveys needed to investigate injuries in abuse cases, consult Monteleone & Brodeur: *Child Maltreatment—A Clinical Guide and Reference*. The cases offered here illustrate both common injuries and injury patterns and lesions that are not abuse. These cases demonstrate the variety and specificity of clinical imaging examinations needed to elicit a specific diagnosis and to ascertain the extent of the pathologic process. In most clinical situations film/screen imaging is the modality of first choice and still accounts for greater than 90% of all the radiographic imaging in the field of medicine. In addition to the relative ease of film/screen radiography, the radiograph provides a generalized scan that guides the specialist to the areas of special interest. Once the area of abnormality is identified, the radiologist can select nuclear, ultrasound, computerized tomography scan, or magnetic resonance imaging for more definitive information with the least expenditure of time. X-ray machines are portable and offer an opportunity for various bedside radiographic projections. Film/screen radiography hastens the identification and extent of the pathologic process and allows the clinician more accuracy in determining which special imaging modalities will elicit the greatest amount of information.

Figure 7-1. This 3 1/2-year-old boy had ruptured hollow viscera after severe blunt trauma to the abdomen. **(a)** Note the subtle outline of the pneumoperitoneum (arrows) in this supine radiograph. **(b)** Cross-table lateral radiograph demonstrates a large amount of free intraperitoneal air.

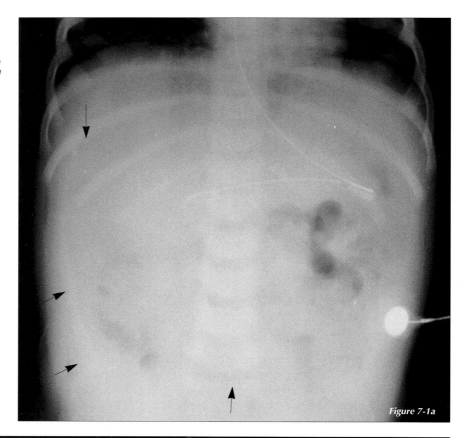

Figure 7-1a

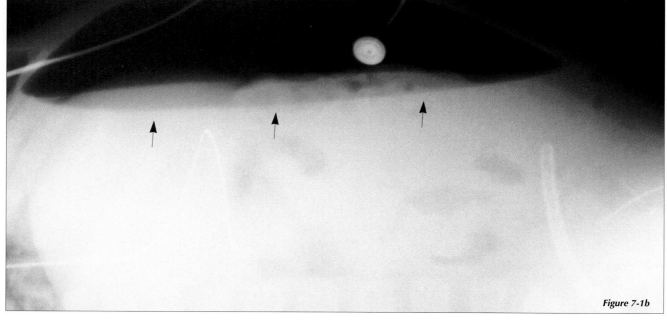

Figure 7-1b

Figure 7-2. Blow-out fracture of the right orbit due to a direct blow to the eye from a blunt object believed to be a fist. A portion of the roof of the maxillary sinus is depressed downward, resulting from increased intraorbital pressure. The rounded soft tissue mass in the roof of the right maxillary sinus is part edema, part hemorrhage, and a portion of the inferior rectus muscle.

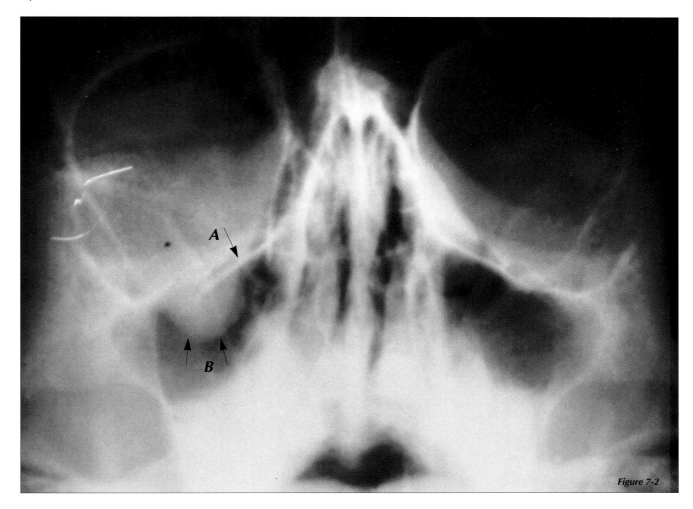

Figure 7-2

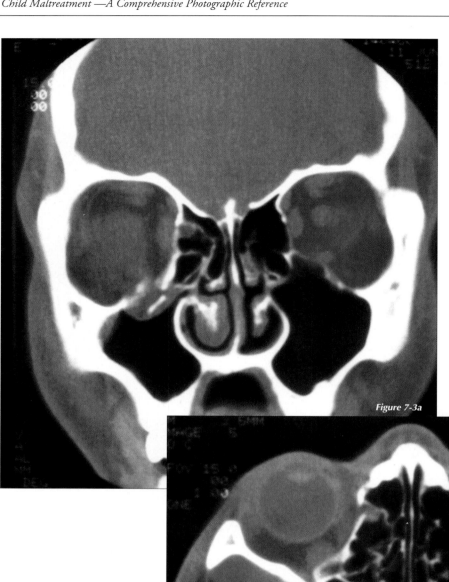

Figure 7-3. *This 12-year-old boy was punched in the right eye. **(a)** CT scan of the face identifies a blow-out fracture of the floor of the orbit projecting downward into the right maxillary sinus. **(b)** The patient also sustained a blow-out fracture of the medial orbital wall projecting into the ethmoid sinuses.*

Figure 7-3a

Figure 7-3b

Figure 7-4. This 6-year-old boy was admitted with vomiting after a severe blow to the mid-abdomen. **(a)** A lateral view of the abdomen shows dilated proximal duodenum above an intramural hematoma (arrows). **(b)** The upper gastrointestinal film shows a partial coil spring sign identified by elongated valvulae conniventes of the duodenum (arrows). This is a classic sign of an intramural hematoma of the duodenum. **(c)** Large intramural hematoma of the transverse colon (arrow). **(d)** Same patient after resolution of the colonic hematoma.

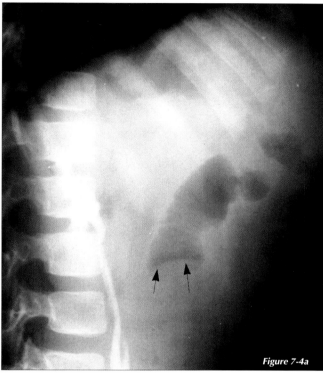

Figure 7-4a

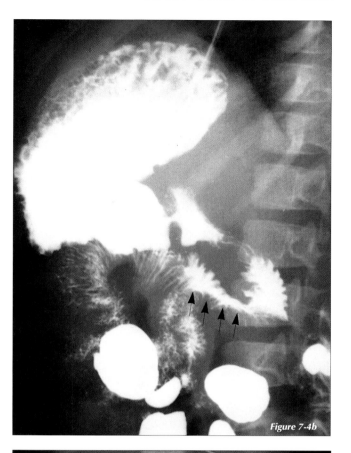

Figure 7-4b

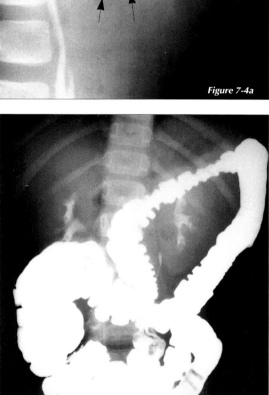

Figure 7-4d

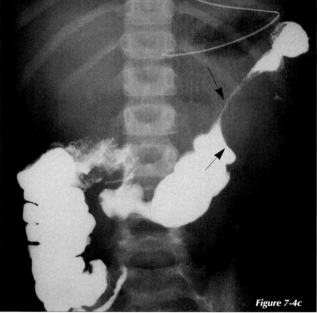

Figure 7-4c

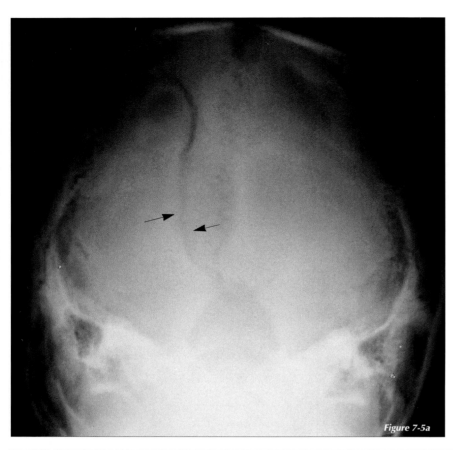

Figure 7-5a

Figure 7-5. *This 3-year-old boy, who was severely malnourished, was admitted because of head injuries. (a) Long linear fracture of the right side of the occipital bone (arrows). (b) Lateral view of the skull is normal. Arrows indicate a film artifact. Note the width of the normal sutures (S). (c) Pseudotumor cerebri 1 month after adequate nutrition. Note the width of the sutures as a result of the rapid brain growth following recovery from malnutrition. (d) Lateral view. The effect of rapid brain growth is greater in the supratentorial area. The coronal suture (C) is wider than the lambdoid suture (L). (e) CT scan of a normal brain in this child after adequate nutrition.*

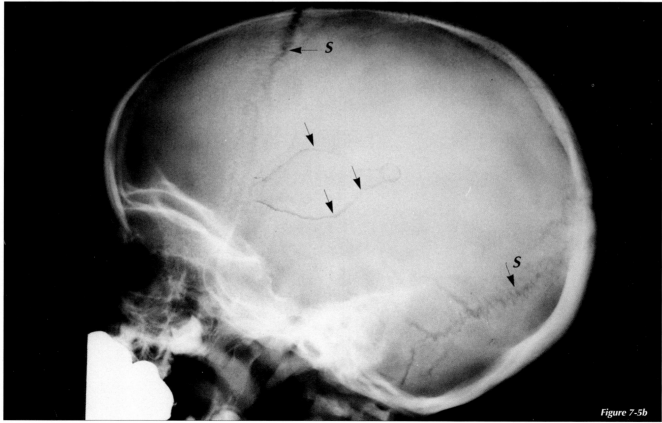

Figure 7-5b

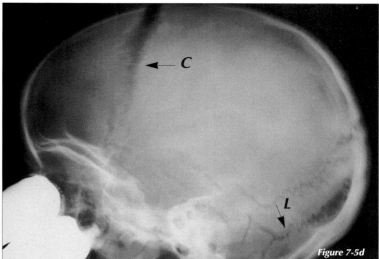

Figure 7-5d

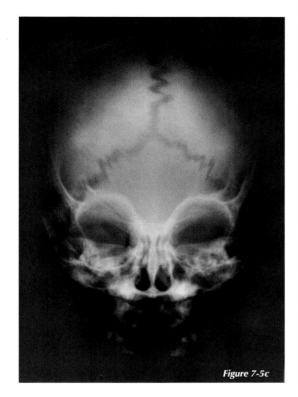

Figure 7-5c

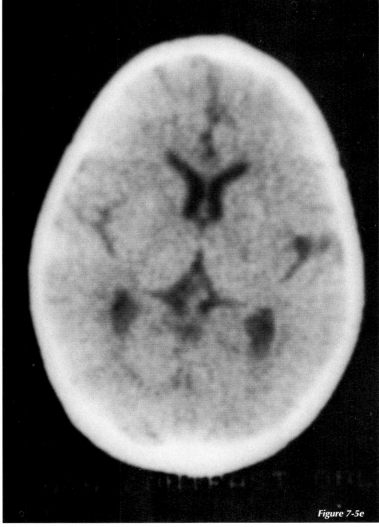

Figure 7-5e

Figure 7-6. *This 7-month-old boy was admitted in shock with a low hemoglobin, rigid abdomen, and multiple bruises. **(a)** CT scan of the upper abdomen shows multiple liver lacerations (large arrows) and peritoneal hemorrhage (smaller arrows). **(b)** CT scan shows peritoneal hemorrhage on the left as well (arrows). **(c)** CT scan of the skull, through bone windows, shows a long linear fracture of frontal bone (arrows); no subdural hematoma was identified. **(d)** Radiograph of the chest shows multiple fractures of the ribs on the left in different stages of healing (arrows) and a moderate left pneumothorax (P). **(e)** There is periosteal reaction along the mid-shafts of both tibia (arrows), an indication of rough handling.*

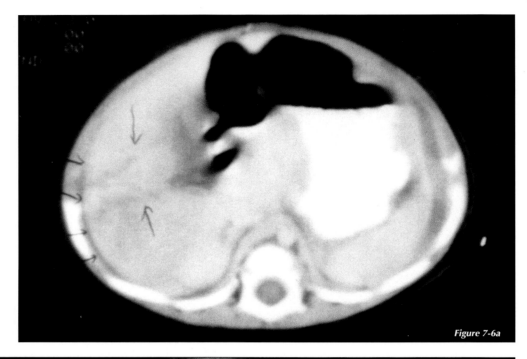

Figure 7-6a

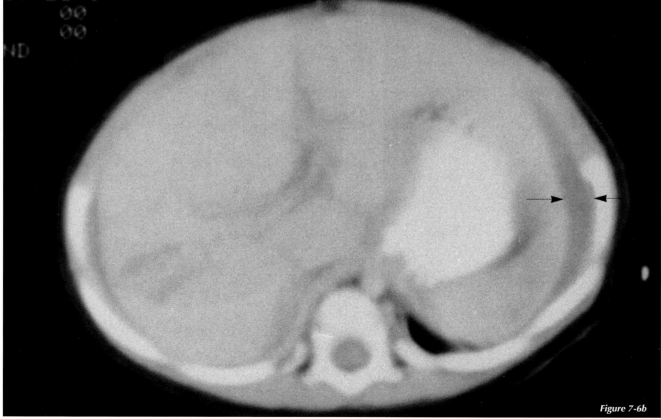

Figure 7-6b

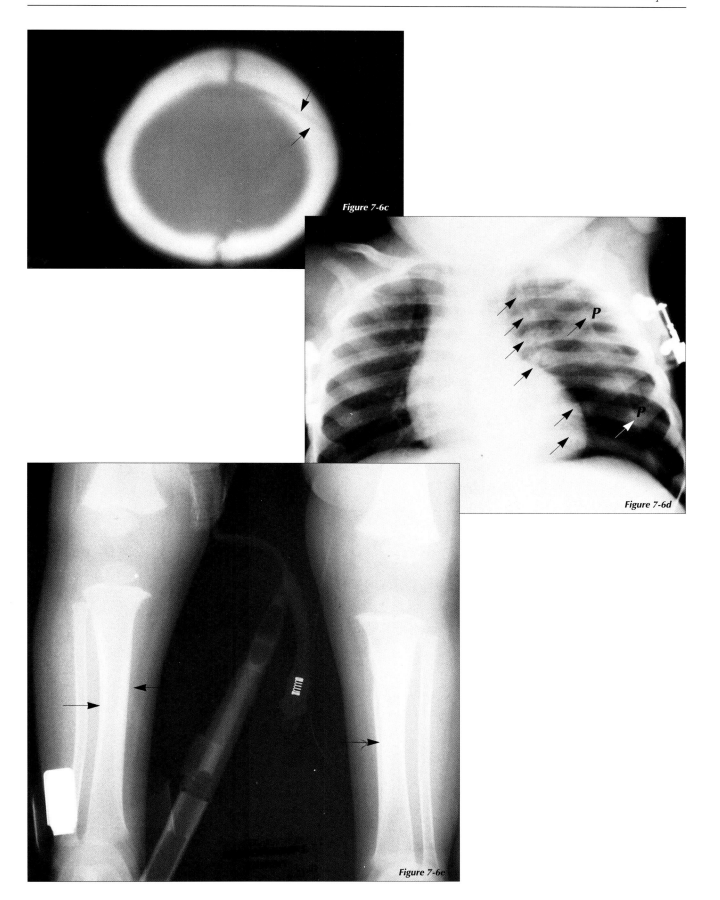

Figure 7-6c

Figure 7-6d

Figure 7-6e

Figure 7-7. This 1-year-old boy was brought, unconscious, to the emergency room after a period of drowsiness and a convulsion. There was no history of trauma. The child was found to have an intraparenchymal hemorrhage on the right and a midline subdural hemorrhage.

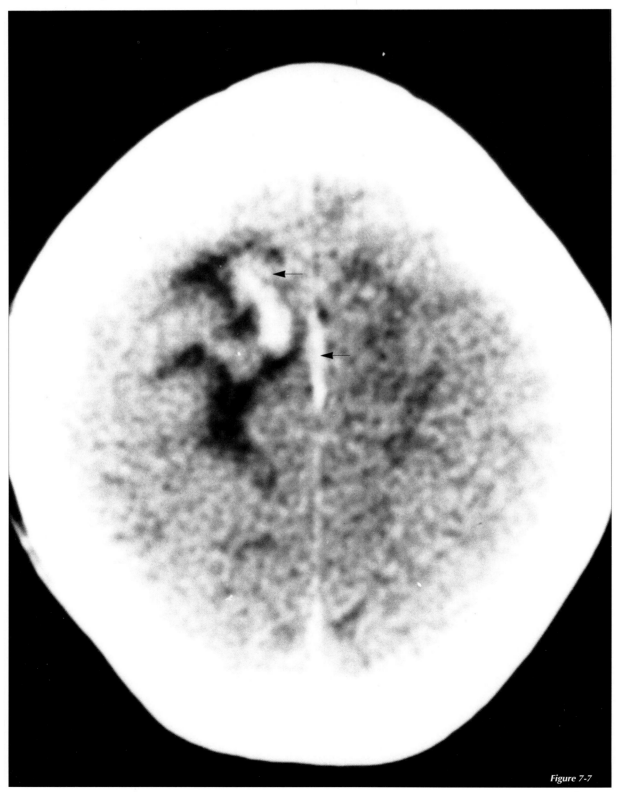

Figure 7-7

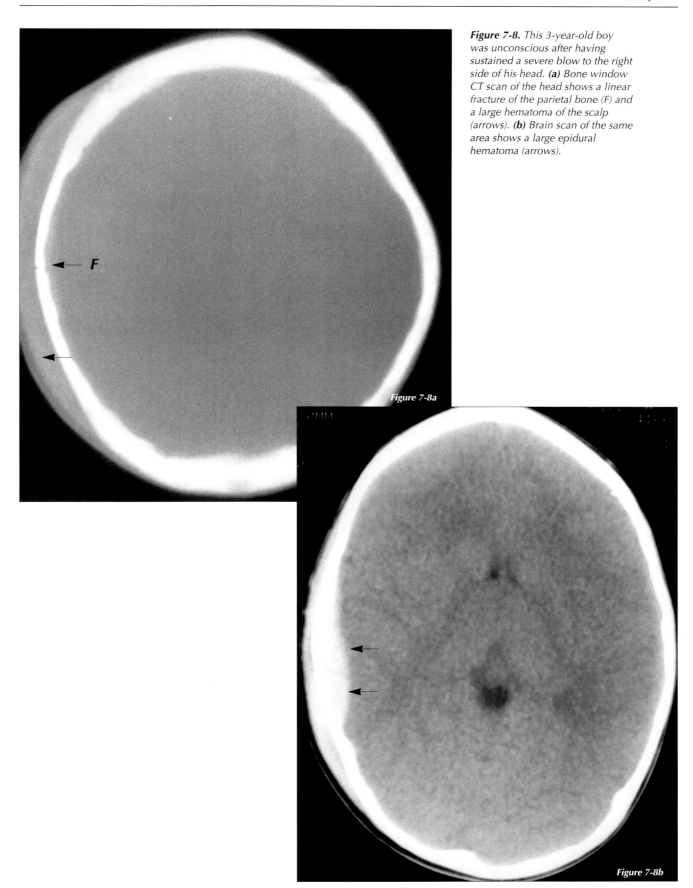

Figure 7-8a

Figure 7-8b

Figure 7-8. *This 3-year-old boy was unconscious after having sustained a severe blow to the right side of his head. (a) Bone window CT scan of the head shows a linear fracture of the parietal bone (F) and a large hematoma of the scalp (arrows). (b) Brain scan of the same area shows a large epidural hematoma (arrows).*

F

Figure 7-9. *This child was seen in the emergency room to evaluate a "soft spot on the head." There was no history of trauma. (a) CT scan (bone windows) reveal multiple fractures of the skull (arrows). (b) Soft tissue hemorrhage of the scalp and small midline subdural hemorrhage associated with the skull fractures. The brain is otherwise normal.*

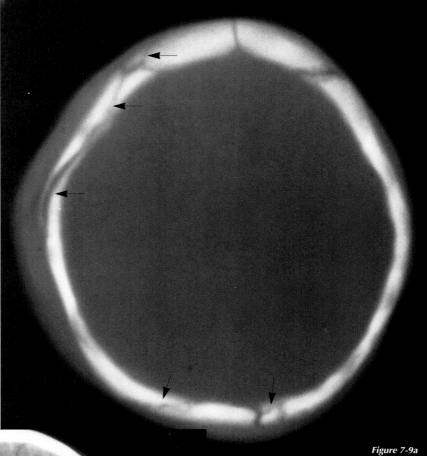

Figure 7-9a

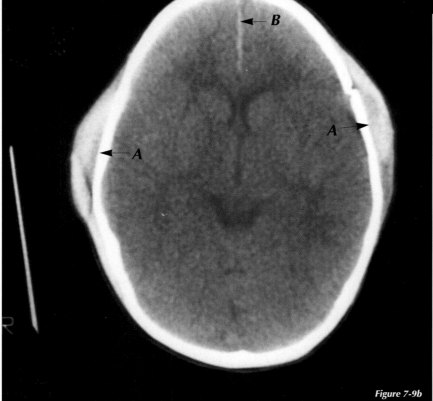

Figure 7-9b

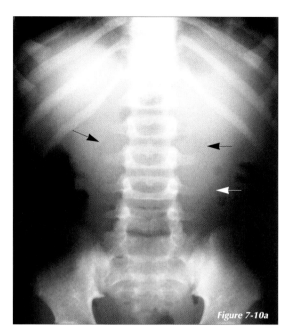

Figure 7-10. This 7-year-old sustained a traumatic rupture of the pancreas secondary to a kick in the abdomen. **(a)** Supine radiograph of the abdomen is generally unremarkable. The psoas muscle shadows are faintly outlined (arrows). Often when the pancreas has been injured the right psoas muscle in particular is obliterated because of edema in the fat line. In this instance, most of the injury was in the tail of the pancreas, but the psoas muscle outline on the left is fairly definite. This abdominal radiograph would not have provided specific localizing information. **(b)** Abdominal ultrasound examination identifies widened tail of the pancreas. The distance between the two cross markers is significantly wider than normal. **(c)** CT scan of the abdomen at the mid-kidney level identifies post-traumatic obstructive hydronephrosis of the left renal pelvis (arrow) secondary to pressure from the hemorrhagic enlargement of the tail of the pancreas. This post-contrast examination identifies a normal right kidney.

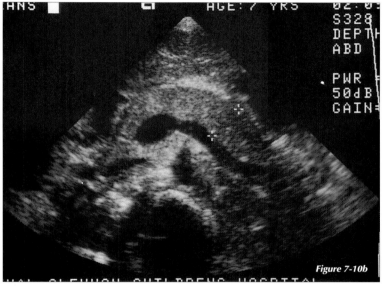

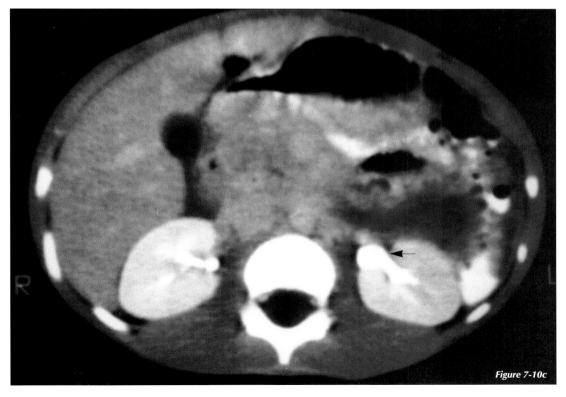

Figure 7-11. *This 13-month-old girl was admitted with irritability, vomiting, and a suspected acute abdomen. She was found to have a traumatic laceration of the liver.* **(a)** *Supine abdominal radiograph was unremarkable. The abdominal shadows are within normal limits. There is no evidence of fluid in the right costophrenic angle and no significant elevation of the right leaf of the diaphragm.* **(b)** *Left lateral decubitus view yields a normal examination. Note the absence of free air, sentinel ileus, or elevation of the right leaf of the diaphragm.* **(c)** *CT scan of the mid-liver reveals a traumatic laceration separating the lobes.*

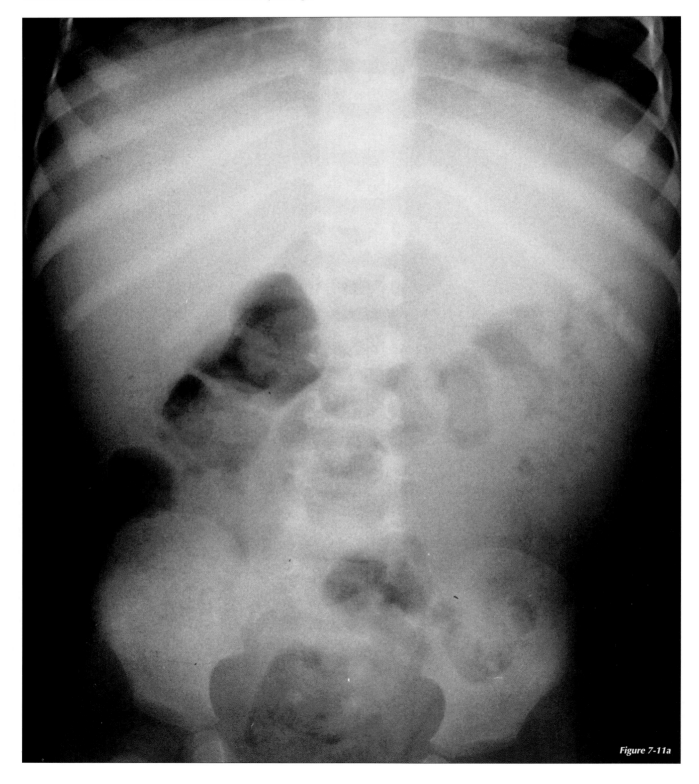

Figure 7-11a

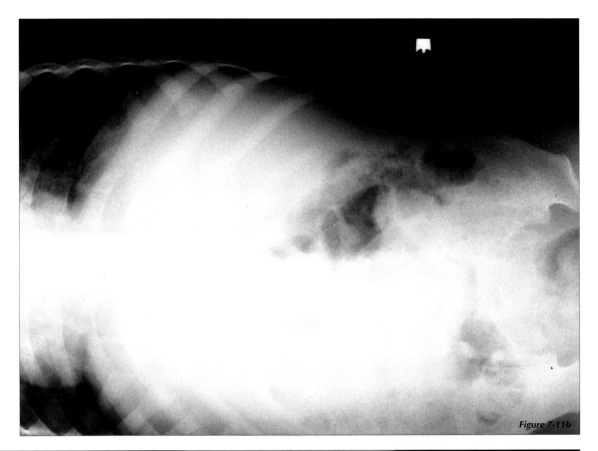

Figure 7-11b

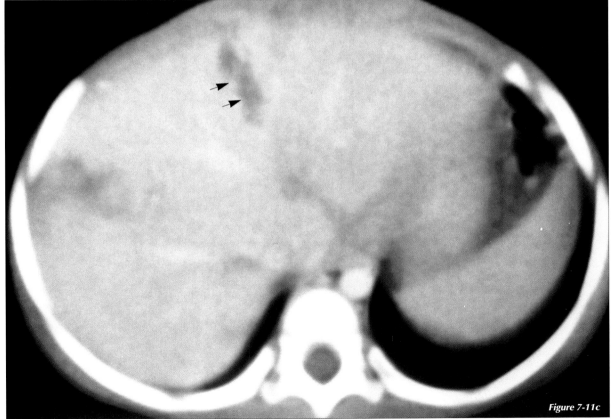

Figure 7-11c

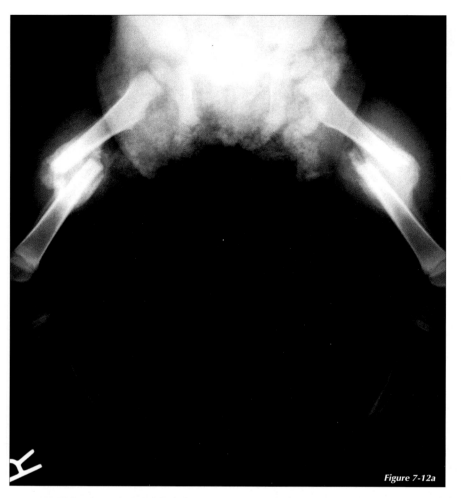

Figure 7-12a

Figure 7-12. *This 14-month-old boy was admitted from an outlying hospital with a diagnosis of child abuse. He presented with redness, swelling, and a mass in both mid-thighs. (a) Fairly well-healed, overlapping mid-femoral fractures. (b) Because of facial bruising, skull radiographs were obtained. No fracture is demonstrated in this projection, but the sagittal suture is in the upper limits of normal in width. In light of the case history, this finding was considered suspicious. (c) Lateral examination shows no fracture, but similarly, the lambdoid suture (arrows) is in the upper limits of normal (or wider). (d) CT scan reveals a normal brain with no hemorrhage.*

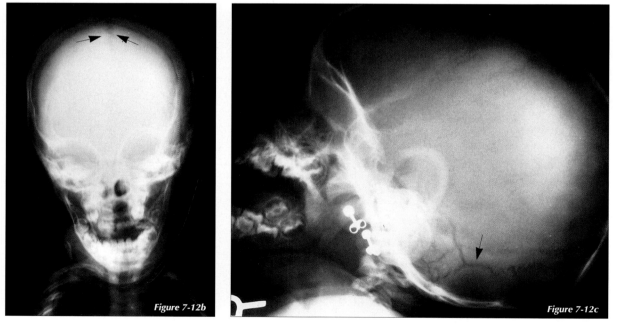

Figure 7-12b

Figure 7-12c

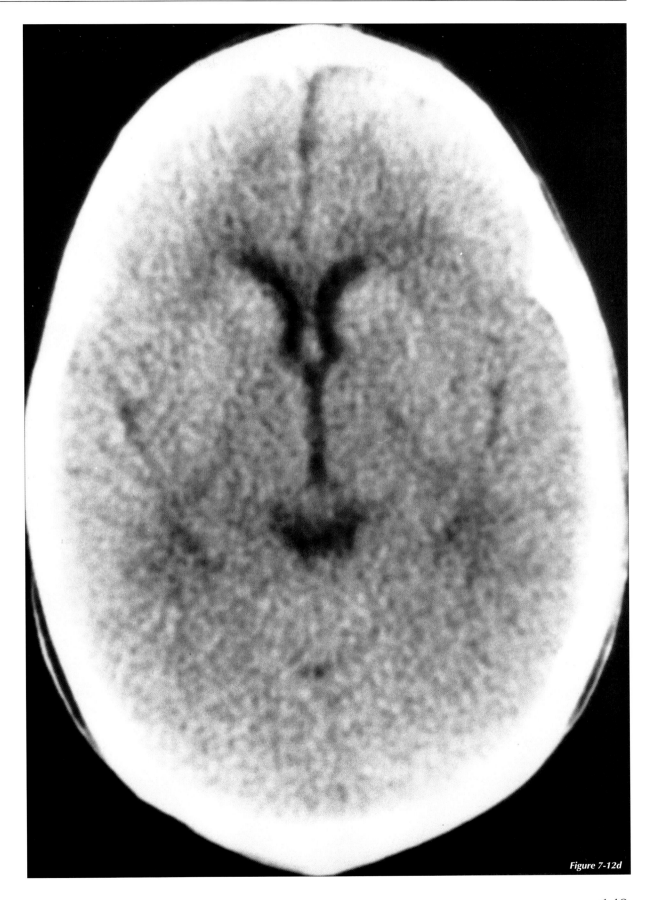

Figure 7-12d

149

Figure 7-13. *This 3-year-old boy was admitted with vomiting, moderately rigid abdomen, and multiple bruises near the midline. The history given was that the child had fallen. (a) CT scan of the upper abdomen shows a wide tail of the pancreas caused by hemorrhage. The history that the father had kicked the boy was subsequently elicited. (b) CT scan in the mid-renal area reveals a widened hydronephrotic left kidney secondary to obstruction. This was a post-contrast examination and there was no excretion on the left. The obstruction was due to the enlarged pancreas. (c) Post-contrast examination of the abdomen reveals moderate adynamic ileus throughout the small intestine (sentinel ileus). A radiograph of the abdomen would not have been sufficient to identify the location or the nature of the injury.*

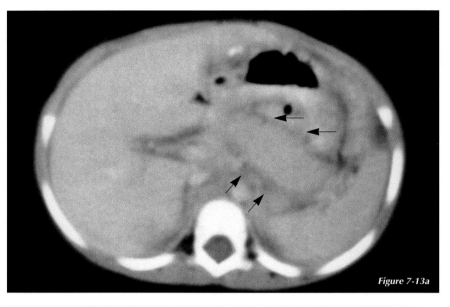

Figure 7-13a

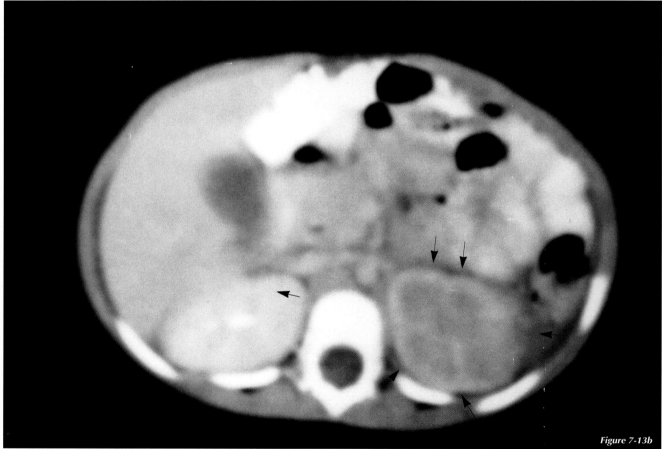

Figure 7-13b

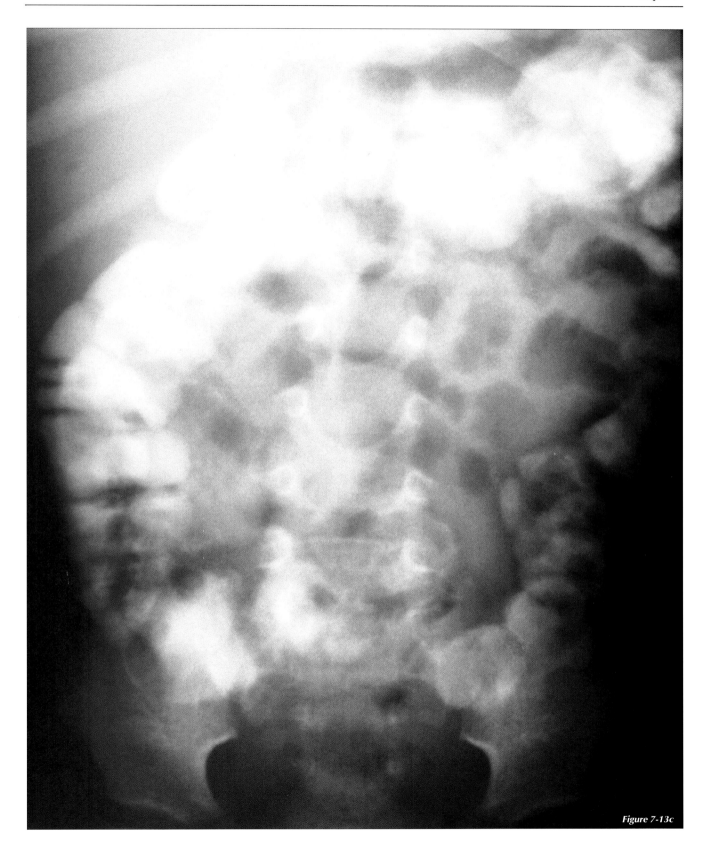

Figure 7-13c

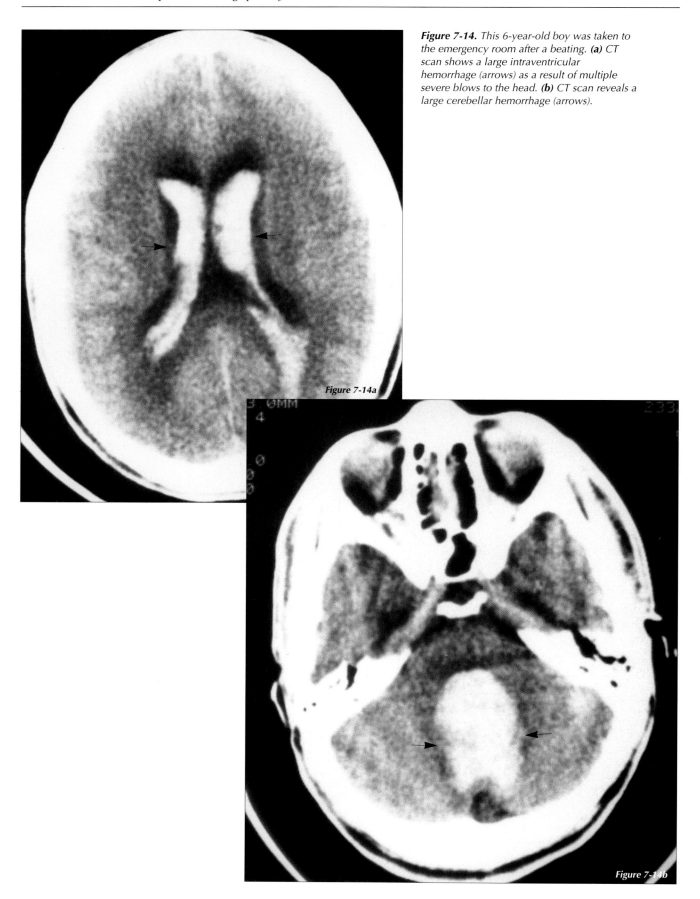

Figure 7-14. This 6-year-old boy was taken to the emergency room after a beating. **(a)** CT scan shows a large intraventricular hemorrhage (arrows) as a result of multiple severe blows to the head. **(b)** CT scan reveals a large cerebellar hemorrhage (arrows).

Figure 7-14a

Figure 7-14b

Figure 7-15. *Left knee showing metaphyseal avulsion fracture. This classically subtle metaphyseal fracture is viewed from the medial side of the distal femur (arrow). It resulted from severe wrenching of the leg. Lateral twisting produces this kind of injury because the capsule is attached to the ring of the femoral and tibial metaphyses. In this instance the medial side was pulled away from its metaphyseal insertion. Commonly, the metaphysis of the proximal tibia will be avulsed as well. If the child had been held by the mid-legs and whipped back and forth in midair, the force of the body would have ruptured the metaphyses of the femur and tibia on both sides.*

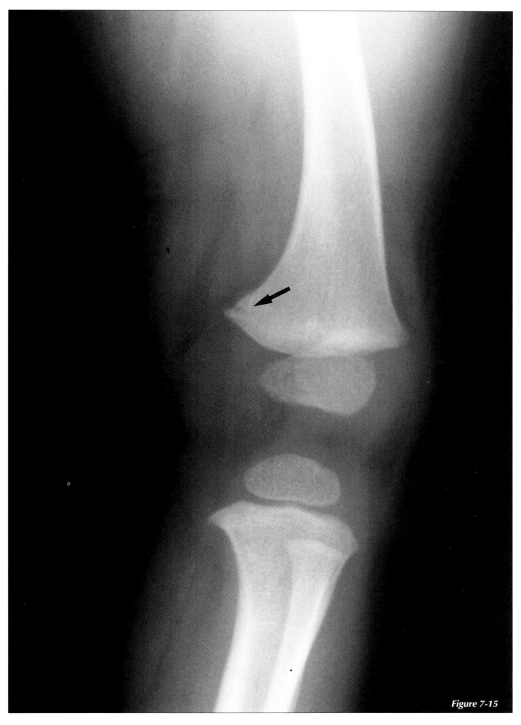

Figure 7-15

Figure 7-16. Rib fracture. With the exception of birth trauma, fractures of the ribs in infants are exceedingly uncommon. The bones of the thoracic cage in a baby are very resilient. A considerable amount of force or pressure is required to fracture the normal ribs. The fifth, sixth, seventh, and eighth ribs on the left (arrows) have been fractured. The rounded densities represent healing new bone. Note that in two locations on the seventh rib the fractures are on the posterior as well as the anterior surface. On the right, the fourth, fifth, and sixth ribs are fractured (ruptured) at the costovertebral junction. The joint ruptures on the right are more recent than those on the left. This finding is evidence of at least two separate incidents of assault. Often the ninth through the twelfth ribs are obscured by abdominal soft tissues on a chest radiograph. A careful search must be made of the lower ribs or the only clue to child abuse may be missed.

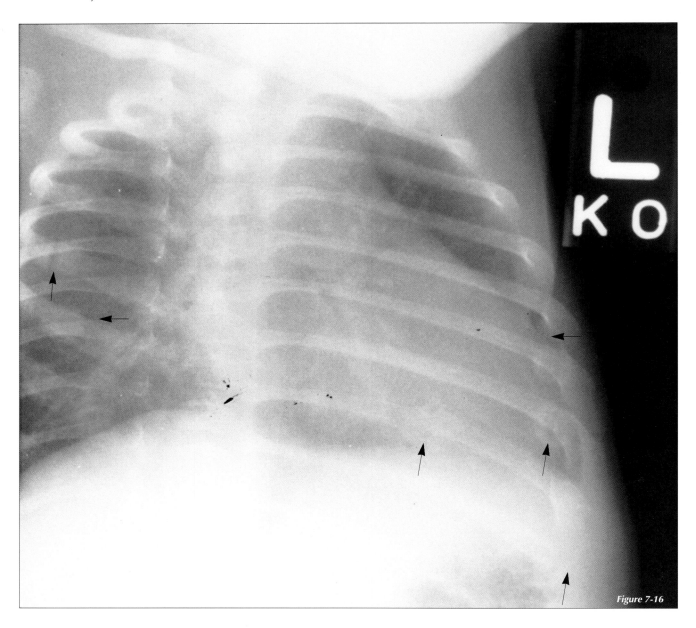

Figure 7-16

Figure 7-17. (a) *Healing rib fracture. With the amount of solid new bone around the fracture site seen here, it is estimated that the injury occurred at least 4 weeks previously, possibly longer. The incident that prompted this examination was the discovery of a compression fracture of the second lumbar vertebra in this 7-month-old infant* **(b)**. *The father confessed to having forcefully seated the baby in a high chair only after the baby had been admitted from the pediatric emergency room with the possible diagnosis of either meningitis or bacterial spondylitis.*

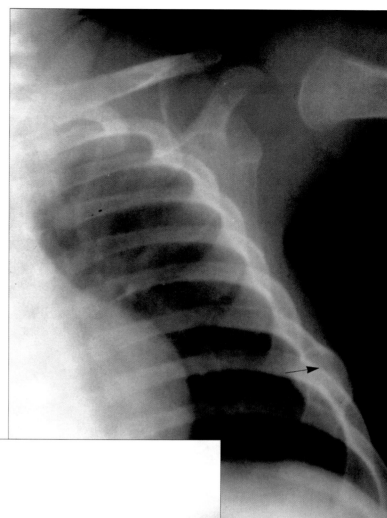

Figure 7-17a

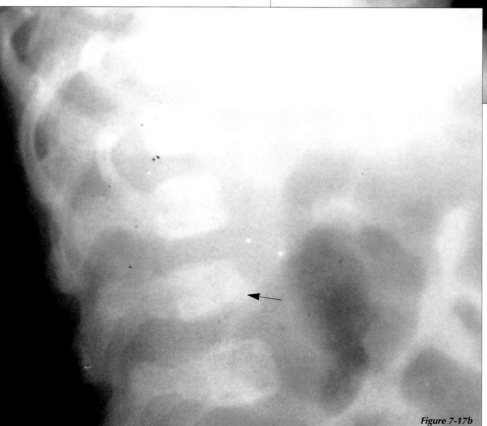

Figure 7-17b

Figure 7-18. *Healing rib fractures. The subtleties of healing rib fractures are such that they may easily escape detection. There are at least 12 healed fractured ribs in this chest radiograph. Several of these are at the costovertebral junction where the changes are slight. Although this example shows injuries of the ribs far greater in number than the average case, this is a classic example of child abuse that occurred 4 to 6 weeks previously. At the time of this examination, the infant displayed no clinical signs and no obvious symptoms. The rib fractures were an incidental finding.*

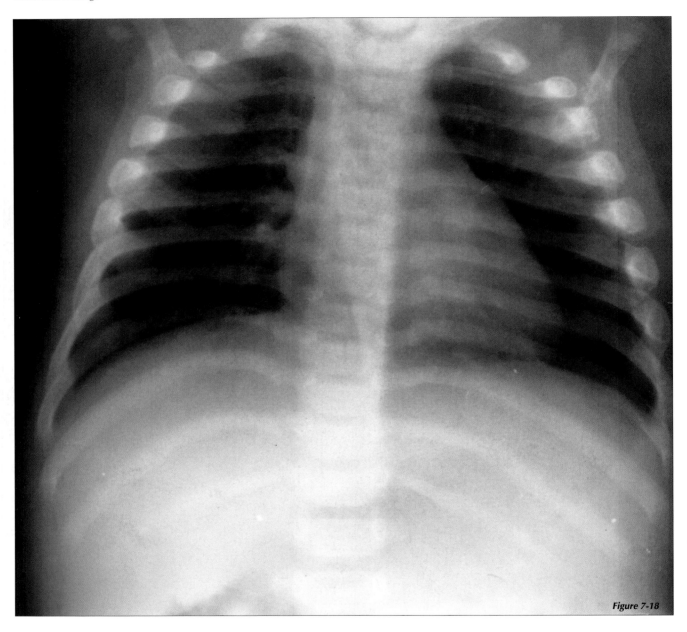

Figure 7-18

Figure 7-19. *Normal clavicle. The small notch on the inferior aspect of the left clavicle at the junction of the middle and lateral thirds is not a healed fracture but the usual site of attachment of the coracoclavicular ligament. The apparent separation of the lower ribs at the costovertebral junction is normal in this age group, particularly in a lordotic radiographic projection such as this. These normal characteristics make it difficult to identify acute separation of the ribs at the costovertebral junction. An examination at a later date would easily have identified any injury that may have been present. Nuclear bone scans are invaluable in instances such as these.*

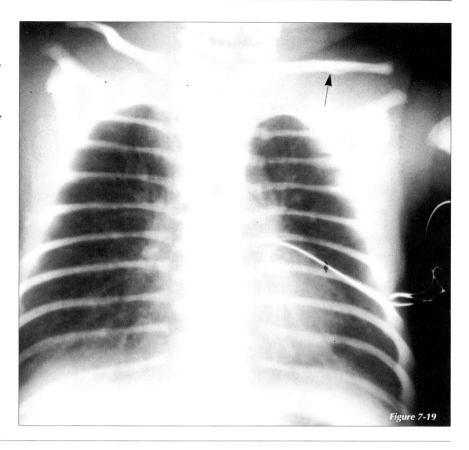

Figure 7-19

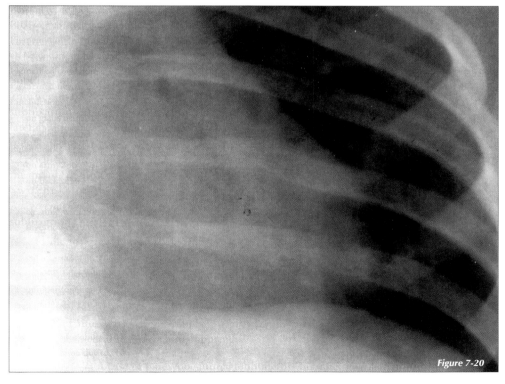

Figure 7-20

Figure 7-20. *Normal costovertebral junctions in infants. Note that the lowest rib in this radiograph appears to be totally separated from the vertebral joint. Radiographic projections are such that the angle of the X-ray beam is in an upward plane, which in effect projects the rib at a higher point in the lower borders of the radiograph.*

Figure 7-21. (a) *Normal knee in a 3-month-old infant. Note the slight "cornering" at the metaphysis in the posterior part of the distal femur. One could not make a positive diagnosis of metaphyseal avulsion on the basis of this view. The examination is not a true lateral view, and you could not determine the knee to be normal based on this single radiographic projection.* **(b)** *Slightly magnified view of same patient in Figure 7-8. On the anteroposterior examination a corner fracture of the metaphysis of the distal femur is readily identified. Disruption of the metaphysis of the proximal tibia on the medial side is easily determined. These types of fractures result from stress on the knee capsule ligaments caused by severe twisting. Note the edema adjacent to the tibial avulsion site. The skin was red, swollen, and tender at the site, and the patient was irritable. This finding is classic for the diagnosis of child abuse. The metaphyseal avulsions common in copper-deficiency syndrome are not isolated incidents on one side of one joint.*

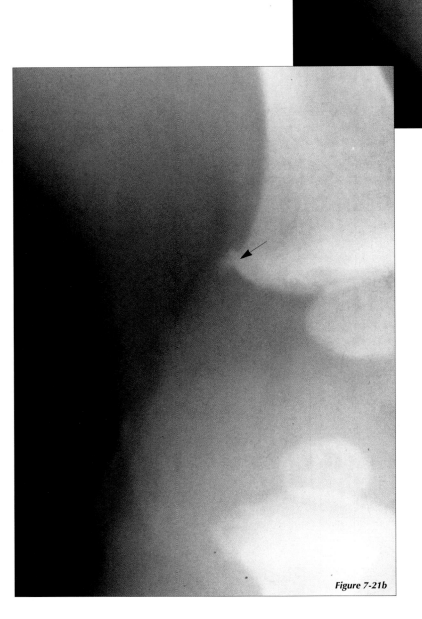

Figure 7-21a

Figure 7-21b

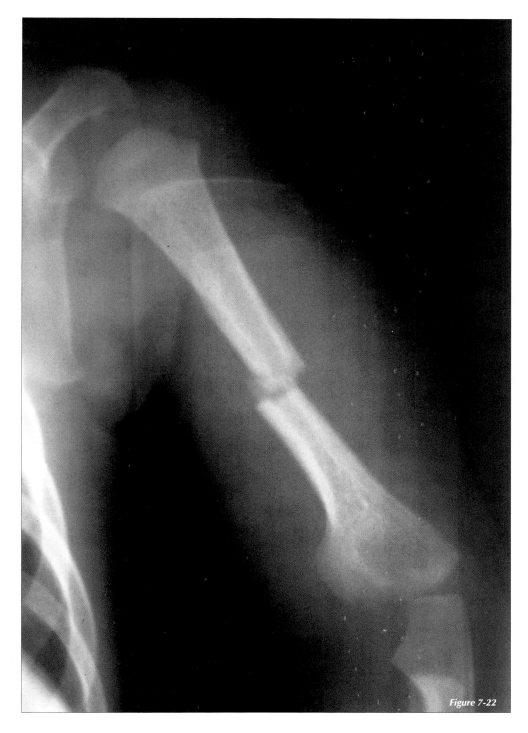

Figure 7-22. *Fractured humerus in 6-week-old infant. The baby was irritable and unwilling to move the left upper limb. A sharp, clean transverse fracture of the humerus was seen. The infant's age was determined by the ossifying epiphysis (arrow) of the humeral head seen just beneath the acromion process. A fracture of this type could only have occurred by a direct blow; a history of a self-generated fall is not possible. Fractures of any of the long limb bones are always highly suspicious for abuse unless the history is precise in explaining the accident.*

Figure 7-22

Figure 7-23. *Multiple fractures demonstrated by infantogram. This 4-week-old girl was brought to the emergency room with poor vital signs, near shock, and multiple bruises. An infantogram revealed a total of 30 fractures. Some are delineated by arrows on this radiograph. Note the number of posterior rib fractures, many at the costovertebral junction, others at the costochondral junction, and still others in between. Nineteen fractures of the ribs were identified. A recent spiral fracture of the left humerus is seen. The stage of healing indicates that this fracture is approximately 2 weeks old. Note the ossifying epiphysis of the proximal humerus on the left side—an indicator of the patient's age of almost 6 weeks.*

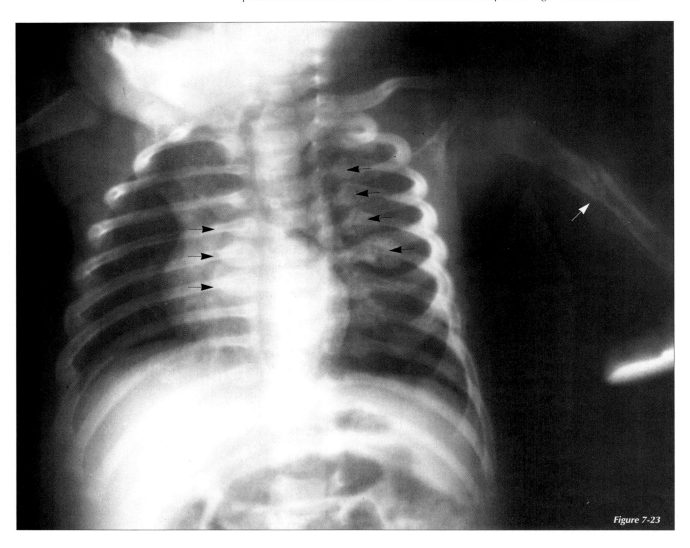

Figure 7-23

Figure 7-24. *Overriding spiral fracture of the midshaft of the femur in a 4-week-old girl. Note the slight metaphyseal irregularity (arrow) on the posterior distal femur, most likely an avulsion related to a twisting injury. The clinical signs included a large amount of swelling and redness. There were no bruises. The baby was irritable and unable to use her left lower limb.*

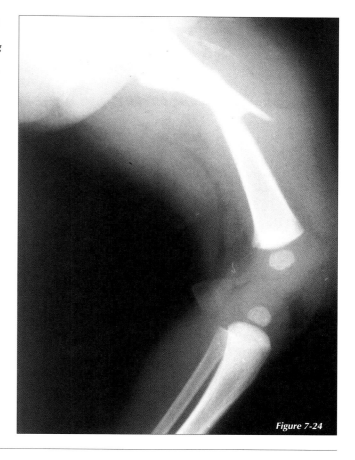

Figure 7-24

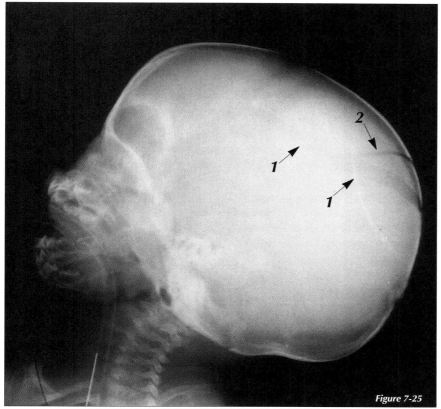

Figure 7-25

Figure 7-25. *Two skull fractures, one on each side. Note the widely separated fracture in the left parietal bone (l), which extends from the sagittal suture to the coronal suture. A second fracture is present in the parietal bone on the right side. The evidence is that of two separate injuries. Their locations are at different sites and could not have occurred simultaneously as alleged by the parents. Note that the coronal suture is widely separated, indicating increased intracranial pressure. The infant was unconscious; there was subgaleal hemorrhage and swelling of the scalp. CT scans identified cerebral edema and subarachnoid hemorrhage. The occipitomastoid suture is separated as well, which is another indication of increased intracranial pressure. This is not a fracture line. The infant is 6 weeks old as revealed by the epiphysis of the proximal humerus that is just beginning to ossify.*

Figure 7-26. *Acute increased intracranial pressure. This infant was admitted to the emergency room in a drowsy state and with neurological signs of concussion. Radiographic examination showed wide separation of the sagittal and lambdoid sutures. Faint evidence of a linear fracture of the left parietal bone is present. Note that the "teeth" of the sutures are short, indicating acute separation. Chronic increasing intracranial pressure allows sufficient time for the edges of the suture to lay down new bone, which results in long serrations with relatively little space in between. Ultimately, it was admitted that this baby was struck on the side of the head with the flat of the hand. The result was cerebral edema and subdural hemorrhage.*

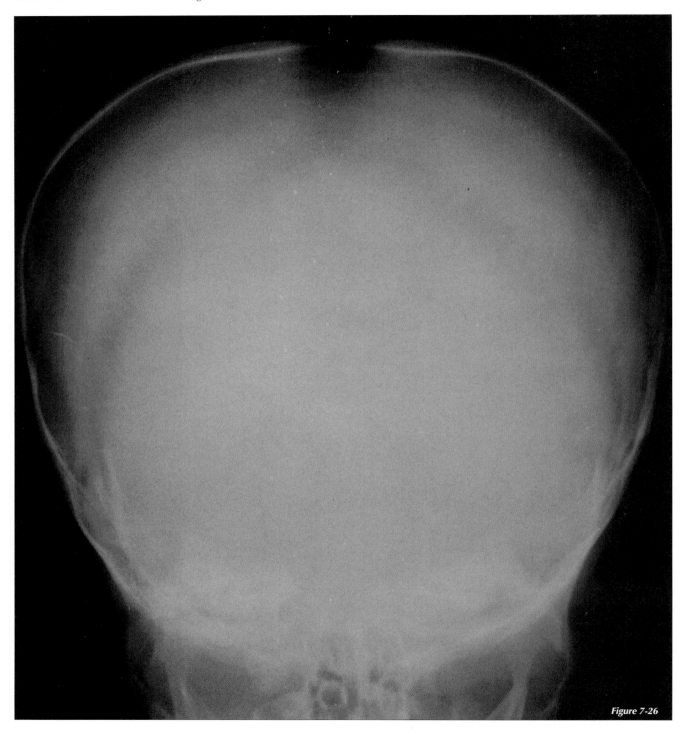

Figure 7-26

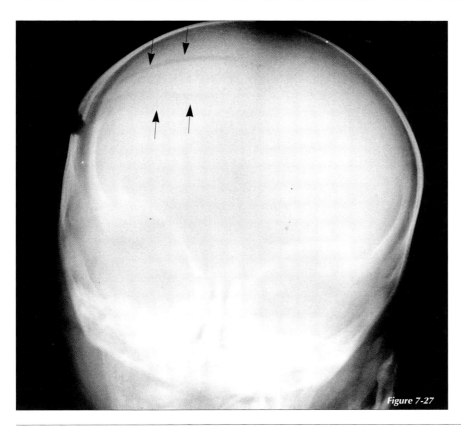

Figure 7-27. *Two fractures of the right parietal bone. It is likely that both of these fractures occurred at the same time. The sagittal suture is widely separated due to cerebral edema and subarachnoid hemorrhage. On the basis of this examination, accidental injury (such as having dropped the child a distance of 3 or 4 feet onto a tile floor) might conceivably have explained this incident. Both fractures are on the same side of the head, but undoubtedly a thorough search of the skeleton for other signs of previous injury would have to be made because abuse is suspected.*

Figure 7-27

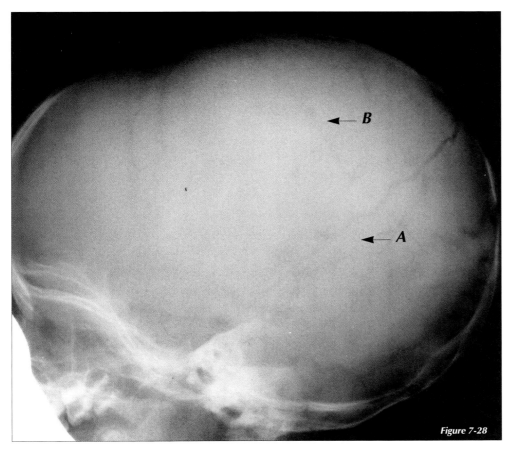

Figure 7-28. *Two linear parietal bone fractures. The longer fracture extends from the sagittal suture downward and anteriorward (a). Note that it crosses the squamous suture line(s) but terminates at the other suture line. Fractures do not cross suture lines. In this instance, the squamous suture from the other side is projected to a position superior to the squamous suture on the injured side. Having been thus superimposed onto the fracture line, it appears to have been crossed. The second fracture (b) extends from the sagittal suture downward and posteriorward, terminating at the lambdoid suture on the same side. There are two other fracture lines. Clearly, the evidence indicates multiple injuries to the skull. The infant was listless; the scalp was swollen. No evidence of fractures was seen elsewhere.*

Figure 7-28

163

Figure 7-29. *Multiple fractures of the skull. Two fractures, (b) and (c), are on opposite sides of the sagittal suture at the vertex. This happens when the blow occurs directly at the midline and each parietal bone sustains a fracture. The fracture line is sharper and clearer at (a) than it is at (b) because (a) is on the right side of the parietal bone in this right lateral view of the skull. The fracture on the left side is less sharp and more magnified because it is further away from the film. Fracture (c) extends from the sagittal suture to the lambdoid suture and appears to have crossed the lambdoid as a result of radiographic superimposition from the opposite side. The vertical line seen at (o.m.) is not a fracture. It is a normal occipital mastoid suture.*

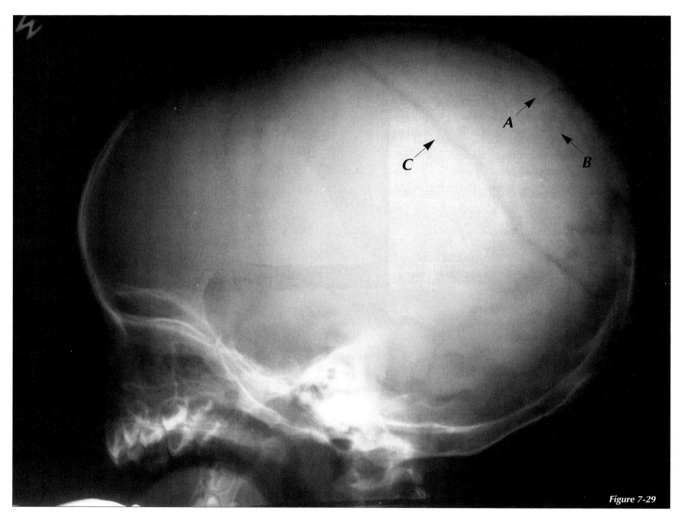

Figure 7-29

Figure 7-30. Two fractures on the same side. Note that the fracture line in the mid-left parietal bone appears to have crossed the squamous suture line (S) and traverses the entire squamous part of the temporal bone, extending into the base of the skull. Since fractures do not cross suture lines, the logical explanation is that the injury occurred directly at the squamous suture line and the fracture extended upward into the parietal bone and downward into the temporal bone.

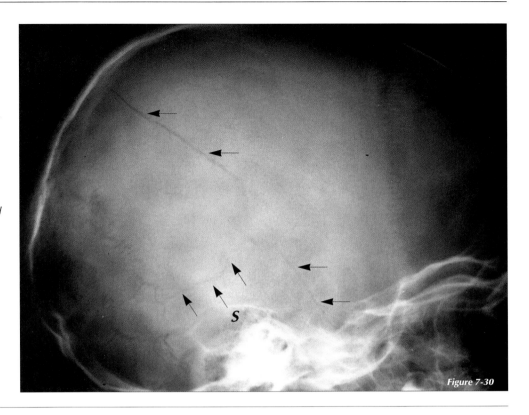

Figure 7-31. Fractured ribs in various stages of healing demonstrated by a nuclear scan. There are three readily identifiable "hot spots": The posterior ninth and tenth ribs on the left and the costovertebral junction of the third rib on the right. Radiographically, a healing fracture of the tenth rib on the left was demonstrable and a nuclear scan was done to search for evidence of fractures elsewhere. The nuclear scan directed attention to the fracture at the costovertebral junction on the right side, which was not evident on a chest radiograph. Injuries in this costovertebral location are subtle and may not become evident until at least 2 weeks later, when new bone becomes visible. A bone scan is helpful in directing attention to the areas of the skeleton that need more definitive detailed radiographic examination.

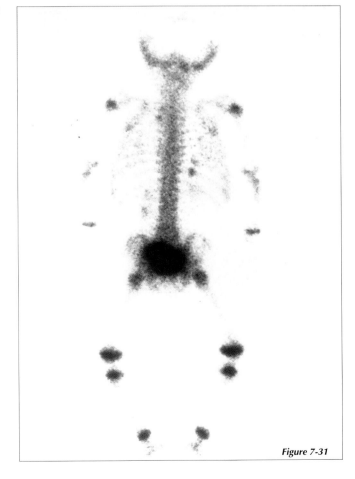

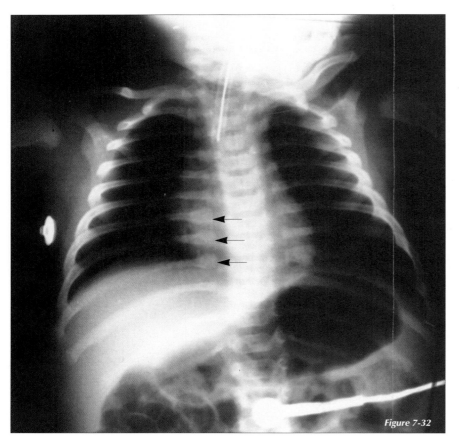

Figure 7-32. *Healing injuries of the seventh, eighth, and ninth costovertebral junctions on the right side. These injuries are greater than 2 weeks' duration. No obvious fracture was involved. The child's chest was apparently squeezed so that these joints were disrupted. Hemorrhage stimulated periosteal repair. Disruption of the costovertebral junction in infants is common and usually the result of a forceful, crushing squeeze.*

Figure 7-33. *Left pleural effusion or hemothorax. The infant had multiple bruises and showed signs of neglect. It was suspected that this might have been the result of a blow to the chest. No fractured ribs or other signs of skeletal trauma were found elsewhere.*

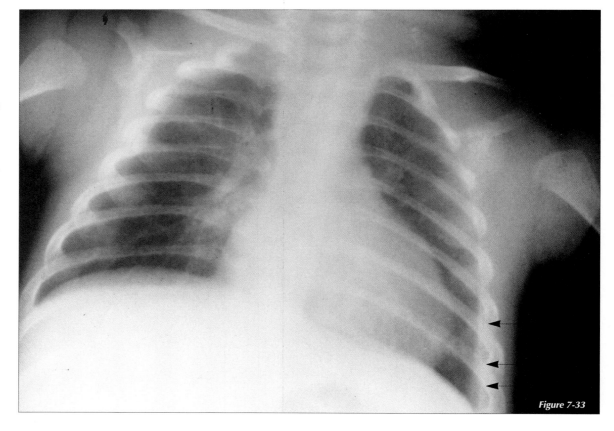

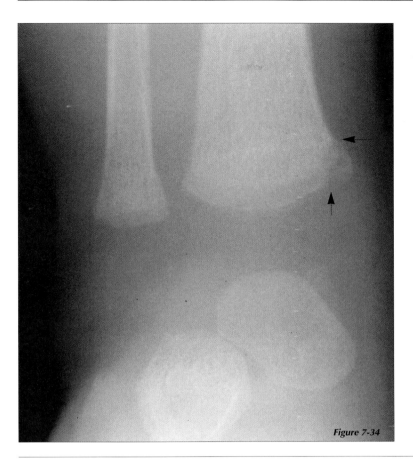

Figure 7-34. *Metaphyseal avulsion fracture of medial distal tibia. This fracture (arrow) is a classic child abuse pattern.*

Figure 7-34

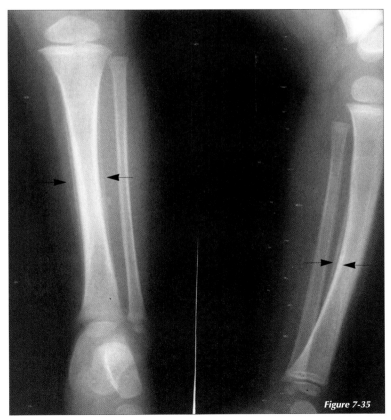

Figure 7-35. *Toddler's fracture. Extensive periosteal reaction midshaft of the left tibia is associated with a "toddler's fracture" in the distal side of the tibia in a 15-month-old boy. Typically the fracture occurs in the distal third of the tibia. Separation of the fragments is so finite that it is often subradiologic. The first and only clinical sign may be limping. Often there are no external signs to give evidence of the broken bone. Toddlers fall frequently, sustaining twisting injuries of a slight nature. Between 11 and 15 months of age the normal infant will fall many times each day. The appearance of a periosteal reaction may require only about 7 or 8 days in these instances because the child continues to use the limb, possibly stimulating a more rapid onset and a greater amount of periosteal reaction.*

Figure 7-35

167

Figure 7-36. *Spiral fracture of the proximal third of the tibia with periosteal reaction on the medial side. A fracture of this type in this location is unusual in a child; this is not a toddler's fracture. The leg was edematous and red, and the child was unwilling to use the limb. Since the radiograph depicted the periosteal reaction around this fracture at the time of the initial examination (**a** and **b**), the fracture had occurred at least 7 to 10 days before the child was seen. This was classified as nonaccidental and most likely child abuse.*

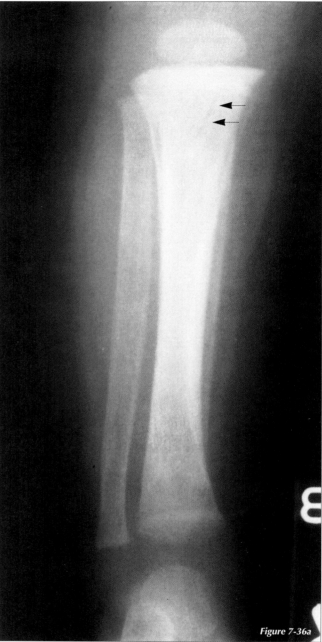

Figure 7-36a

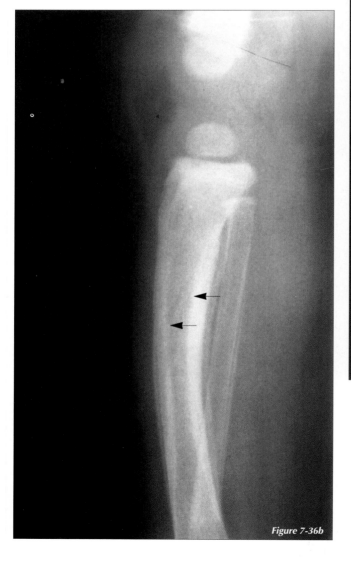

Figure 7-36b

Figure 7-37. *Classical metaphyseal avulsion fracture of the distal tibia. When the entire metaphysis is pulled off (arrow), it has the characteristic appearance of a "bucket handle" and is so named.*

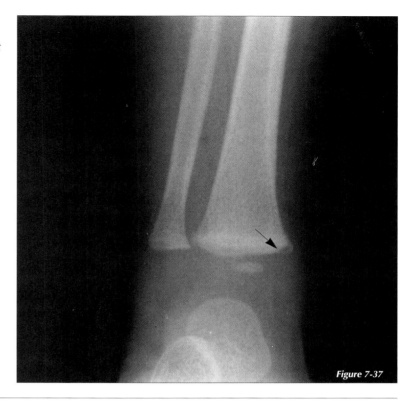

Figure 7-38. *Toddler's fracture of the mid-tibia, left leg. The oblique radiolucent fracture line (arrow) is faint, which is part of the classical picture. Toddler's fractures ordinarily occur in the distal third. In this case there was a faint line in the distal third of the tibia that extended into the middle third. The absence of periosteal reaction and the slight soft tissue swelling noted on the original radiograph confirm the diagnosis. This was not child abuse.*

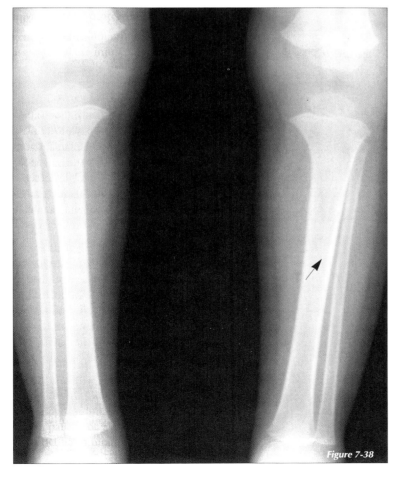

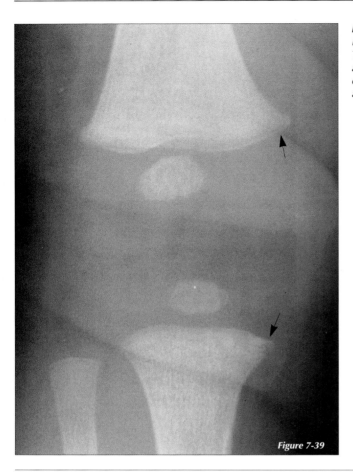

Figure 7-39. *Metaphyseal avulsion fractures. These can be subtle. Note the distal femur and proximal tibia of the right knee (arrows). The baby was admitted to the emergency room with multiple bruises and injuries believed to be cigarette burns. These tiny fractures were discovered on a routine skeletal survey. There were no clinical signs around the knee.*

Figure 7-39

Figure 7-40. *Transverse fracture, midshaft, of the left femur in a 4-week-old infant. The child was admitted to the emergency room with marked swelling and redness of the left thigh and was extremely irritable. The history given by the parents was that the baby had gotten the leg caught on the side of the mattress and apparently rolled over, fracturing the femur. This fracture was likely the result of a severe blow—sufficient to separate the fragments—and the ensuing muscle spasm resulted in the overriding of fragments noted. The absence of sharp edges on the fracture surfaces suggest that this injury is more than 24 hours old. (This would have given time for the osteoclasts to begin the fracture surface preparation process for healing, which results in less sharpness of the fracture fragments.)*

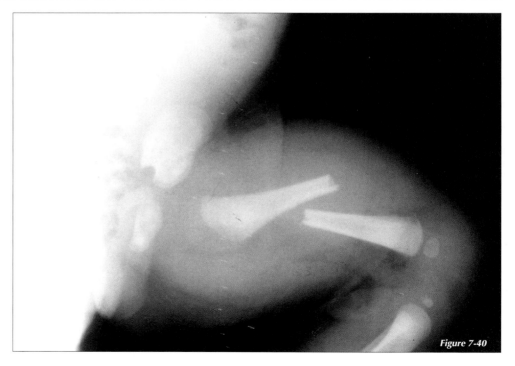

Figure 7-40

Figure 7-41. *Multiple rib fractures in different stages of healing. There are at least 14 rib fractures in different stages of healing, some subtle and hardly recognizable. This radiograph emphasizes the fact that had there been but two of these subtle fractures (for example, the third and fourth ribs on the right side), they might not have been detected. Another important point is the fact that the tenth, eleventh, and twelfth ribs are usually well hidden beneath the diaphragm, obscured by liver shadow, and small deformities of a healing fractured rib in this area are readily overlooked. Surprisingly, there was no evidence of costovertebral disruption in the process of healing anywhere along the thoracic spine.*

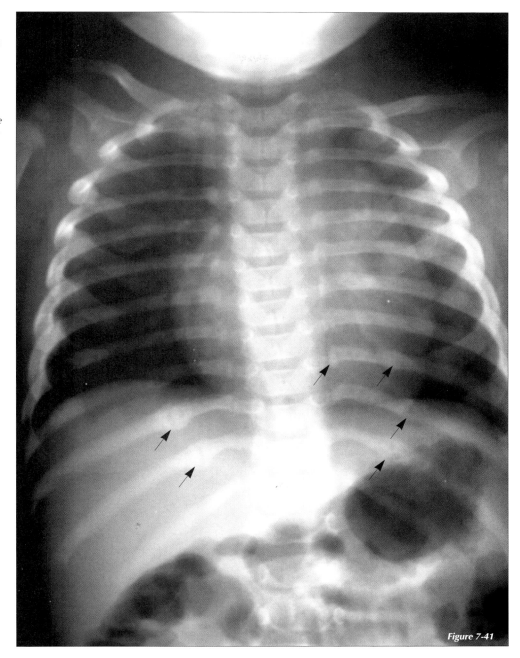

Figure 7-41

Figure 7-42. *(a)* *Transverse fracture of the surgical neck of the humerus. This 6-month-old infant presented with irritability, swelling and hemorrhagic discoloration of the right shoulder, and unwillingness to use the right upper limb. A fracture of this severity in the third strongest bone in the skeleton is unique at this age from any cause. The parents stated that the baby was simply found crying. The father later admitted striking the child across the shoulder with his fist.* *(b)* *A similar, unlikely fracture in a 9-month-old infant. The history of a self-inflicted twisting injury is not acceptable.*

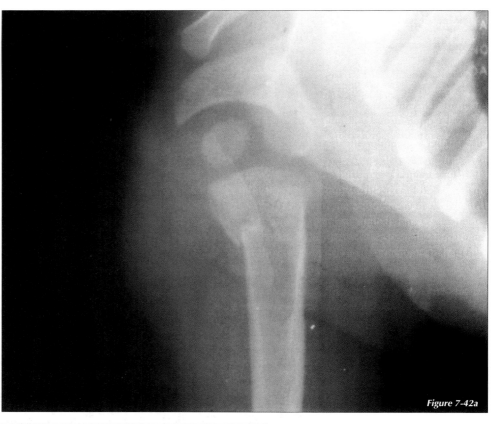

Figure 7-42a

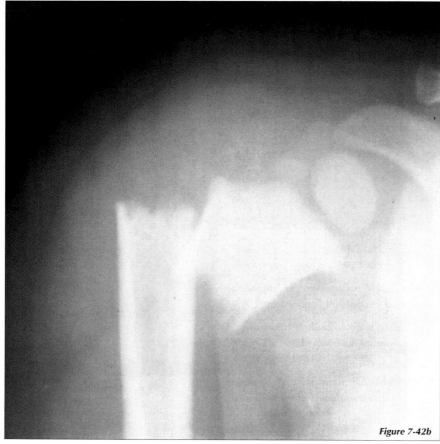

Figure 7-42b

Figure 7-43. *Transverse fracture of the shaft of the right femur in a 1-year-old child. This child was admitted with fever, listlessness, marked swelling and redness of the right thigh, unwillingness to use the right lower limb, moderate deformity, and shortening of the thigh. The parents' story was that the child had gotten her foot caught in the side of the bed between the mattress and the footboard. This is a transverse and not a spiral fracture and was not caused by a twisting force but by a direct blow.*

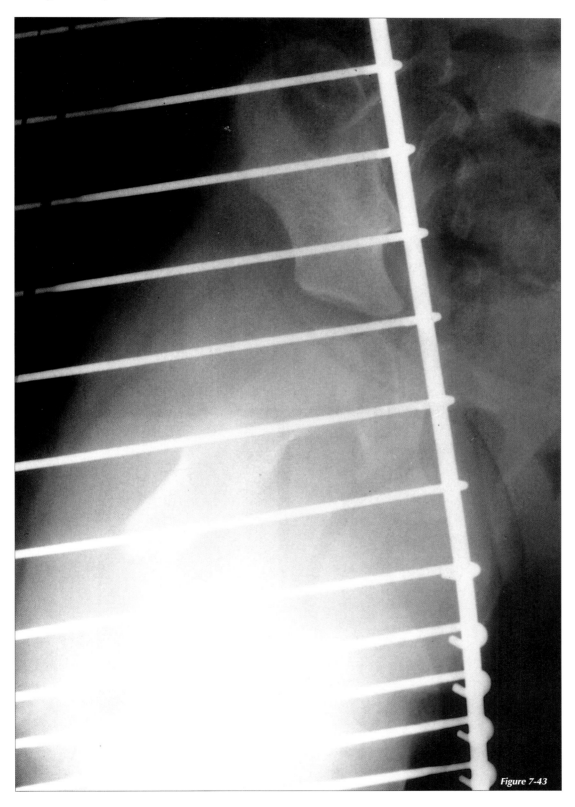

Figure 7-43

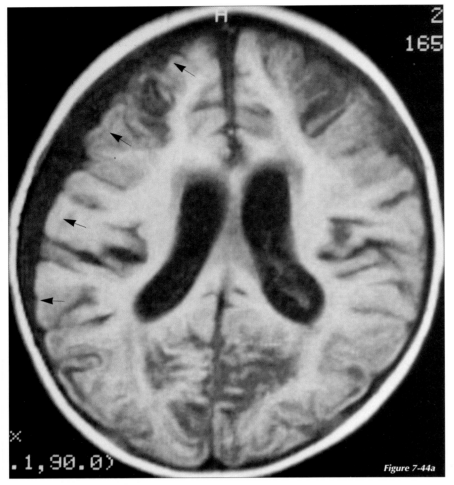

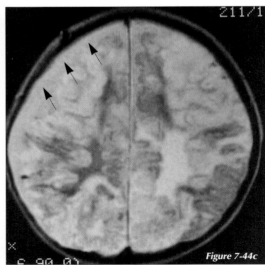

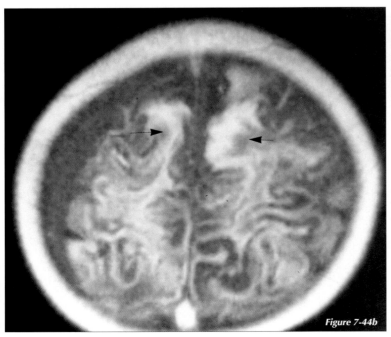

Figure 7-44. Magnetic resonance images of a 1-year-old infant admitted via the emergency room where he had been taken by his mother because of lethargy and convulsions. He was found to have multiple bruises and ecchymotic areas, in various stages of healing, on the face and chest. **(a)** The T-1 weighted image identifies chronic subdural hematoma (arrows). **(b)** Acute intraparenchymal hemorrhage (arrows) shown on T-1 weighted image. **(c)** Chronic subdural hemorrhage on the right in T-2 weighted image. Late subdural hemorrhage appears as a brighter band.

Figure 7-44a

Figure 7-44b

Figure 7-44c

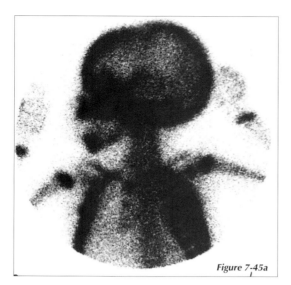

Figure 7-45a

Figure 7-45. *This infant was admitted with a severe closed head injury, retinal hemorrhages, and CNS bleeding. A skeletal survey looking for other evidence of trauma was unremarkable. A bone scan was done using 2 mCl of Tc-99m MDP. Numerous abnormalities were noted (**a** through **d**). There was increased activity in both anterior rib cages and a series of 2 or 3 rib lesions on the left anteriorly, presumably in the left third through fifth ribs. There are also lesions in the upper right anterior ribs. Increased activity is seen in the right parietal skull, best illustrated on a posterior image. Increased activity extends at least two-thirds of the way up the right tibia. These findings are compatible with multiple sites of very recent bony trauma. The areas of increased uptake at the wrists, elbow, shoulder, knees, and hips are growth centers.*

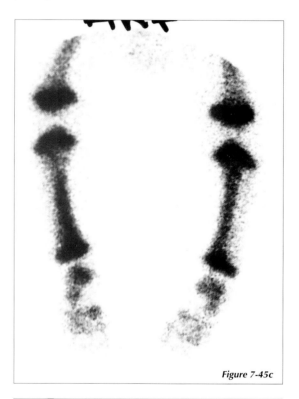

Figure 7-45c

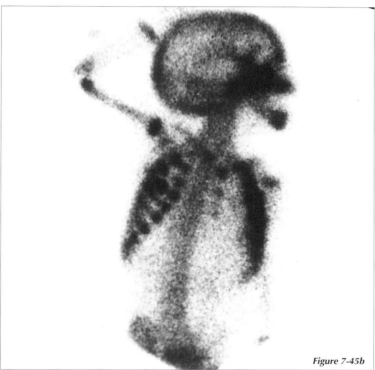

Figure 7-45b

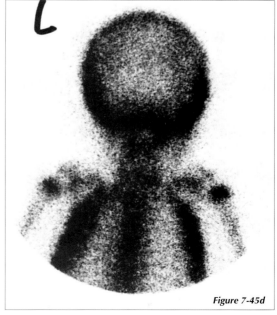

Figure 7-45d

Figure 7-46. Infant with history similar to that in Figure 7-45. This bone scan revealed three recent left lateral rib fractures.

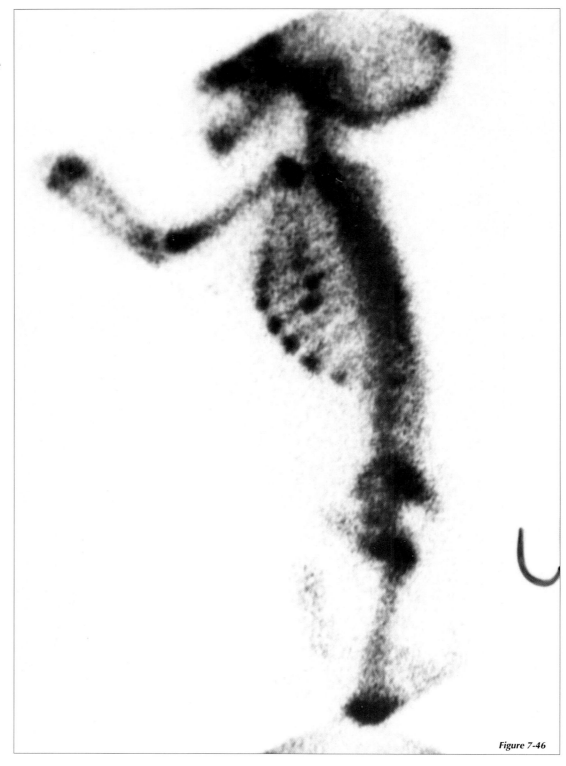

Figure 7-46

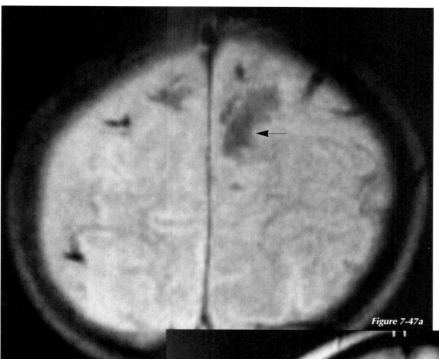

Figure 7-47a

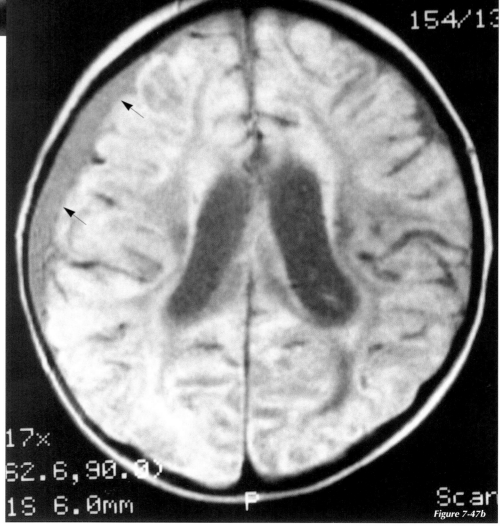

Figure 7-47. (**a**) *Intracerebral hemorrhage (arrows) shown on T-2 weighted MRI.* (**b**) *Subdural hematoma (arrows) on proton-density MRI. Note that the subdural hematoma has a higher density than the cerebrospinal fluid in the ventricle.*

Figure 7-47b

Figure 7-48. *Magnetic resonance images of an 18-month-old boy seen in the emergency room with a history of having fallen out of bed. The child was unconscious and unreactive to painful stimuli.* **(a)** *Day of admission. Acute parenchymal hemorrhage was noted on a sagittal T-1 weighted cranial MRI without contrast as a hypo-intense wedge-shaped area of abnormal signal (arrows).* **(b)** *Six days after admission, note the subacute parenchymal hemorrhage.* **(c)** *Sagittal T-1 weighted MRI without contrast reveals large areas of signal hyperintensity, indicating extracellular methemoglobin.* **(d)** *Six days after admission note the appearance of the subacute parenchymal hemorrhage. This axial T-1 weighted cranial MRI without contrast reveals an area of signal hyperintensity that represents the region of extracellular methemoglobin (single arrow = parenchymal hemorrhage; double arrow = parafalcine hemorrhage).* **E,** *Six days after admission a coronal T-2 weighted cranial MRI reveals bilateral subdural hemorrhages larger on the right.*

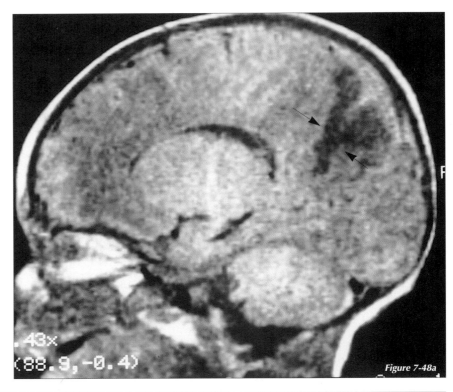

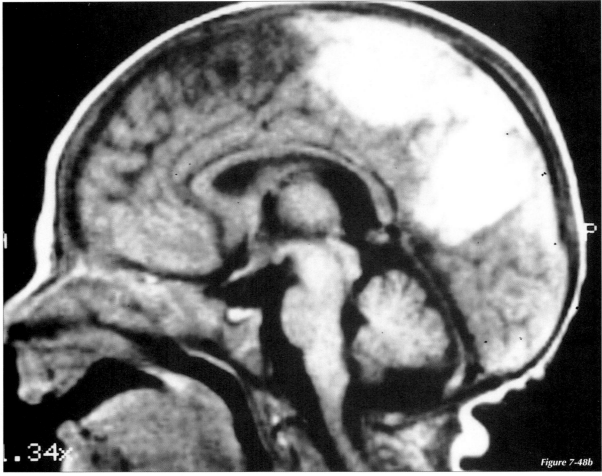

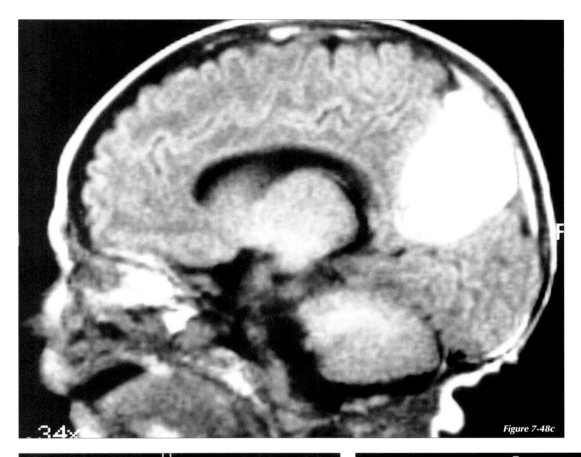

Figure 7-48c

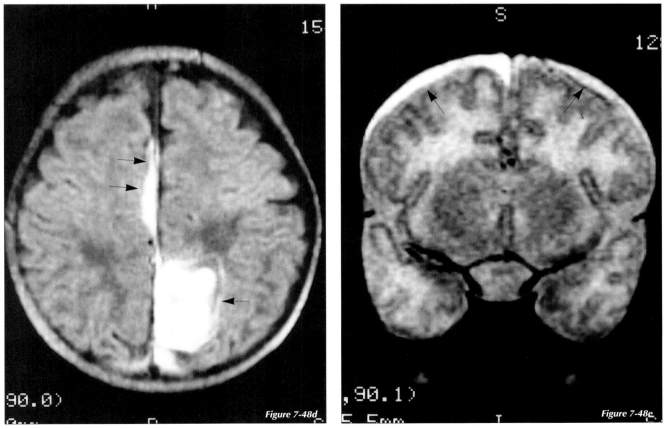

Figure 7-48d

Figure 7-48e

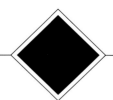

PART THREE

Sexual Abuse Cases

CASES WITH A HISTORY OF POSSIBLE SEXUAL ABUSE

JAMES A. MONTELEONE, M.D.
JOHN R. BREWER, M.D.
TIMOTHY J. FETE, M.D.

Three-fourths of the crimes against children are sex crimes. Too much emphasis has been placed on the physical examination because most sexually abused children show no physical findings, so if you conclude that only those children with positive physical findings are credible, a great disservice will be done to 60% to 70% of children claiming to be abused. Several physical findings, such as pregnancy in a child under 12 years of age and semen in the vagina, clearly diagnose abuse, but without a credible statement from the child identifying the perpetrator, the investigation can be stymied. The child may even deny abuse. A good interview of the child suspected to have been sexually abused is critical. The physical findings, although important, can only support what the child says.

The following outline summarizes the various findings in cases suspected to involve sexual abuse:

I. **Normal appearing examination**

The majority (60% or more) of abused children fall into this category.
Examination reveals no distinctive changes involving mounds, clefts, bands, remnants, or urethral dilation (or only mild dilation).

II. **Nonspecific findings of sexual abuse**

These are often found in children who have not been sexually abused. A nonspecific finding can become a specific finding when a child gives a clear history of recent sexual abuse, especially describing pain.

Condylomata (caused by human papillomavirus [HPV]) in children under 2 years of age (may be upgraded to specific for sexual abuse if there is a strongly suggestive history or supportive physical findings such as hymenal tear or attenuation).

Hymenal thickening or edema*

Infection, erythema, vaginitis (nonspecific), areas of increased vascularity*

Rounding of hymenal edges

Labial adhesions (depending on the history, this could be a specific finding)

Urethral dilation (moderate)

Narrowing of hymen (greater than 2 mm)

Enlargement of the hymenal opening (with no other findings)*

Thickening of the perianal tissue

Increased pigmentation

Venous pooling (after prolonged knee-chest position)

Funneling or fat atrophy

III. Specific for sexual abuse

Hymenal scars (usually retracted) or mounted linear avascular areas

Herpes II

Chlamydia trachomatis†

Trichomonas vaginalis infection

Reflex anal dilation in the absence of stool in the antrum and greater than 20 mm

Hymenal transections

Hymenal narrowing or flattening (less than 2 mm)

Synechiae (lower pole, 3 to 9 o'clock; may be confused with bands of tissue extending from the vaginal wall caused by stretching with labial traction)

Severe rounding of hymenal margin with loss of vascularity

Perianal skin tags or folds (normal midline structures can be mistaken for skin tags)

Anal scars (normal midline structures can be mistaken for scars)

Marked irregularity of the anal orifice during dilatation

Persistence of a prominent anal verge

Urethral dilation (severe)

Pelvic inflammatory disease (PID)

IV. Conclusive of sexual abuse

These are considered conclusive of abuse only in children under 12 years of age; older children may be sexually active.

HIV infection* (no history to explain)

Neisseria gonorrhoeae infection†

Treponema pallidum infection (syphilis)†

Sperm, seminal fluid, or acid phosphatase activity in discharge (must be very high if nonspecific assay or prostatic specific)

Pregnancy

Finally there are conditions that can be mistaken for abuse. *These are as follows:*

Lichen sclerosis et atrophicus

Accidental straddle injuries

Accidental impaling injuries

Nonspecific vulvovaginitis and proctitis

Group A streptococcal vaginitis and proctitis

Diaper dermatitis

Foreign bodies

Lower extremity girdle paralysis (as in myelomeningocele)

Defects that cause chronic constipation—Hirschsprung disease, anteriorly displaced anus

Chronic gastrointestinal disease—Crohn disease

Labial adhesions

Anal fissures

Nonspecific finding that becomes specific when the child gives a clear history of recent sexual abuse, especially involving pain.

†Nonneonatal.

Figure 8-1. *A 35-month-old girl with a history of digital vaginal penetration. On simple labial separation the injury is seen under the colposcope (**a**). Erythema is present around the lesion. It was not visible with the naked eye. With labial traction the lesion becomes more obvious (**b**).*

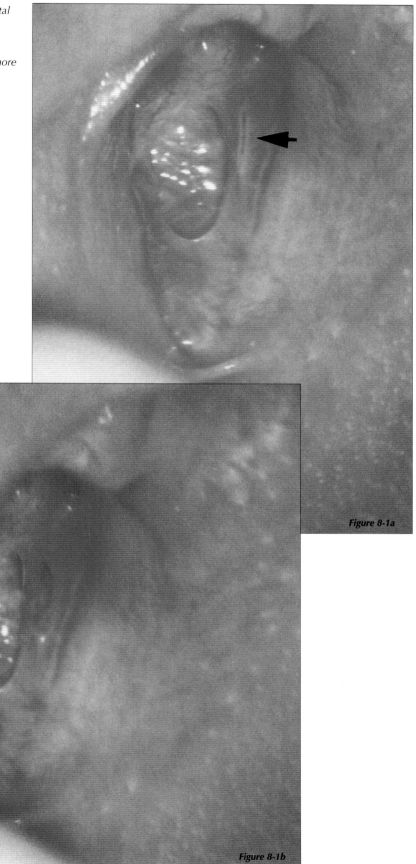

Figure 8-1a

Figure 8-1b

Figure 8-2. This 9-year-old girl gave a credible history of vaginal penetration and possibly anal penetration. On simple labial separation the vaginal examination was not remarkable **(a)**. With labial traction the hymen initially appeared normal **(b)**. With coaxing a separation became obvious at the anterior column **(c** and **d)**. Whether this represented a tear or a band was debatable. The individual viewing it under colposcopy felt that it was a tear. Those viewing the photos thought it was a band. The child was found to have moderate anal dilation, which was considered to be a nonspecific change **(e)**.

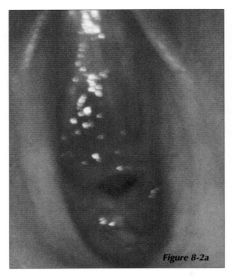

Figure 8-2a

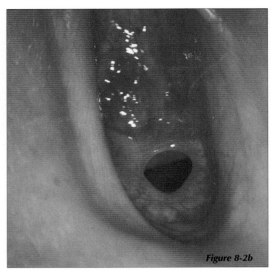

Figure 8-2b

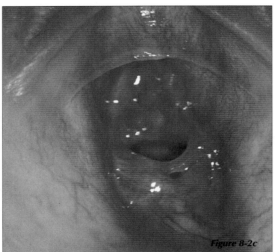

Figure 8-2c

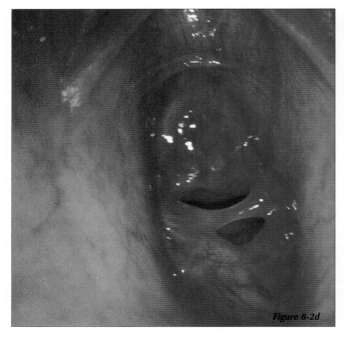

Figure 8-2d

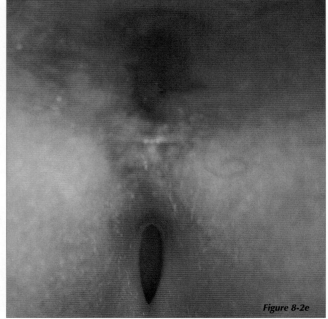

Figure 8-2e

Figure 8-3. This 7-year-old girl described digital penetration. With labial separation the examination is not remarkable **(a)**. The tear, at nine o'clock, is seen after labial traction **(b)**.

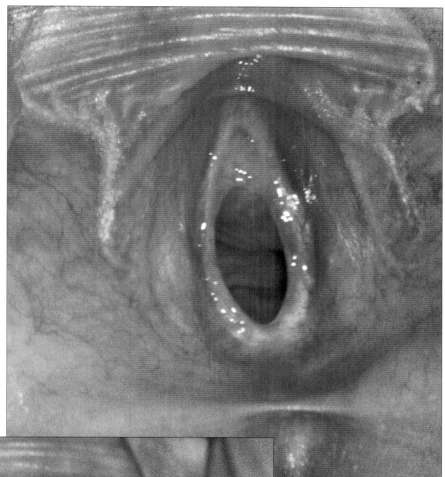

Figure 8-3a

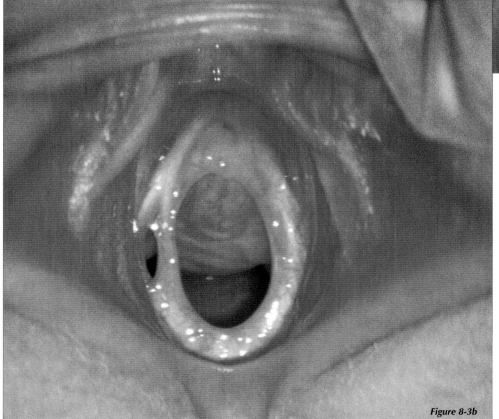

Figure 8-3b

Figure 8-4. *Examination in this 13-year-old girl (Tanner Stage 2) showed a break in the hymen at 3 o'clock (**a** and **b**). The rest of the hymen appeared normal.*

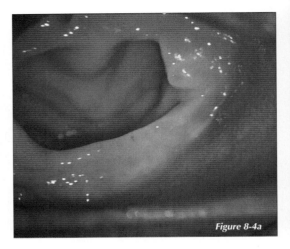

Figure 8-4a

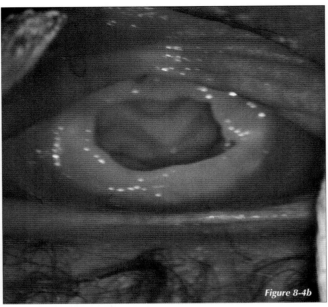

Figure 8-4b

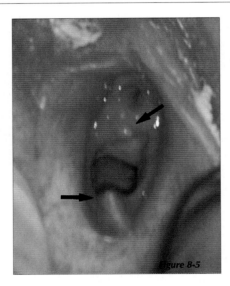

Figure 8-5

Figure 8-5. *This 19-month-old girl had remnants of a hymenal band. Two days earlier the child was seen in the emergency room with vaginal bleeding. The two ends were ragged and appeared to be freshly severed (arrows). The child was preverbal, and no history of how the injury occurred was obtained. Abuse was suspected.*

Figure 8-6. *Healing perineal injury in a 35-month-old boy believed to be the result of dry intercourse.*

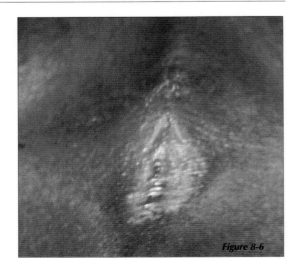

Figure 8-6

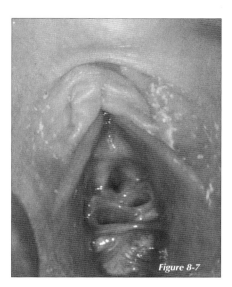

Figure 8-7. *This 3-year-old girl was seen by her private physician for vaginal irritation and itching. The physician thought she had been sexually abused and referred her to the sexual abuse management clinic. She denied any abuse. The child had an unusually shaped hymen that was boggy and erythematous. The mucosa was irritated. It was determined that the vaginal irritation was due to an allergic reaction to shampoo. The hymen was irritated but was a normal variant of a cribriform hymen. She was told to discontinue shampooing in the tub and not to use bubble bath.*

Figure 8-8. *This 7-year-old girl gave a credible history of vaginal manipulation. The vaginal examination was abnormal. The hymen from 1 to 6 o'clock was normal in appearance, but from 6 to 12 o'clock it was distorted, with raised scar tissue that was avascular. The edge was convoluted and irregular in that area.*

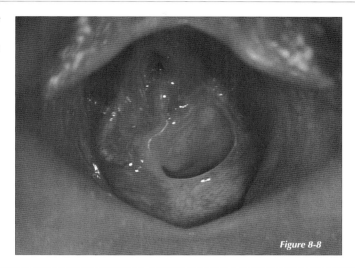

Figure 8-9. *This 3-year-old girl was reported as suspected of having been sexually abused. She was seen by her family physician for a painful blood-tinged discharge. On physical examination she was found to have a prolapsed ureter (**a**). The hymen was intact and normal (**b**). She denied abuse.*

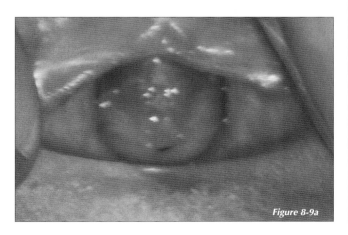

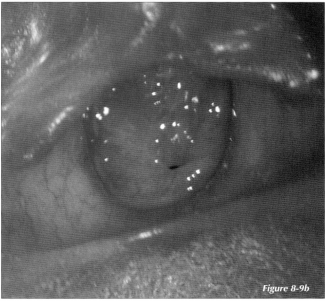

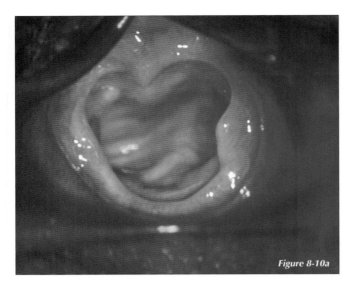

Figure 8-10a

Figure 8-10. Colposcopic examinations of a 4- **(a)**, 5- **(b)**, 6- **(c)**, and 7- **(d)** year-old, respectively, who had been chronically sexually abused. The openings are enlarged and the hymens rudimentary. They afford a good view of the lower vaginal anatomy demonstrating the transverse rugae and the anterior and posterior columns. Note how the structures vary and how at times the columns can be obliterated by the transverse rugae.

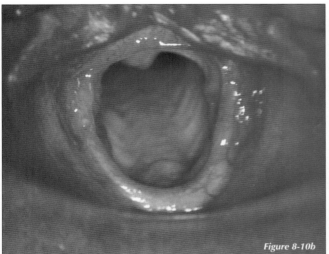

Figure 8-10b

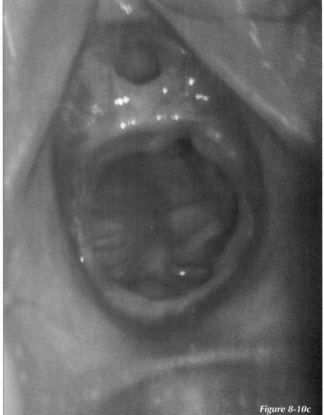

Figure 8-10c

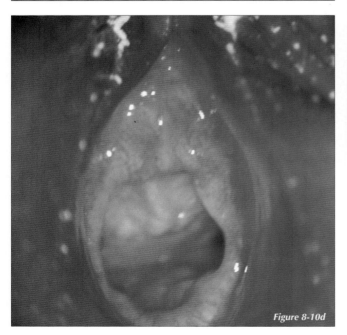

Figure 8-10d

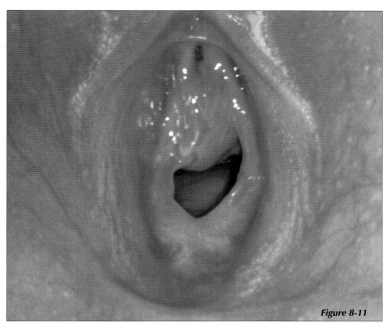

Figure 8-11. *This 9-year-old child gave a credible history of digital penetration. Colposcopic examination was abnormal. The hymen was asymmetrical with a disruption anteriorly and hymenal remnants from 10 to 12 o'clock. There is also angulation at 6 and 9 o'clock.*

Figure 8-11

Figure 8-12. *This 7-year-old girl was seen in the emergency room for vaginal bleeding. The attending physician reported her to the hotline as sexually abused, stating that she had a severe vaginitis with bloody purulent discharge. The mucosa was described as edematous and the hymen and hymenal opening obliterated (**a** and **b**). The child denied abuse. Chlamydial and gonorrheal cultures 24 hours after admission were negative. Routine cultures taken when the colposcopic photographs were taken grew Shigella flexneri. Two weeks after antibiotic therapy, the vaginal mucosa were boggy but otherwise normal.*

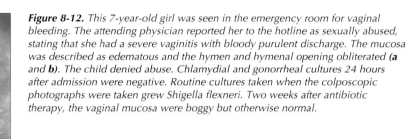

Figure 8-12a

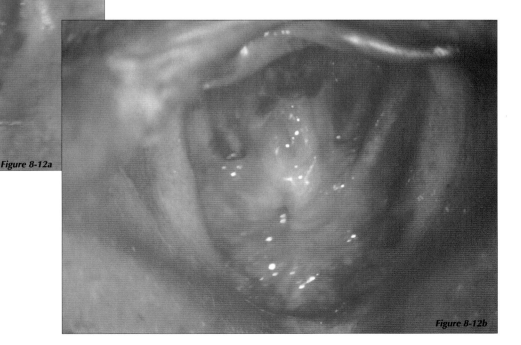

Figure 8-12b

Figure 8-13. *This 5-year-old girl was seen in the sexual abuse management clinic suspected of having been abused. Her mother had noted a bloody discharge in the girl's panties. The child had mild behavioral indicators but denied abuse. On physical examination, a bluish colored mass was noted behind the hymen. A vaginal polyp was removed at surgery.*

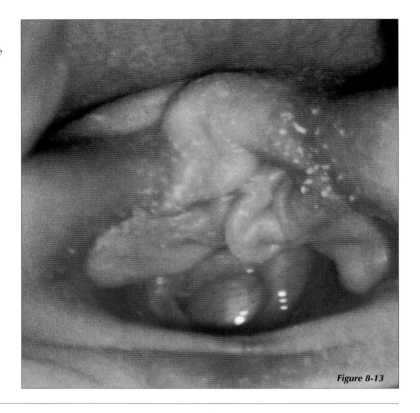

Figure 8-14. *This 30-month-old girl was walking "funny" after returning from the babysitter. She complained that it hurt to sit down. The mother noted a foul odor and, when examining the child's diaper, noted a mucous and bloody discharge. There was a rectal tear (not seen in the photograph). The girl stated that a 19-year-old boy at the sitter's home had hurt her. The anus was markedly dilated with loss of landmarks, and the mucosa was erythematous (a). The vaginal examination showed boggy mucosa. There was a septated vaginal band (b). There was no evidence of acute vaginal trauma.*

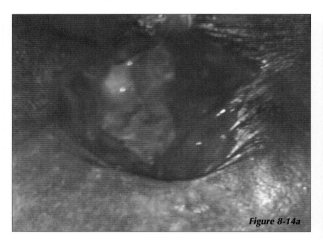

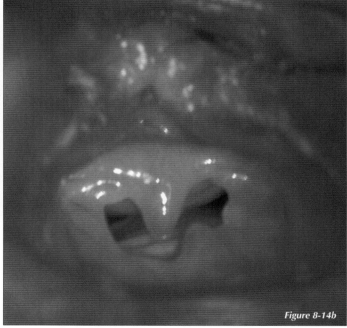

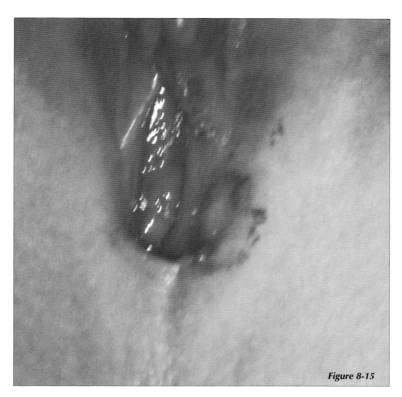

Figure 8-15. This 4-year-old girl was taken to the emergency room for possible sexual abuse. The staff there described genital trauma and referred the child to the sexual abuse management clinic. She had lichen sclerosis. She denied sexual abuse.

Figure 8-15

Figure 8-16. This 14-year-old girl complained of vaginal pain and itching and pain on urination. She gave a credible history of sexual abuse. Other than having candidal vulvovaginitis, physical findings were not remarkable. The candidal infection was not related to her abuse.

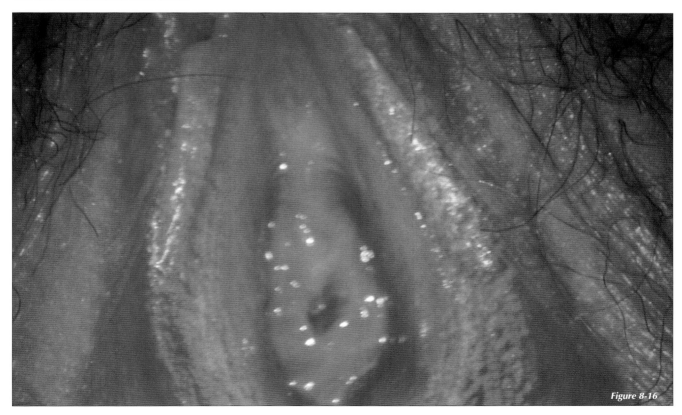

Figure 8-16

Figure 8-17. This 8-year-old girl had a bloody discharge. She gave a credible history of sexual abuse. The hymenal opening was enlarged, with narrowing of the hymen throughout. She had a urethral prolapse.

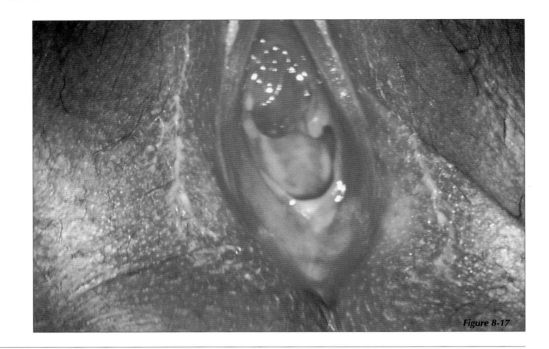

Figure 8-17

Figure 8-18. This 6-year-old girl gave a credible history of sexual abuse. The vaginal findings were nonspecific. She shows marked labial adhesions, but this is nonspecific for sexual abuse.

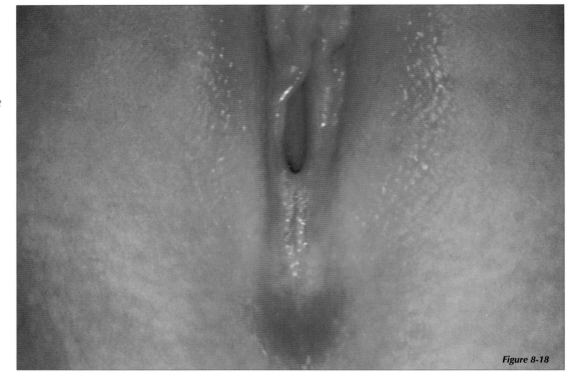

Figure 8-18

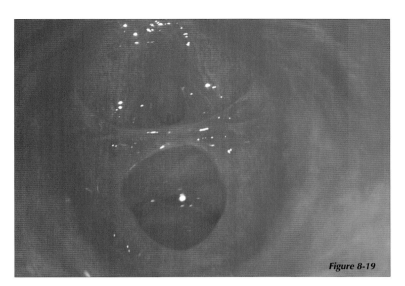

Figure 8-19. *This 8-year-old girl was referred from an adolescent psychiatric unit. While on the unit she gave a history of sexual abuse by both parents and complained of acute vaginal pain. On examination, she had acute vaginitis, but no other remarkable physical findings. She had a history of playing in a sandbox and taking bubble baths. No specific cause for the vaginitis could be determined. This is a nonspecific finding of sexual abuse.*

Figure 8-19

Figure 8-20. *This 11-year-old girl gave a history of digital penetration. She shows early pubertal changes. There is a questionable notch at 10 o'clock on the hymen.*

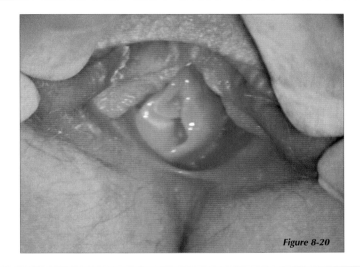

Figure 8-20

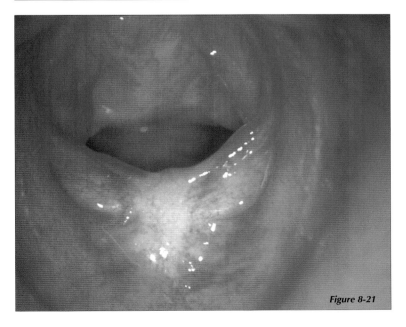

Figure 8-21. *This 11-year-old girl was referred to the clinic for evaluation of rectal bleeding. She denied abuse. The anal examination was not remarkable, but vaginal examination revealed a raised avascular midline area, believed to be a healed scar. She stated that she had recently had some blisters in the genital area. Cultures for specific vaginitis and herpes were not remarkable. The child was referred for counseling.*

Figure 8-21

Figure 8-22. This girl (3 years and 5 months old) was seen in the sex abuse management clinic with a credible history of ongoing sexual and physical abuse. Her genital examination was consistent with chronic sexual abuse (*a*). She had multiple curling iron burns to her left shoulder (*b*) and right calf (*c*). The shoulder wound was older than the calf wounds. She had a healed cigarette wound to the right shoulder (*d*). There were healed human bite wounds to her back (*e*) and left inner leg (*f*).

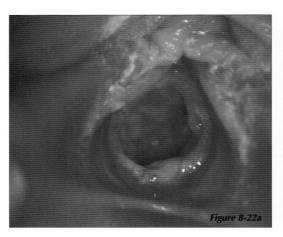
Figure 8-22a

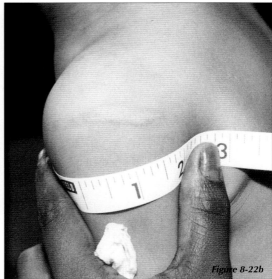
Figure 8-22b

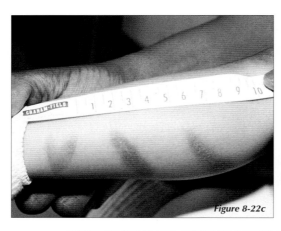
Figure 8-22c

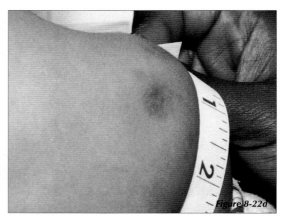
Figure 8-22d

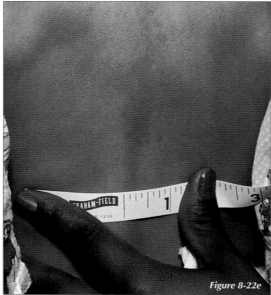
Figure 8-22e

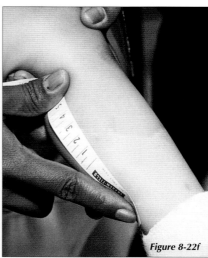
Figure 8-22f

Figure 8-23. *This 4-year-old girl gave a history of sexual abuse. The depigmented area* **(a)** *is vitiligo; lichen sclerosis et atrophicus can present with similar depigmentation and can be mistaken for vitiligo. A biopsy is needed to distinguish between the two. The vaginal examination was otherwise normal with a midline defect that was a septum* **(b)**. *Anal findings were also normal* **(c)**.

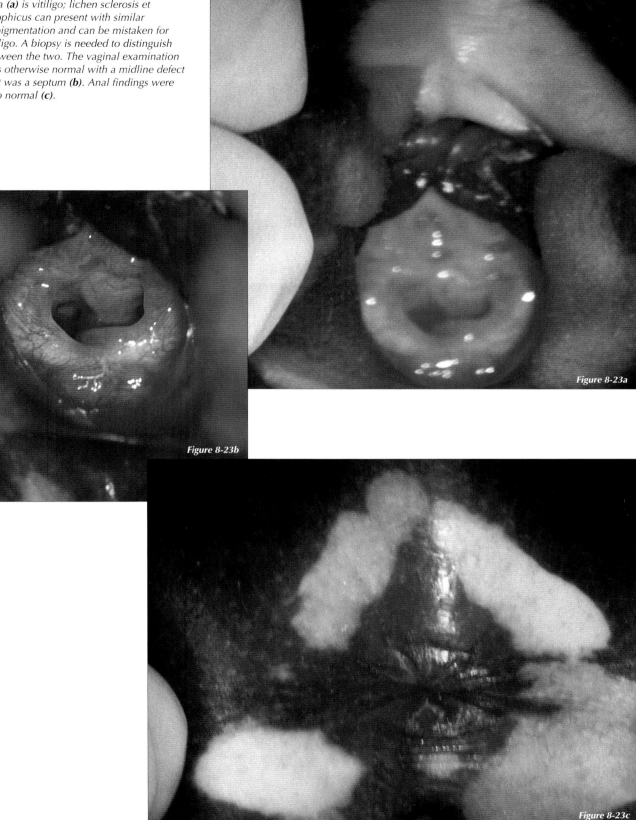

Figure 8-23a

Figure 8-23b

Figure 8-23c

Figure 8-24. This 9-year-old boy described fondling. The lesions, found at the base of the penis, are molluscum contagiosum (**a** and **b**). Although molluscum can be sexually transmitted, in children it is usually not. These lesions are not typical, with a less prominent umbilicated center than is usually seen.

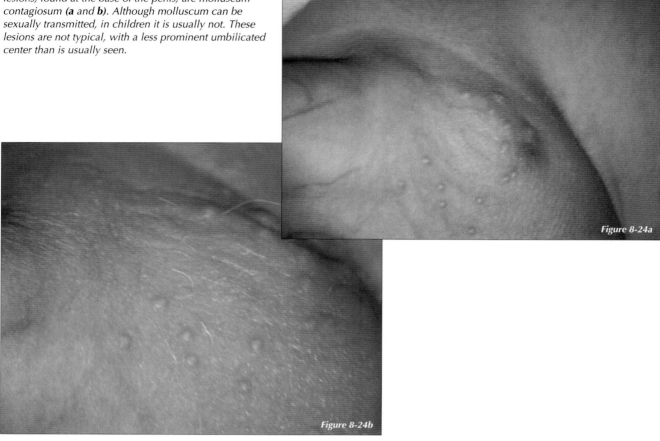

Figure 8-24a

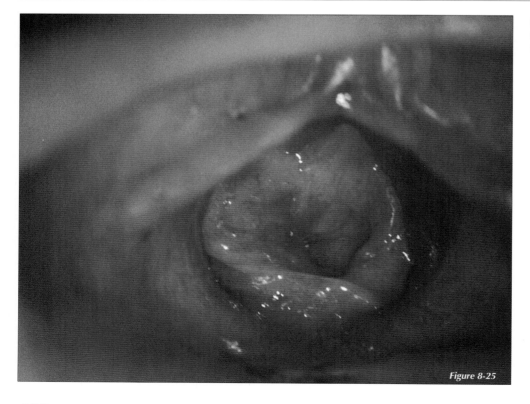

Figure 8-24b

Figure 8-25. Normal redundant hymen in a 6-year-old girl.

Figure 8-25

Figure 8-26. *Narrowed annular hymen in a 9-year-old girl. She described penile penetration on several occasions.*

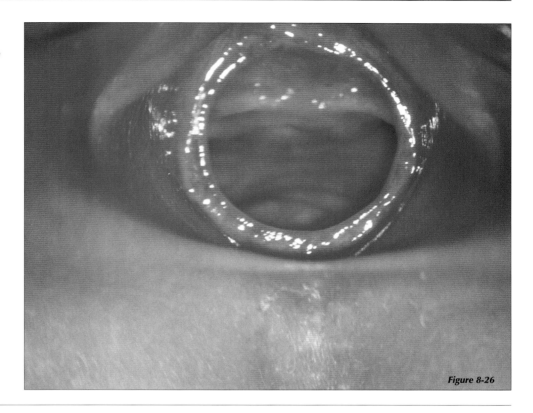

Figure 8-26

Figure 8-27. *Iatrogenic tear in a 4-year-old girl. The child had labial adhesions, but, with labial separation, the friable adhesions broke down.*

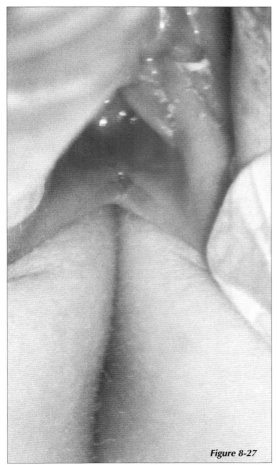

Figure 8-27

Figure 8-28. Acute injury in a chronically sexually abused 11-year-old girl following a painful rape. There is a raised red blistered area at 12 o'clock. This injury may be caused by oral sex.

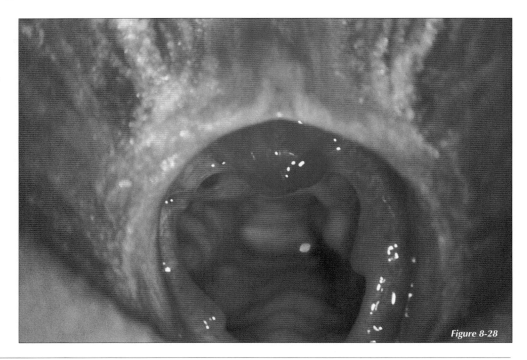

Figure 8-29. This 5-year-old girl was referred by her family physician for vaginal trauma and was suspected to have been sexually abused. The genital examination of areas other than the vascular area was normal. The child had lichen sclerosis et atrophicus.

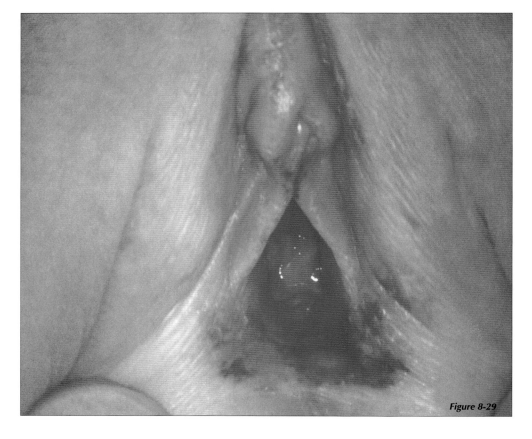

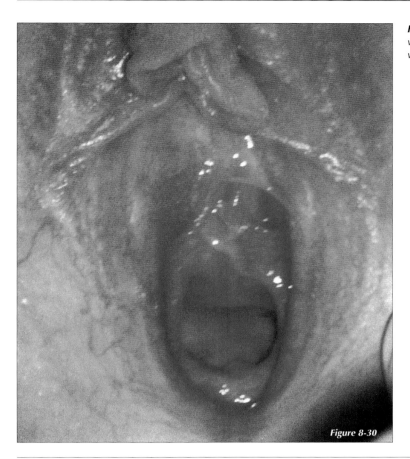

Figure 8-30. *Acute vaginitis in a 10-year-old girl who was chronically sexually abused. Cultures were positive for Chlamydia trachomatis.*

Figure 8-31. *Annular hymen with redundant tissue from 10 to 5 o'clock. The area described projects outward toward the viewer. This was considered a normal variant. There is also separation of labial adhesions at the bottom of the photograph. The child described digital penetration.*

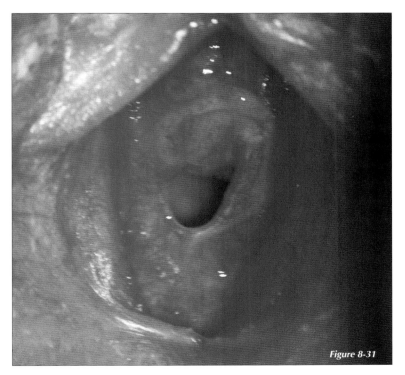

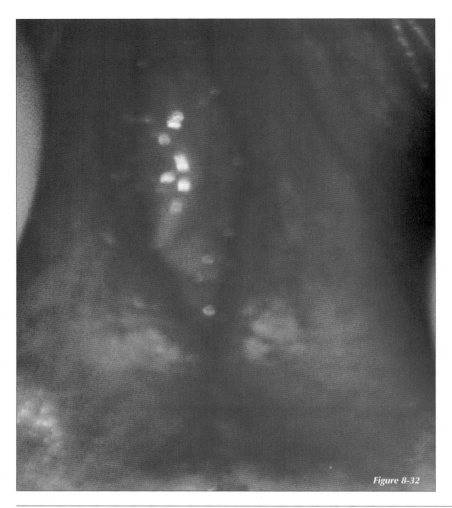

Figure 8-32. *Severe labial adhesions in an 11-year-old girl who described chronic digital manipulation and masturbation. The hymenal examination was normal. Although labial adhesions are a nonspecific finding, in this case the severity indicated that this was probably related to the abuse.*

Figure 8-33. *This 4-year-old girl gave a credible history of sexual abuse by her father. She described digital penetration. The vaginal mucosa was infected, a nonspecific finding, and the labia minora had areas of increased pigmentation. The hymen was redundant. These findings are normal variations.*

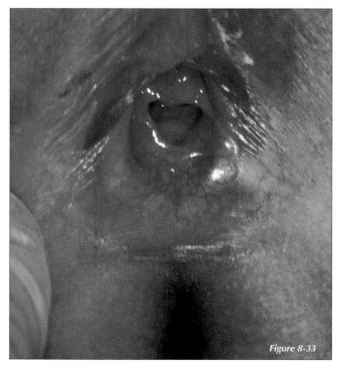

Figure 8-34. *This 3-year-old girl arrived home from the babysitter's house complaining of vaginal pain. Her panties were blood soaked. She said that an older boy at the babysitter's house had hurt her. Her vaginal mucosa was edematous, and she had hymenal vaginal mucosa tears.*

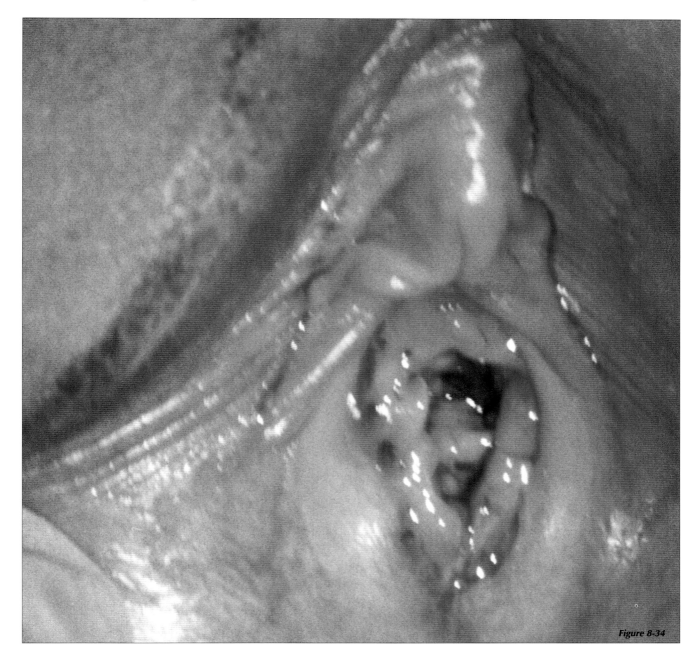

Figure 8-34

Figure 8-35. *This 8-year-old girl described vaginal penetration and fondling. (a) This gives the false impression of an imperforate hymen. (b) The same child after relaxation. The angulation at 6 o'clock is an artifact caused by the technique. The protrusions at the base of the urethral opening are periurethral polyps, which are normal variants.*

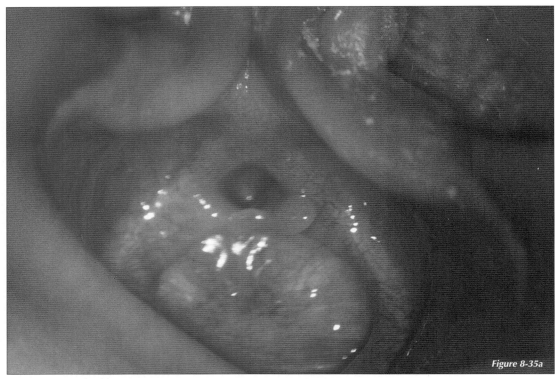

Figure 8-35a

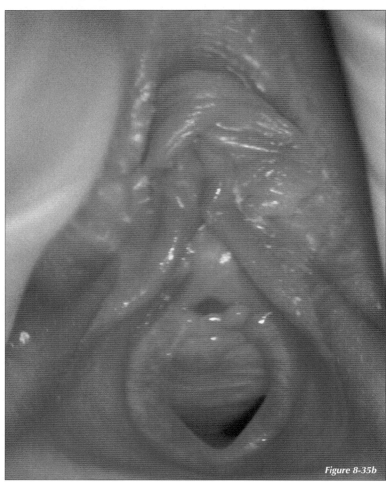

Figure 8-35b

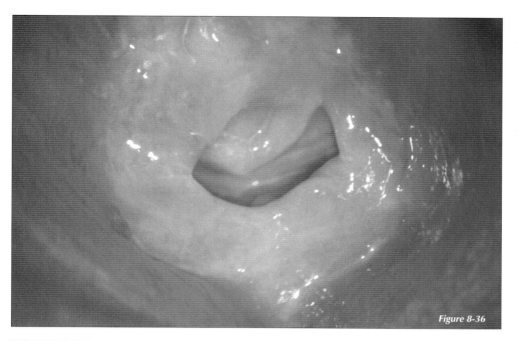

Figure 8-36. Normal early pubertal changes of an annular hymen in a 13-year-old girl. There is a hint of angulation at 2 o'clock. This is an artifact of the technique of examination. Exploration of the edge of the hymen with a cotton-tipped swab showed no defect.

Figure 8-36

Figure 8-37. This 9-year-old girl described numerous incidents of digital fondling by her father. **(a)** On low power there is angulation at the midline. **(b)** On high power, the hymen is flattened on the viewer's right of midline with angulation at 3 o'clock and attenuation of the hymen above it. Note the patulous urethral opening that gives the illusion of another hymen. The viewer is looking into the urethra, and the "other hymen" is the anterior column. These are artifacts of the examination technique.

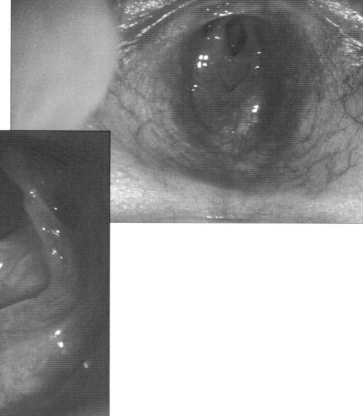

Figure 8-37a

Figure 8-37b

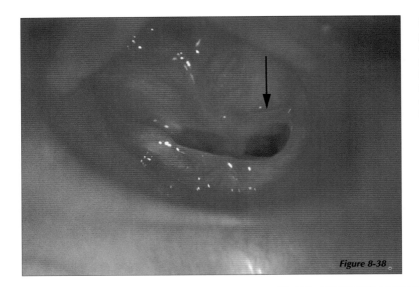

Figure 8-38. *This 8-year-old girl described painful penetration in the past. The hymen was distorted with narrowing of the hymen on the (viewer's) right. There was a thin band of hymenal tissue extending inwardly from the hymenal edge to the midline of the anterior column. This was believed to be the result of a faulty repair of an old tear.*

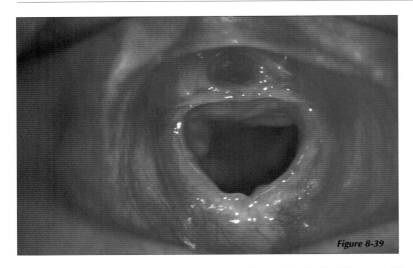

Figure 8-39. *This 9-year-old girl described painful penetration several weeks before this examination. She had an angular notch at the midline surrounded by boggy, avascular hymenal tissue. This was believed to be a healing hymenal tear.*

Figure 8-40. *This 3-year-old girl gave a history of fondling and digital penetration. The examiner was concerned about the hymenal attachment at 10 o'clock. This is probably a normal crescentic hymen with redundant tissue at that location. There is a similar configuration on the opposite side.*

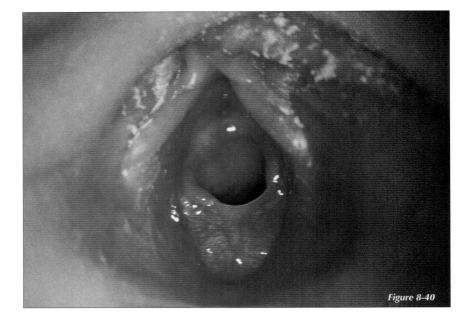

Figure 8-41. Separated hymenal septum in an 11-year-old early pubertal girl.

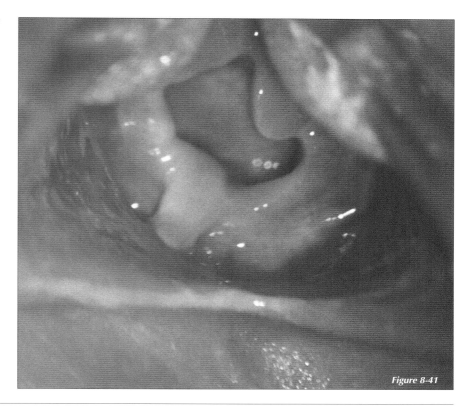

Figure 8-42. Genital examination of a chronically sexually abused 12-year-old girl.

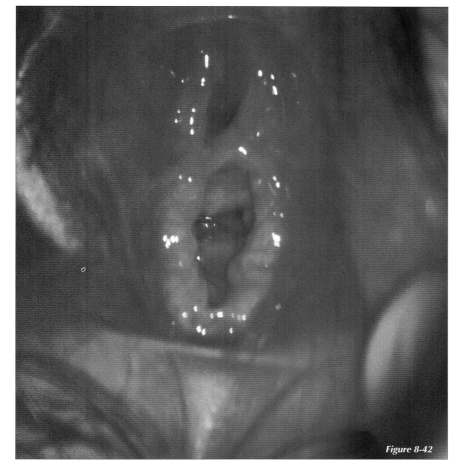

Figure 8-43. *Penile injury in a 22-month-old boy found to have blood in his diaper while at a daycare center. The urethral opening was irritated with a blood stain (**a**). There was also a small laceration of the glans (**b**). Urinalysis was normal. Cultures, including viral cultures for herpes, were not remarkable. The injury was reported to the hotline, but the cause was not determined.*

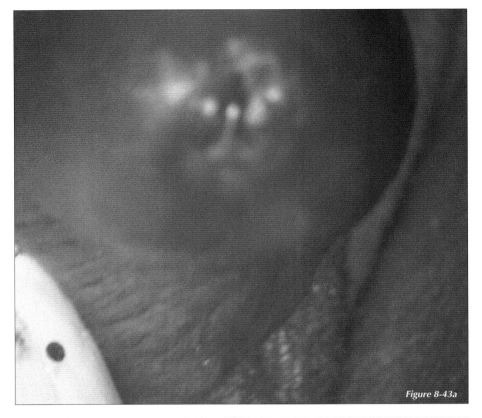

Figure 8-43a

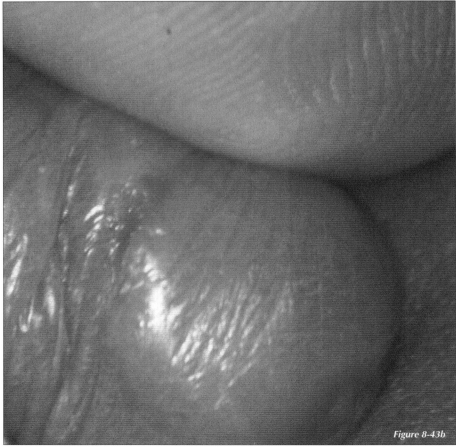

Figure 8-43b

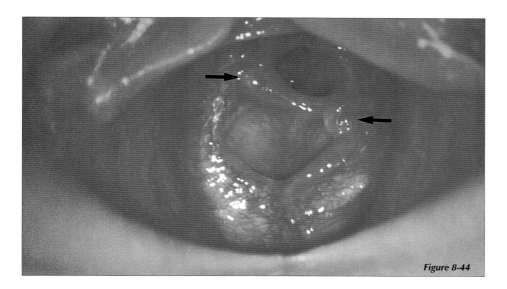

Figure 8-44. Normal crescentic hymen in a 5-year-old girl. Note the redundant hymenal tissue at 11 and 2 o'clock. The latter gives the false impression of angulation and a tear, but if you follow the hymenal edge at the tip of the right arrow, it is contiguous.

Figure 8-45. Healed old penile laceration in a 9-year-old boy.

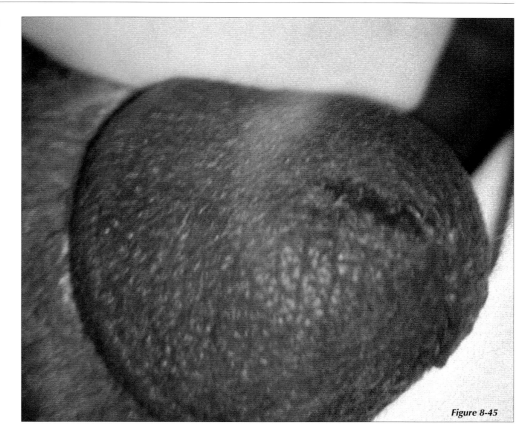

Figure 8-46. *Two sisters, ages 4 and 7 years, were raped and mutilated by their mother's live-in boyfriend. He killed the mother and left them all for dead. The children survived and identified their attacker. The older child (**a** through **g**), after the rape, was slashed several times with a knife. The knife was run, midline from below the anus, through the perineum and into the vagina. (**a**) Before surgery; (**b**) just before surgery. She sustained a puncture wound to her arm (**c** and **d**), a small laceration to her mid-chest (**e**), a laceration of her left arm (**f**), and defense wounds of her left hand where she tried to ward off her attacker (**g**). It is important to note that the palmar wounds can be abuse injuries because children often defend themselves palm outward against their attackers. The younger child (**h** and **i**) had a knife slash across her throat (**h**) and evidence of anal abuse (**i**). She probably suffered the same abuse as her mother, who was anally penetrated with a broom handle. Compare the vaginal injury in the older child with cases of accidental injury, specifically with the child doing the splits and the child impaled on a light fixture (Figures 8-47 and 8-48).*

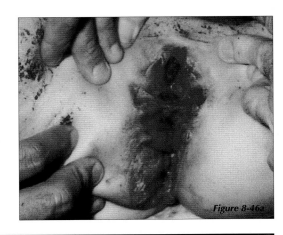

Figure 8-46a

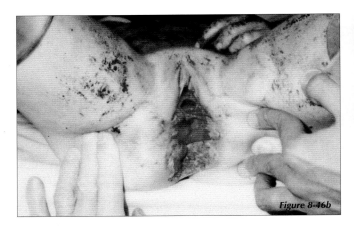

Figure 8-46b

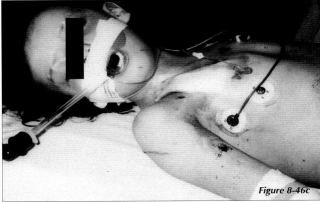

Figure 8-46c

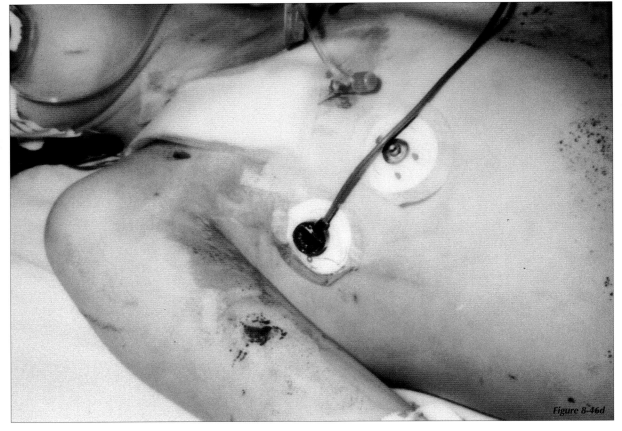

Figure 8-46d

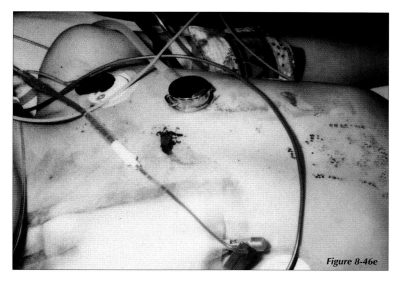

Figure 8-46e

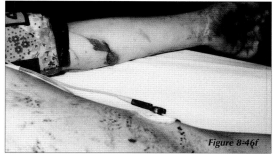

Figure 8-46f

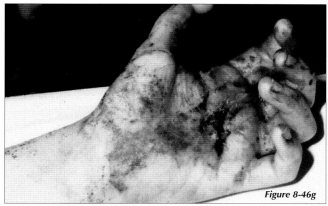

Figure 8-46g

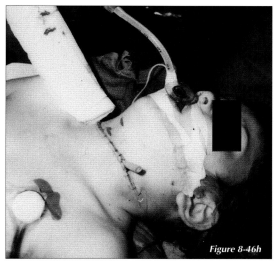

Figure 8-46h

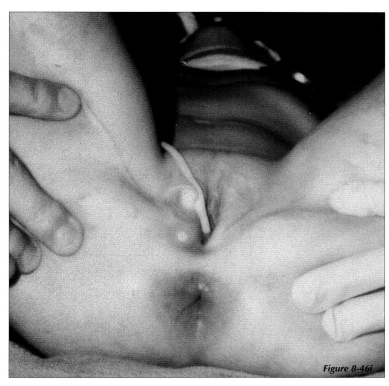

Figure 8-46i

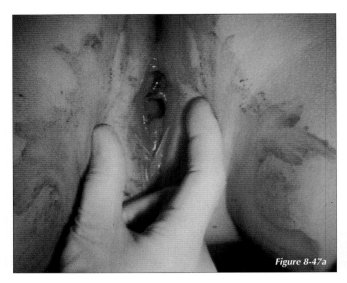

Figure 8-47a

Figure 8-47. This 13-year-old girl was seen in the emergency room with a third-degree laceration of the vagina extending from the base of the vagina to the rectum (**a** and **b**). The rectum was not affected. She stated that she was alone in her room and her father was in another part of the house. She was listening and dancing to music and tried to do the splits. She suddenly slipped to the floor and was injured. Because of the location of the injury, the hotline was called. The police investigated the home and the family, which was not known to child protection authorities. The home was well kept and the girl's room had a highly polished hardwood floor that could have explained the injury. The injury was therefore determined to be accidental. It is important to note that this is a midline injury, limited to the perineal area. The police investigated the scene and found the highly polished surface necessary to produce such an injury.

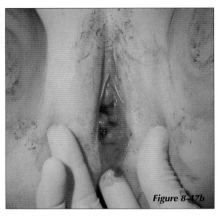

Figure 8-47b

Figure 8-48. This 6-year-old girl was riding on the handlebars of a bike when the bike suddenly stopped and she fell forward, landing on a broken light fixture on the front fender. The injury was midline and did not involve the labia majora (**a** and **b**). Impaling injuries usually involve external structures. The police investigated the scene, and witnesses verified the story.

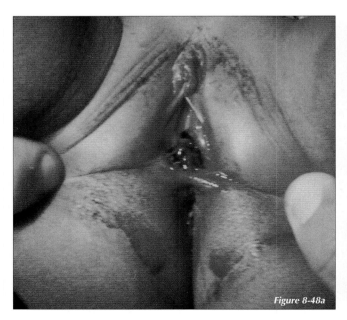

Figure 8-48a

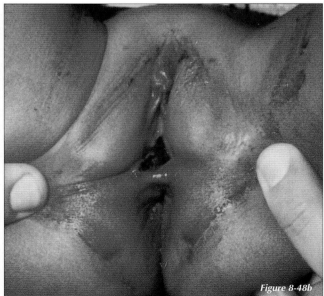

Figure 8-48b

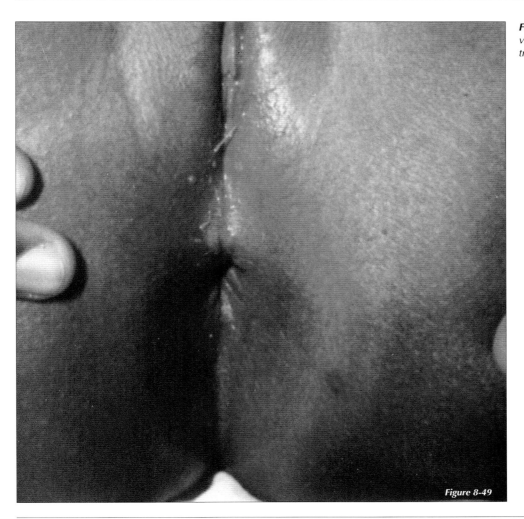

Figure 8-49. *Nine-year-old rape victim whose only evidence of trauma was a perineal tear.*

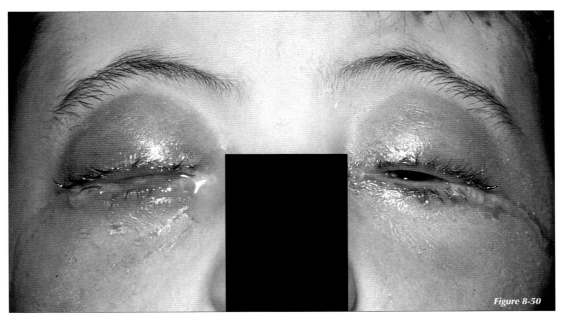

Figure 8-50. *Ocular gonorrhea in a 12-year-old girl. She had vaginal gonorrhea and probably inoculated herself. She disclosed that she had been sexually abused. (Courtesy J. Giangiacomo)*

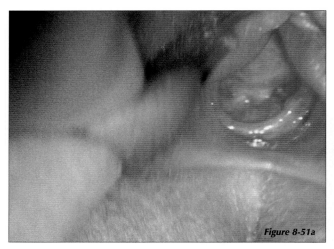

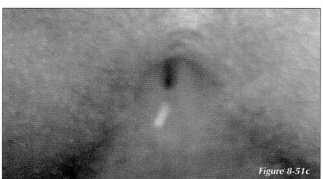

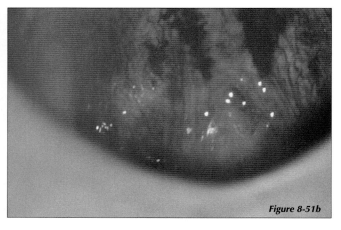

Figure 8-51. *Gonorrheal pelvic inflammatory disease in a 6-year-old girl. She had an enlarged vaginal opening with hymenal narrowing **(a)** and anal findings. The anterior column was injected and edematous **(b)**, and the perineal area was scarred and retracted **(c)**. This examination was performed 3 days after therapy began. On admission, the landmarks were barely discernible. She denied abuse.*

Figure 8-52. *This 5-year-old girl injured herself while climbing out of a wooden toy box. She was momentarily hung up while straddling the front side. The child spontaneously told emergency personnel of the incident. She had no other injuries or genital abnormalities.*

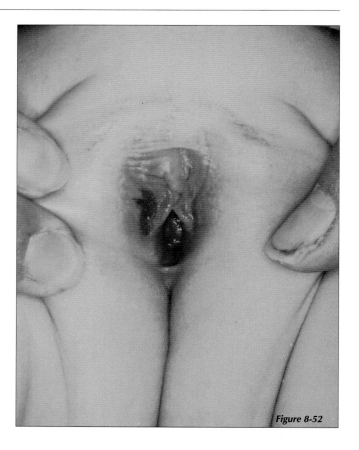

Figure 8-53. Pseudoabuse. This 10-year-old boy was taken to the emergency room for genital swelling and suspected penile injury. The child was in renal failure, with the edema and unusual penile configuration **(a)** secondary to the renal condition. This can be mistaken for penile injury caused by tying the penis with a string (see Chapter 3). Note that he also had ascites **(b)**.

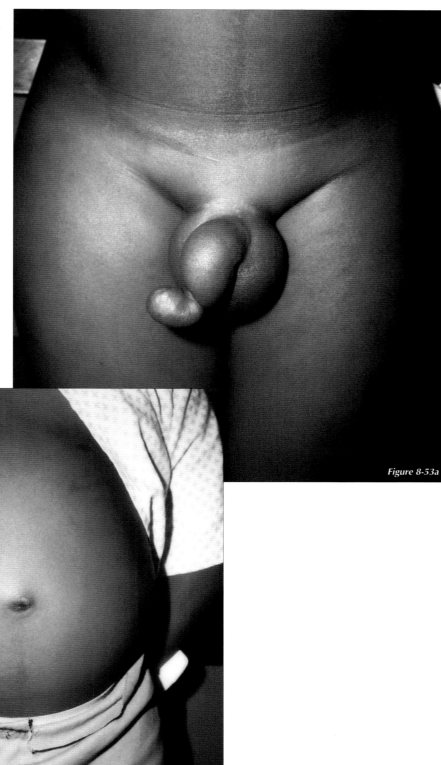

Figure 8-53a

Figure 8-53b

Figure 8-54. *Primary type 2 herpes in a 3-year-old girl who gave a credible history of sexual abuse.*

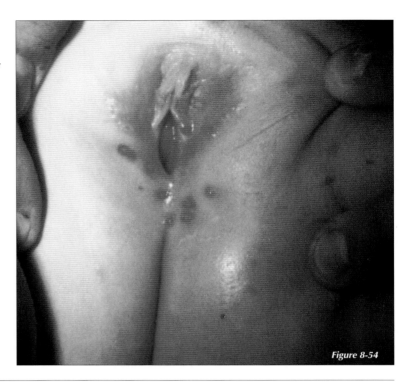

Figure 8-54

Figure 8-55. *The uncle of this 3-year-old girl had been recently released from prison for sexual abuse and had moved in with the family. When the child's mother noted blood in the girl's panties and saw the vascular changes, she asked the child if anyone had hurt her. The child said that her uncle had done it. On examination, the child was found to have lichen sclerosis; other vaginal findings were normal. Whether the uncle had abused her was uncertain. Note the pale "halo" effect at the periphery of the vascular changes, a characteristic of lichen sclerosis.*

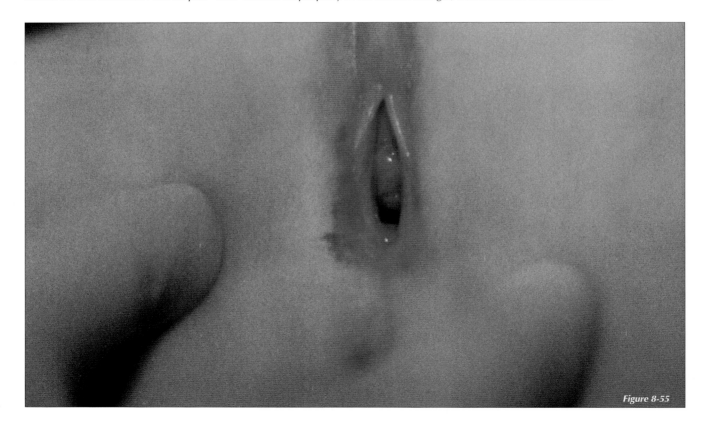

Figure 8-55

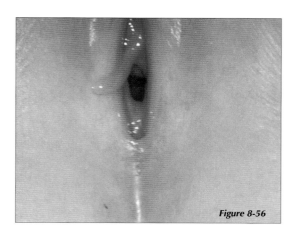

Figure 8-56. This 4-year-old girl was taken to the emergency room by her mother, who was concerned that she might have been abused because "she had something hanging out of her." This was a septal remnant. The rest of the examination was not remarkable, and the child denied abuse.

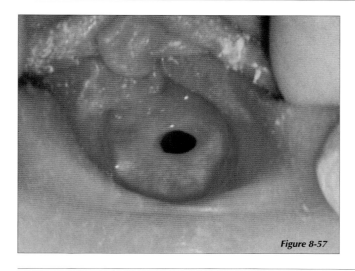

Figure 8-57. Normal annular hymen in a 3-year-old girl who gave a credible history of digital penetration.

Figure 8-58. Six-year-old girl with a mound of tissue at 8 o'clock, a normal variant.

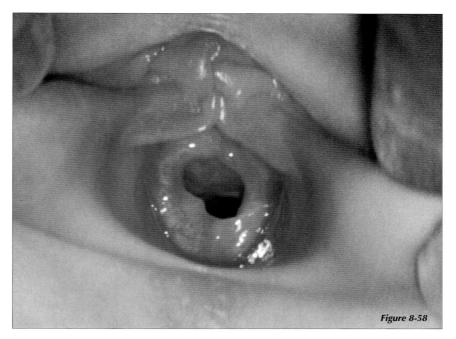

Figure 8-59. (a and **b)** Bilateral contusions along the labia minora in a 4-year-old girl. The child described masturbatory action by the caregiver. **(c)** Stain to enhance the lesions. The rest of the genital examination was not remarkable, and the three examiners disagreed as to the findings. Although the interviewer felt that the child gave a credible history of abuse, one of the examiners believed that the lesions were secondary to a monilial infection, even in the absence of any other evidence of monilia.

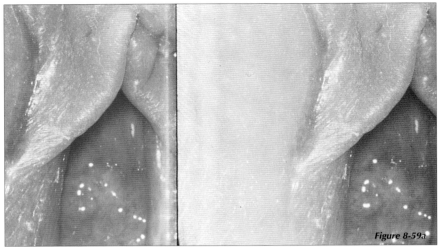

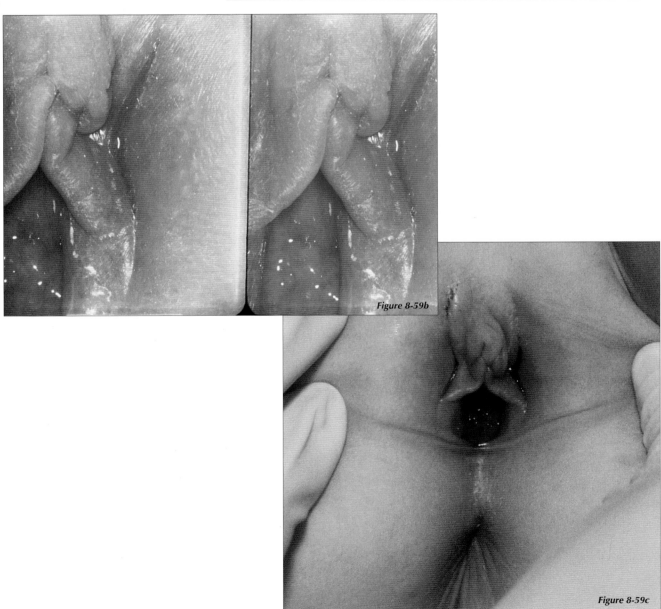

Figure 8-60. *This 12-year-old girl was referred by her private physician as possibly abused. She complained of a severe vaginal and anal infection and denied abuse. On physical examination, the hymen, although boggy, was intact (**a**). The skin along the linea was friable and weeping, as was the anal sphincter (**b**). Cultures grew group B Streptococcus. Cultures were negative for salmonella and shigella organisms. She responded to ampicillin.*

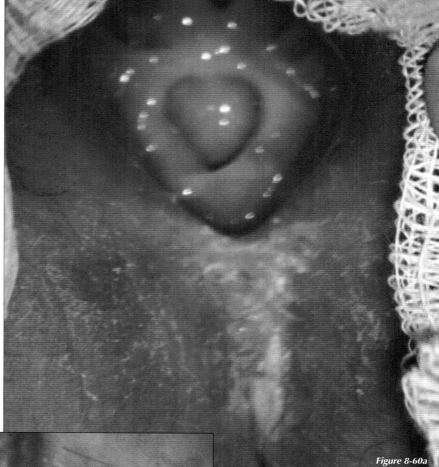

Figure 8-60a

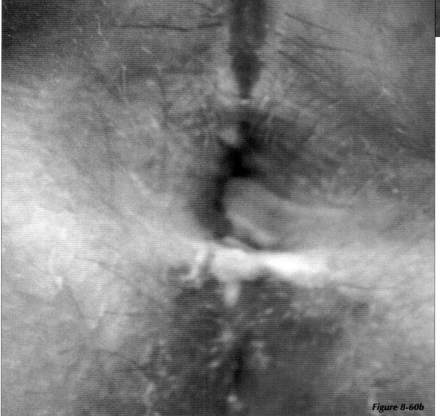

Figure 8-60b

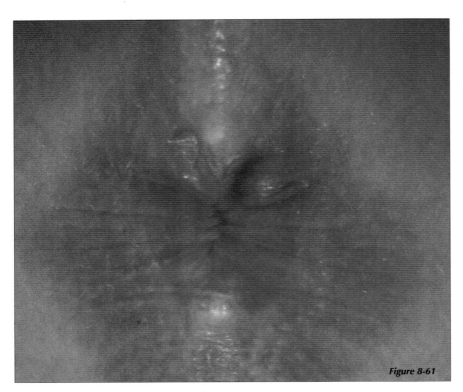

Figure 8-61. This 12-year-old boy, along with his younger brother, described several episodes of anal penetration. Note the small anal tag at 11 o'clock and the venous defect at 1 o'clock. The younger brother had no physical findings suggestive of sexual abuse.

Figure 8-61

Figure 8-62. Healing rectal tear in a 4-year-old girl (a and b).

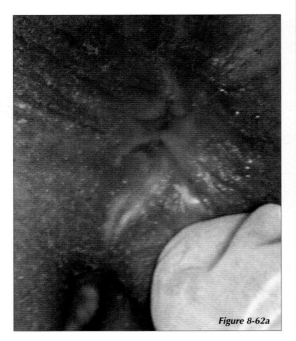

Figure 8-62a

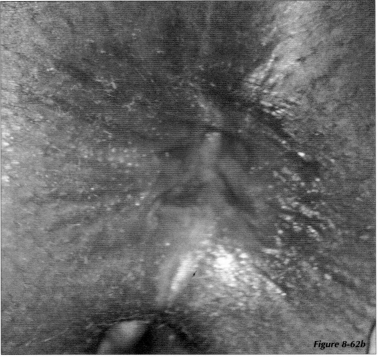

Figure 8-62b

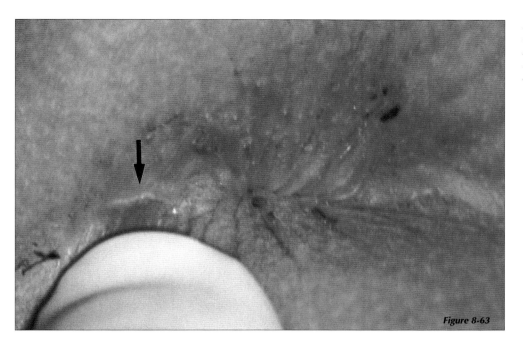

Figure 8-63. Healed perineal tear. This was located just below the anal sphincter and not in the usual location for an anal fissure.

Figure 8-63

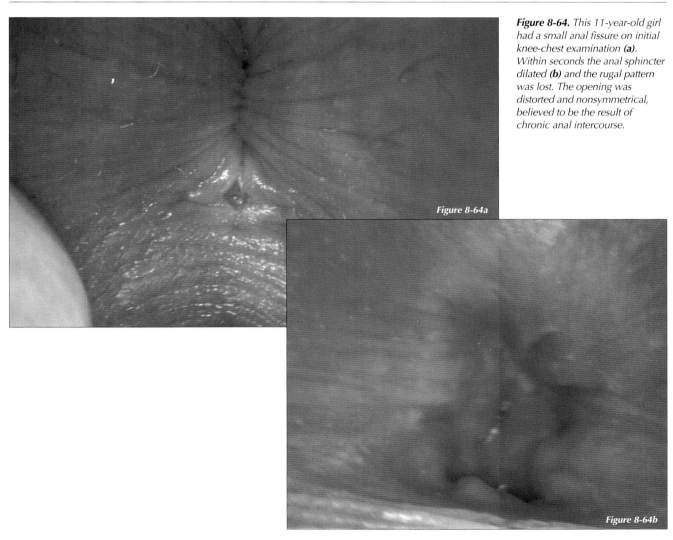

Figure 8-64. This 11-year-old girl had a small anal fissure on initial knee-chest examination **(a)**. Within seconds the anal sphincter dilated **(b)** and the rugal pattern was lost. The opening was distorted and nonsymmetrical, believed to be the result of chronic anal intercourse.

Figure 8-64a

Figure 8-64b

Figure 8-65. *Anal tear in an 11-year-old girl. She gave a history of vaginal penetration and denied anal penetration.*

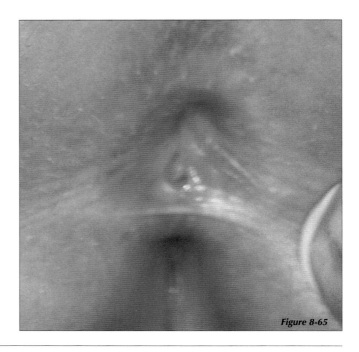

Figure 8-65

Figure 8-66. *This 11-year-old girl gave a credible history of sexual abuse that involved digital vaginal and rectal contact. She denied penetration. The vaginal examination was not remarkable. She had an unusual midline raphe that was thickened at rest (**a**). With gluteal separation, the thickening expanded into a large broad scar, the end of which was irregular and contiguous with a hemorrhoid at 11 o'clock (**b**). Whether this was the result of abuse could not be determined.*

Figure 8-66a

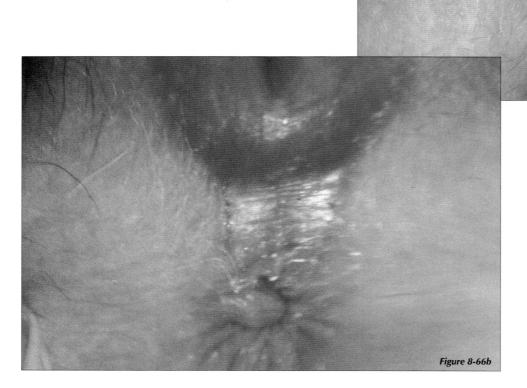

Figure 8-66b

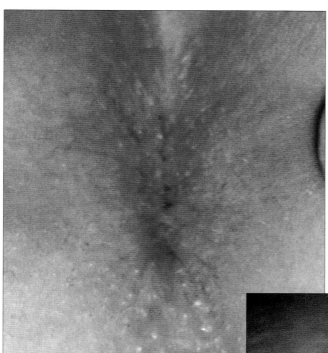

Figure 8-67a

Figure 8-67. This 6-year-old boy described multiple episodes of anal intercourse over a 2-year period of time. The last abuse occurred several months before this visit. The anus showed normal tone and rugal pattern. There were numerous raised lesions at 6 o'clock in the knee-chest position along the gluteal fold and several larger raised lesions in the perianal area (**a** through **c**). The lesions were diagnosed as condyloma.

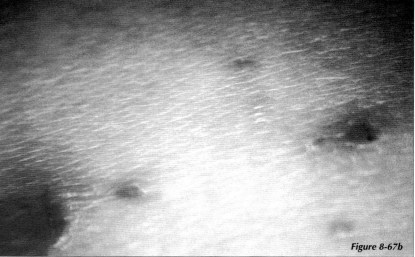

Figure 8-67b

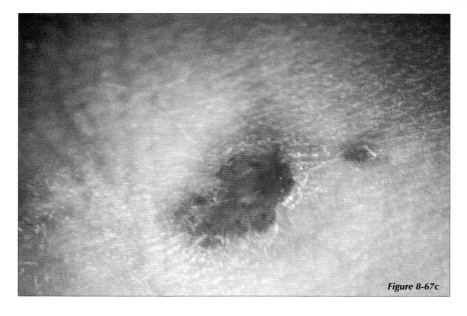

Figure 8-67c

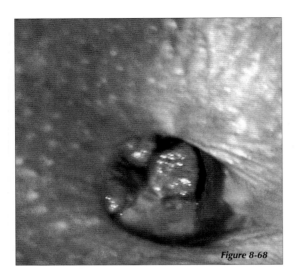

Figure 8-68. *Anal dilation due to stool in the anal canal.*

Figure 8-69. *Eighteen-month-old boy with pigmented nevus. These lesions must be distinguished from condylomas. A biopsy is needed.*

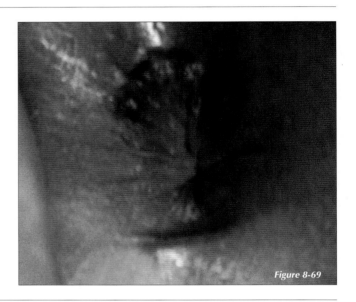

Figure 8-70. *Anal tear in a 12-year-old girl who described sodomy.*

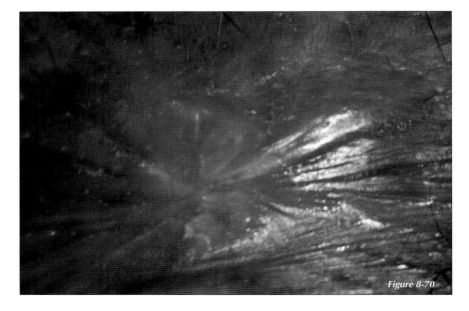

Figure 8-71. *Venous pooling or laking in a 12-year-old boy who described anal penetration. This is an artifact of the examination.*

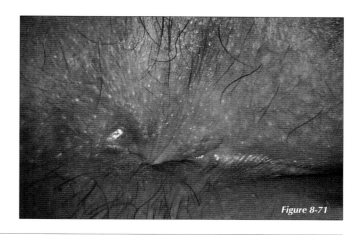

Figure 8-72. *Healing anal tear in a 9-year-old girl who had described anal penetration occurring several days before this examination.*

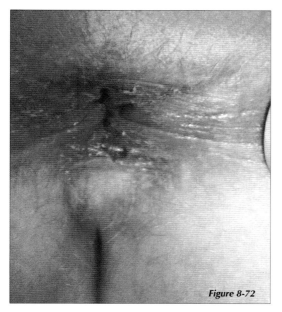

Figure 8-73. *Anal examination of 6-year-old boy who was found to have blood in his underwear following a visit with his father. The mother suspected sexual abuse, although the child denied it. The child was found to have a small nick of the anus, probably self-inflicted while scratching.*

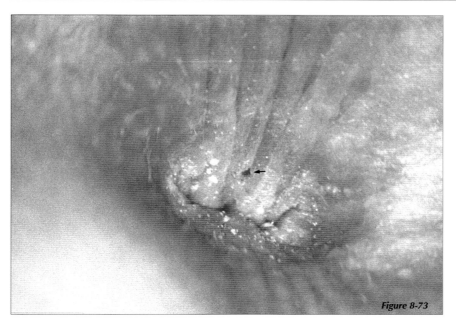

Figure 8-74. Anal tag in a chronically sexually abused 9-year-old boy.

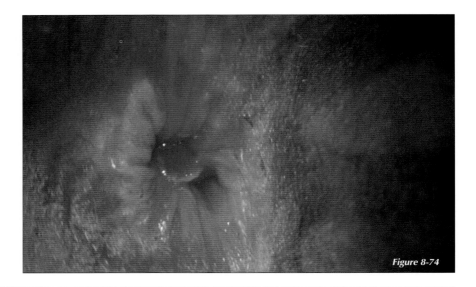

Figure 8-75. Acute streptococcal anal cellulitis in a 3-year-old boy.

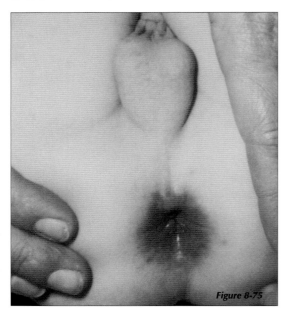

Figure 8-76. This 3-year-old boy was sexually abused by his older brother. Note the ecchymotic area from 10 to 12 o'clock.

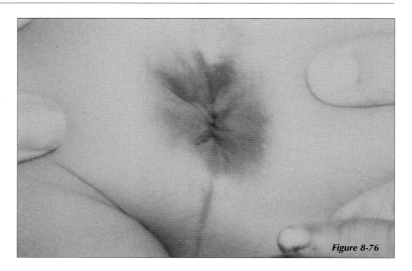

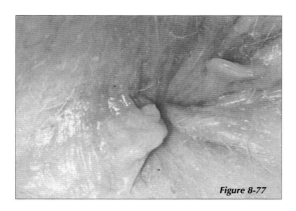

Figure 8-77. *Anal tags in a 6-year-old girl who described anal penetration.*

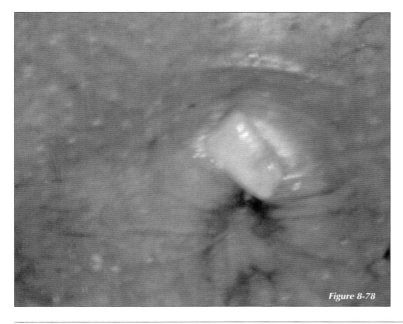

Figure 8-78. *Anal tag in a 5-year-old girl who described vaginal penetration but denied anal abuse.*

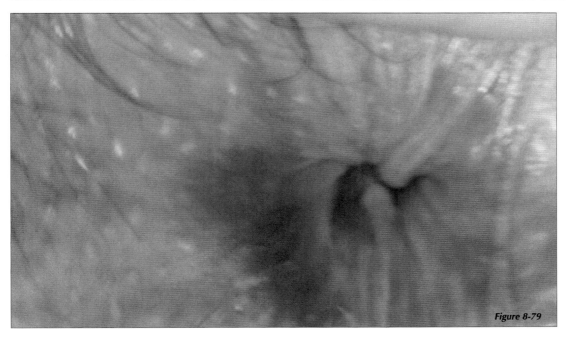

Figure 8-79. *Anal trauma in a 16-year-old following forced anal penetration.*

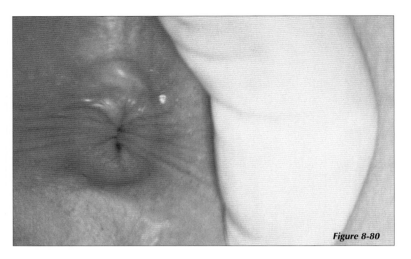

Figure 8-80. *Anal examination in a 3-year-old boy who described anal penetration. The child had anal spasm, which might explain the tire-like appearance of the sphincter. The smooth area of mucosa at 12 o'clock was believed to be a normal variant.*

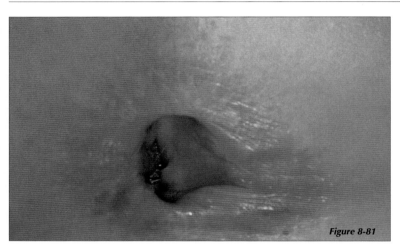

Figure 8-81. *Anal trauma after sexual abuse in a 5-year-old girl. Note the bruising and loss of tone at 3 to 6 o'clock.*

Figure 8-82. *This 3-year-old boy was seen in the emergency room after complaining to his mother of anal pain. He disclosed anal penetration by his father. Note the increased pigmentation, funnelling, and moderate dilation. These are all nonspecific findings of abuse. With the history given, assuming that it is credible, they become stronger.*

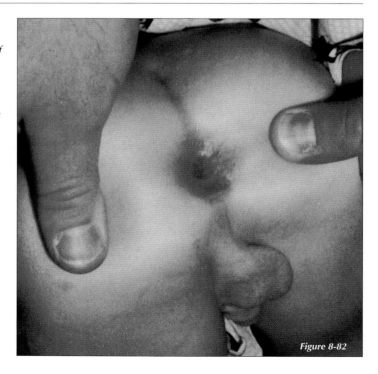

Figure 8-83. Crab louse (Phthirus pubis) found in the eyebrows of a 4-year-old girl. Although this parasite is usually sexually transmitted, it can also be transmitted by nonsexual means. The child's mother also had an infestation. The crab louse must be distinguished from the head and body louse. Head and body lice are larger and have an elongated body.

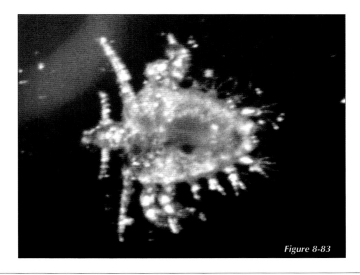

Figure 8-83

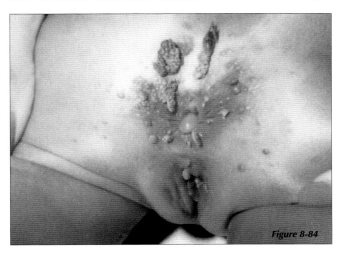

Figure 8-84

Figure 8-84. Condyloma in a 9-month-old child. Although the anal findings were suspicious, the mother also had a history of condyloma and no report was made. Condyloma first appearing before 2 years of age are usually congenital, especially with a positive family history. In congenital cases, the child should have no other physical findings consistent with sexual or physical abuse.

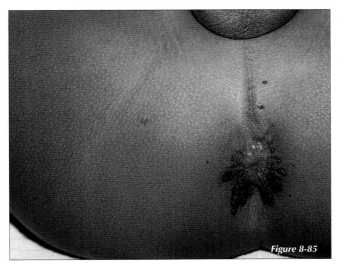

Figure 8-85

Figure 8-85. Condyloma in a 3 1/2-year-old boy. This was reported because of the child's age. The child denied abuse, and there were no other findings suggestive of abuse.

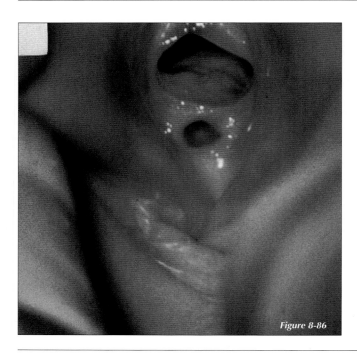

Figure 8-86. *Healing midline hymenal tear. Note the angulation and discoloration.*

Figure 8-86

Figure 8-87. *Secondary syphilis in a 14-year-old girl. Note the areas of patchy increased pigmentation on the palms (a), soles (b), and feet (c).*

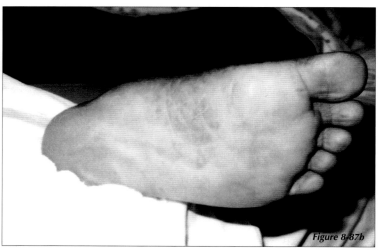

Figure 8-87b

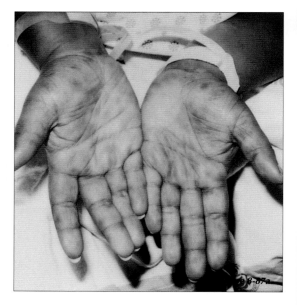

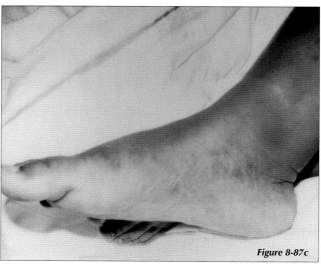

Figure 8-87c

Figure 8-88. *This 10-year-old girl was sent by her private physician to the emergency room because he suspected this "injury" to be sexual abuse. The child denied abuse. This is not abuse, but instead is lichen sclerosis et atrophicus. Compare this with Figure 8-29, which is also lichen sclerosis. Note the labial adhesions, which can be very friable. Also note that the ecchymotic area of the labia minora can be seen in this condition.*

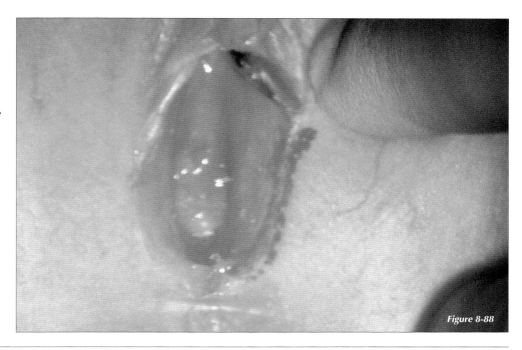

Figure 8-88

Figure 8-89a

Figure 8-89. *An adolescent rape victim who was seen several days after the attack. Note the healing injury to the posterior fourchette. (Courtesy D. St. Germain, D.O.)*

Figure 8-89b

Figure 8-89c

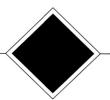

PART FOUR

Forensics

Chapter

THE MEDICAL EXAMINER PART 1

MARY E. S. CASE, M.D.

The medical examiner determines the cause and manner of death and provides expert evaluation of the presence, absence, nature, and significance of injuries and disease. He or she collects and preserves evidence and correlates clinical and pathologic findings. The forensic pathologist evaluates the deaths of children who die because of accidental injuries, nonaccidental trauma, or neglect.

The involvement of the medical examiner in child abuse and neglect begins at the time of death. Any sudden and unexpected death or any death suspected to be caused or contributed to by any injury or nonnatural condition must be reported to the medicolegal authority having jurisdiction where death was pronounced.

The medical examiner's role does not begin and end in the autopsy room. To be most effective, the medical examiner must work closely with law enforcement personnel and the clinicians involved with the case. Once an opinion is rendered, he or she must communicate with the prosecuting attorney, as appropriate.

The cases shown in this chapter illustrate the types of injuries that fall into the jurisdiction of the medical examiner.

Figure 9-1. *This 4-month-old living child was examined for the Department of Family Services to provide an interpretation of the marks found on the child's body. The child has multiple pinch marks on his back and arms. These pinch marks consist of two centrally placed, narrow, vertical reddish clusters of petechiae surrounded by contusion.*

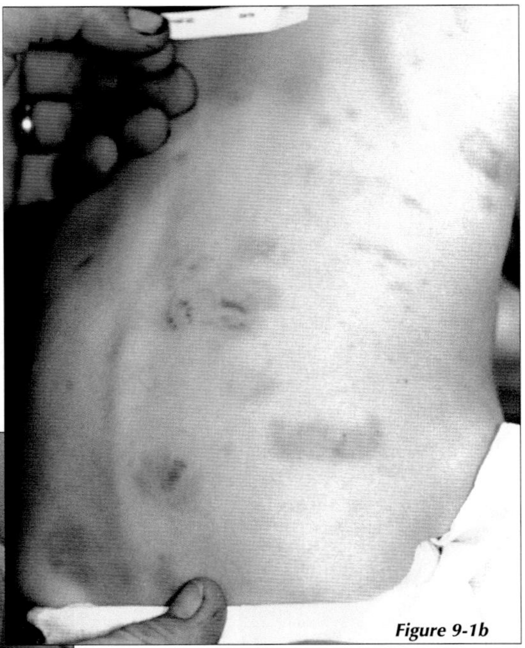

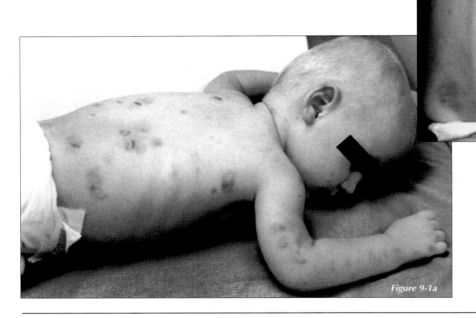

Figure 9-1b

Figure 9-1a

Figure 9-2. *This 2-year-old child had a fatal head injury and evidence of old traumatic chipping of the anterior enamel of the upper central incisor that is thought to result from abuse.*

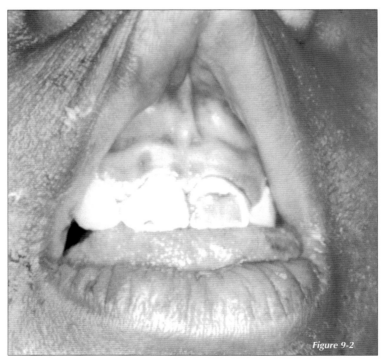

Figure 9-2

Figure 9-3. *This 27-month-old boy, left in the care of the 23-year-old boyfriend of his mother, became suddenly ill, vomited, and stopped breathing. There was no history of trauma. The child was taken to the hospital and resuscitated. He underwent surgery to remove a lacerated portion of distal duodenum **(a)** and died 2 days later. Photographs demonstrate contusions of the buttocks with deep subcutaneous bleeding **(b)**, a contusion and laceration of the duodenum removed at surgery **(a)**, and peritonitis found in the abdomen at autopsy **(c)**. The boyfriend in this case had been arrested 2 years before for beating and burning with cigarettes another girlfriend's child.*

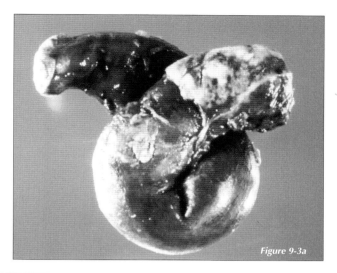

Figure 9-3a

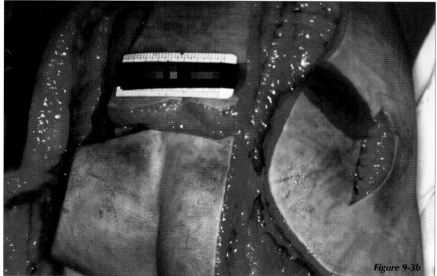

Figure 9-3b

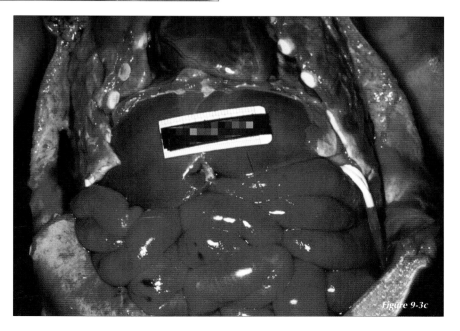

Figure 9-3c

Figure 9-4. *This 16-month-old girl was admitted to the hospital with a closed head injury. Her mother eventually admitted that her boyfriend beat the child and threw the child against the metal headboard of the bed. Photographs demonstrate a large contusion of the right forehead (**a**), multiple areas of bruising in the scalp seen as subgaleal (**b** and **c**), and thin layers of subdural blood over both cerebral convexities (**d**). There were bilateral retinal hemorrhages. Note that on the surface the bleeding is not readily detected (**a**).*

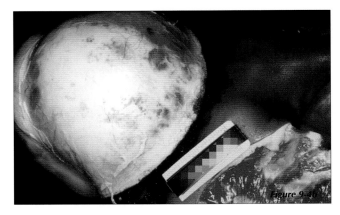

Figure 9-4b

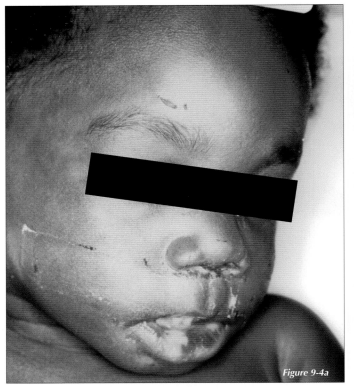

Figure 9-4a

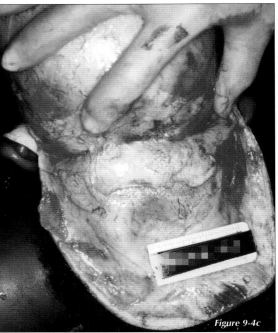

Figure 9-4c

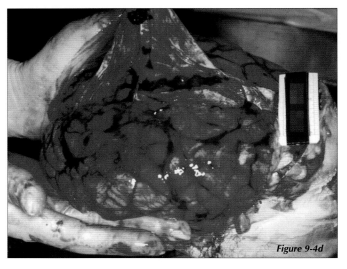

Figure 9-4d

Figure 9-5. *This 11-week-old boy was left in the care of his teenage father who said he found the child unresponsive. He called the mother to come home. They took the child to the hospital where he survived 2 days, although he was brain dead. Autopsy demonstrated a contusion of the penis (**a** and **b**), a large contusion of the frontoparietal scalp seen as subgaleal hemorrhage (**c**), small amounts of subdural hemorrhage over the cerebral convexities (**d**), and healing fractures of left ribs 3, 4, 5, and 6 posteriorly (**e**) (arrows). Three of the excised ribs (**f**) show early callous formation.*

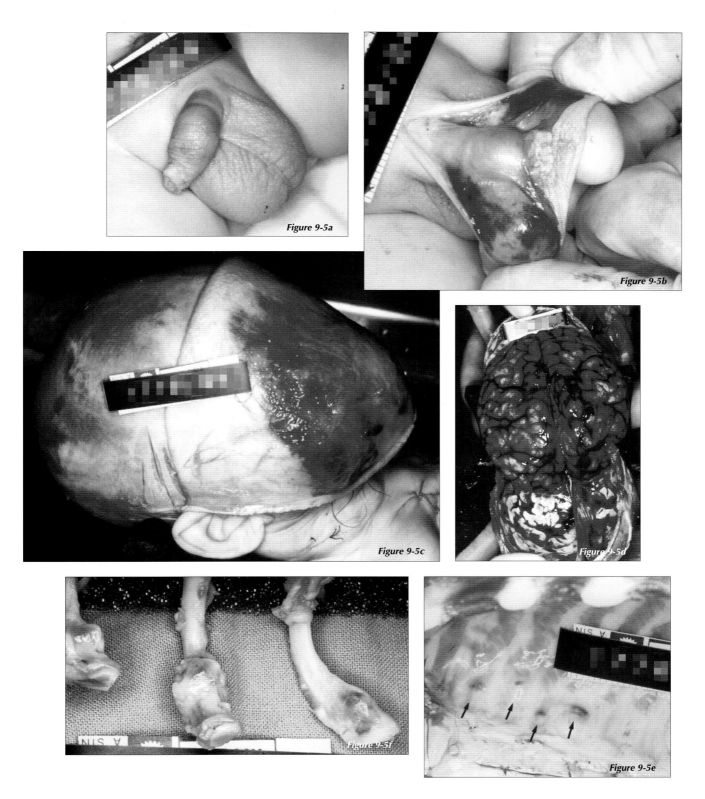

Figure 9-6. *This 26-month-old girl was reported by her mother to have just suddenly died. At autopsy the child weighed 19 pounds (well below the 5th percentile) and had multiple contusions about her face, neck, scalp, extremities, abdomen, back, and buttocks. Photographs demonstrate multiple bruises of the face* **(a)**; *a large healing laceration of the frenulum* **(b)** *(arrow) above the tooth line; a fresh loop mark on the inner thigh* **(c)** *from a belt, which is also shown* **(d)**; *old scars related to previous belt marks* **(e** *and* **f)**; *and incisions of the lower extremities to show contusions of soft tissues* **(g).** *The cause of death was blunt soft tissue trauma.*

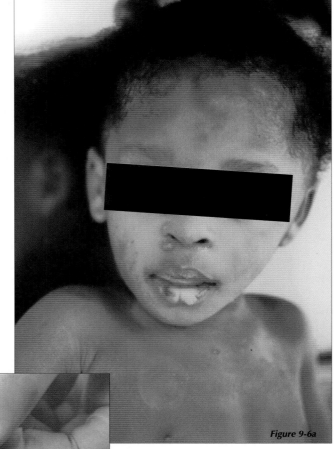

Figure 9-6a

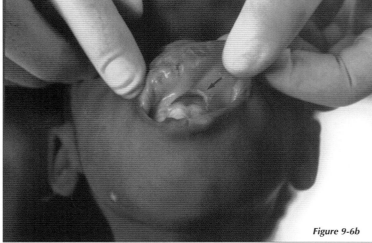

Figure 9-6b

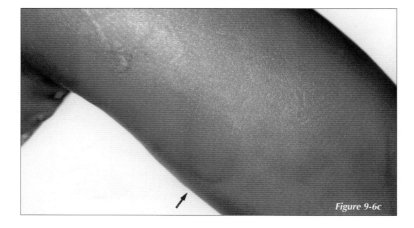

Figure 9-6c

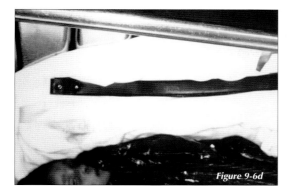

Figure 9-6d

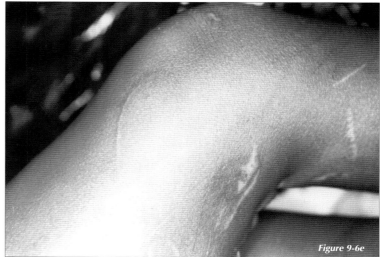

Figure 9-6e

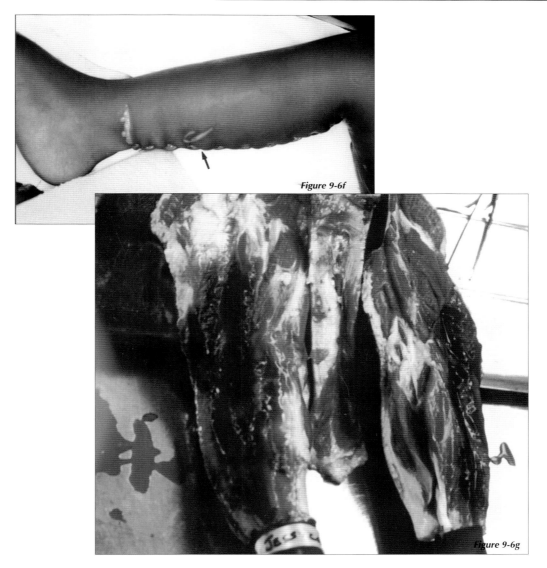

Figure 9-6f

Figure 9-6g

Figure 9-7. *This 5-year-old girl was beaten by her father with a variety of instruments, including a cord, a belt, a paddle, a fan belt, and tree branches, as shown in the photograph* **(a).** *The child was dead on arrival at the hospital. Injuries included multiple abrasions and contusions of head, face, neck, chest, abdomen, back, and extremities, as shown in photographs* **b** *through* **g.** *Patterned injuries of loops from belt marks and notches from the fan belt are recognizable. The cause of death was blunt soft tissue trauma* **(h** *and* **i).**

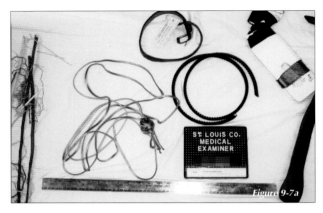

Figure 9-7a

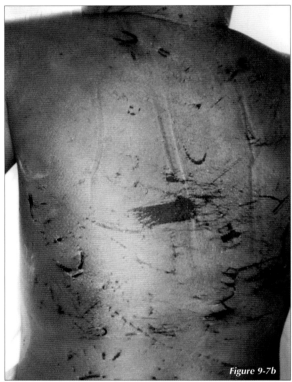

Figure 9-7b

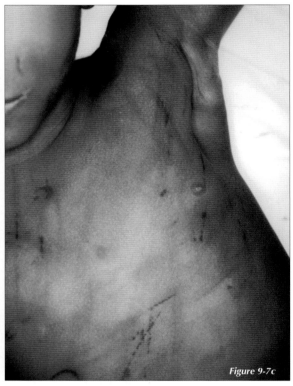

Figure 9-7c

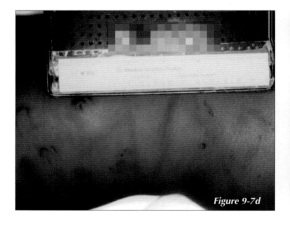

Figure 9-7d

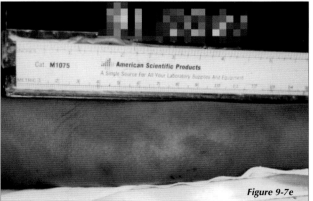

Figure 9-7e

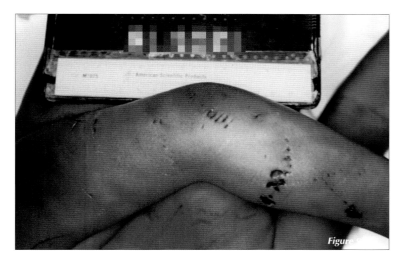

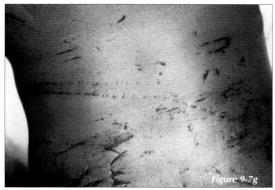

Figure 9-7g

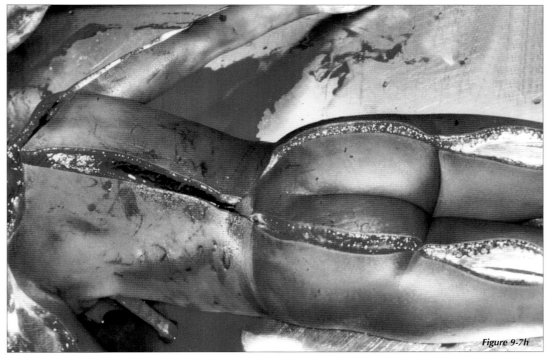

Figure 9-7h

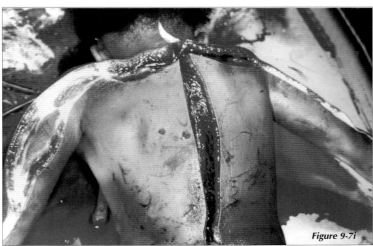

Figure 9-7i

Figure 9-8. This 2-year-old girl and her mother were visiting from another city and staying with friends. The child was sleeping on a couch in the living room and was found dead in the morning. The photographs demonstrate petechial hemorrhages over the eyelids and beneath the eyes **(a)**, on the palpebral conjunctivae **(b)**, on the gingiva of the upper gum **(c)**, and along the left side of the neck **(d)**. A male member of the host family eventually admitted to lying down on top of the child to keep her from crying, and he said that after about 15 minutes the child appeared to be sleeping. The cause of death was traumatic asphyxia.

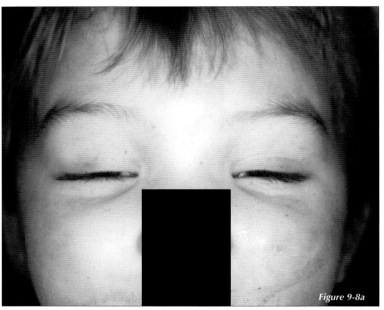

Figure 9-8a

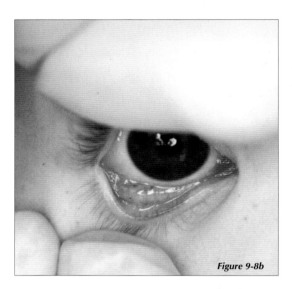

Figure 9-8b

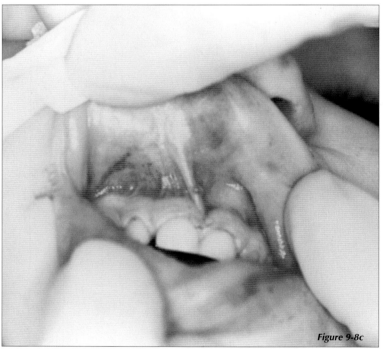

Figure 9-8c

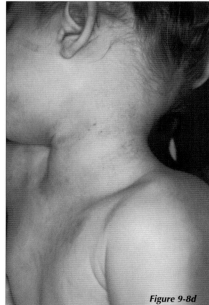

Figure 9-8d

Figure 9-9. This 6-month-old boy was found dead in a crib at the babysitter's home with no history of trauma. Photographs demonstrate a 5 cm contusion in the right occipital scalp (*a* and *b*), a linear fracture of the adjacent right posterior fossa, epidural hemorrhage of 6 to 8 ml in the right posterior fossa (*c* and *d*), and marked flattening of the adjacent right occipital pole (*e*).

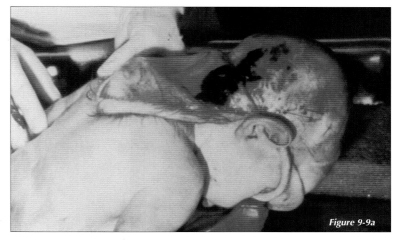

Figure 9-9a

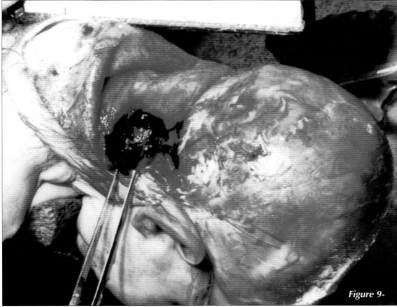

Figure 9-

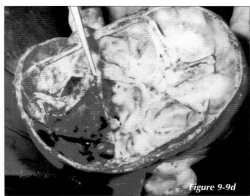

Figure 9-9d

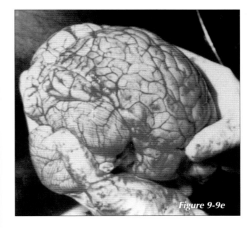

Figure 9-9e

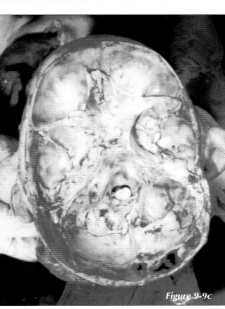

Figure 9-9c

Figure 9-10. This 7-month-old boy was admitted to the hospital with a history that he fell from a mattress 8 inches to the floor, had seizures, and became unresponsive. Photographs demonstrate bruising of the right forehead **(a)**, right frontal subgaleal hemorrhage **(b)**, and contusion of the inner lower lip **(c)**. Not shown is a thin layer of subdural hemorrhage over both cerebral convexities and small retinal hemorrhages.

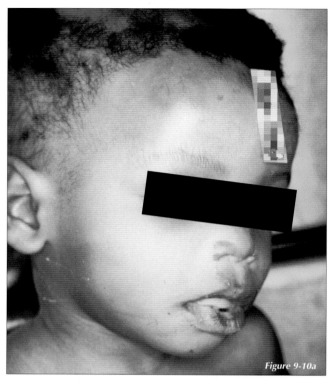

Figure 9-10a

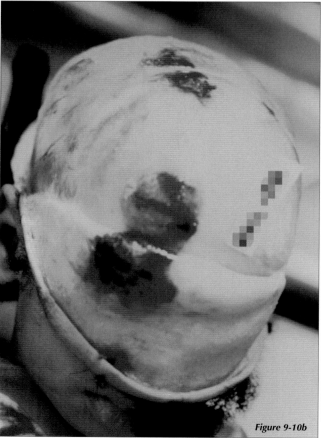

Figure 9-10b

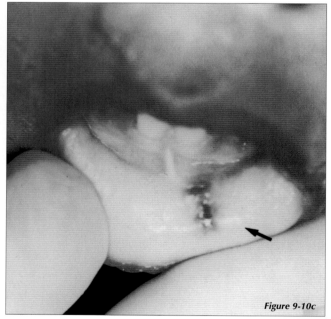

Figure 9-10c

Figure 9-11. *This 23-month-old boy was left with the mother's boyfriend who said the child "disappeared." The child was found in a plastic bag on the roof of the apartment building the next day and was frozen from the subzero weather. Shown in the photographs is the child in the plastic bag (a), large subgaleal hemorrhages (b), and small amounts of subdural hemorrhage over both cerebral convexities (c).*

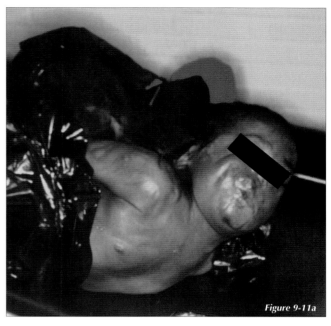

Figure 9-11a

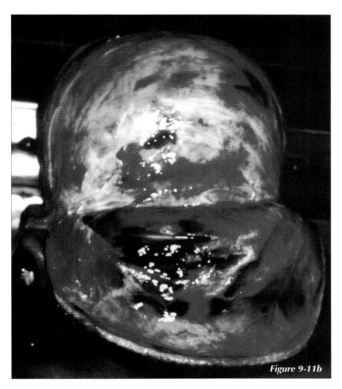

Figure 9-11b

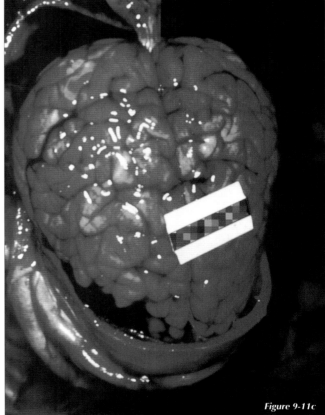

Figure 9-11c

Figure 9-12. This 3-year-old boy was said, by his mother, to have been found dead in his bed. Shown in the photographs is hemorrhage in the right temporalis muscle (broad arrow), a linear fracture of the right parietal calvarium (arrow in **a**), 80 ml of epidural blood lying over the right cerebral lateral convexity (**b** and **c**), fracture contusion of the right temporal gyri, and marked concave compression of the right cerebral hemisphere (**d** and **e**).

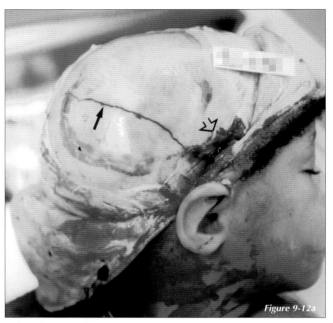

Figure 9-12a

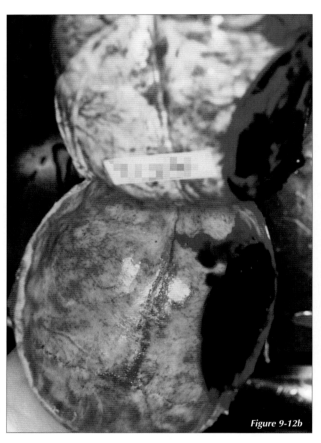

Figure 9-12b

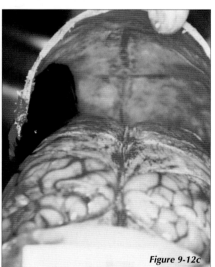

Figure 9-12c

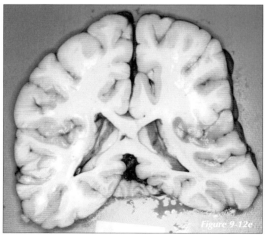

Figure 9-12e

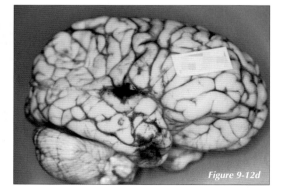

Figure 9-12d

THE MEDICAL EXAMINER PART 2

MICHAEL GRAHAM, M.D.

Figure 9-13. Scalp injuries inflicted with a hair brush.

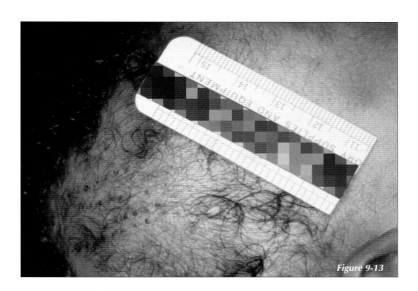

Figure 9-14. This 7-month-old boy was found dead in his crib. He had multiple bruises to his head and face. Note grab marks on his chest.

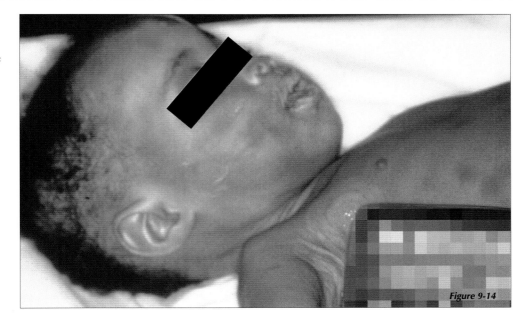

Figure 9-15. *This 5-month-old child was found dead at home (**a**). He has a torn frenulum. Note the separation of the mucosa at the gum line. This is caused by jamming an object such as a spoon or nipple into the child's mouth. These injuries can also be caused by a blow to the mouth. The other photographs (**b** to **e**) demonstrate other oral injuries that gave little external evidence of their existence.* **This emphasizes the need to examine the mouth in suspicious deaths. Oral lesions such as these can occasionally be the only injury seen in suffocation homicides.**

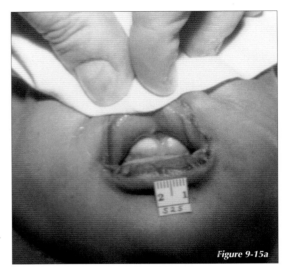

Figure 9-15a

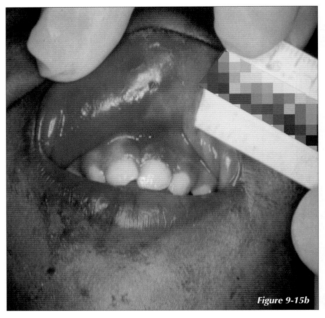

Figure 9-15b

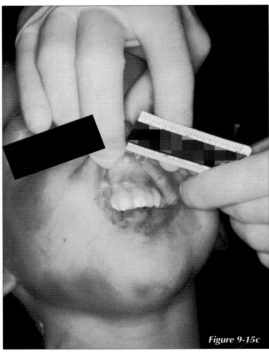

Figure 9-15c

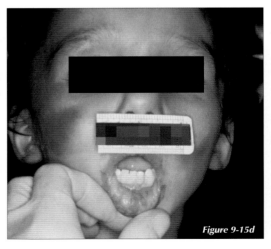

Figure 9-15d

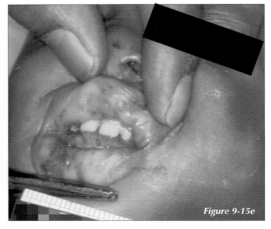

Figure 9-15e

Figure 9-16. *This battered toddler died of a fresh closed head injury. Many bruises antedate the head injury. These could not be explained by a single incident.*

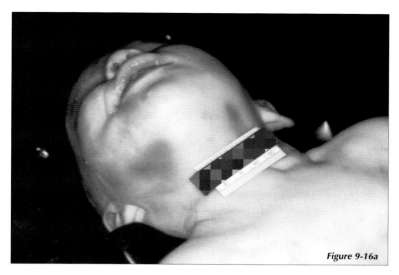

Figure 9-16a

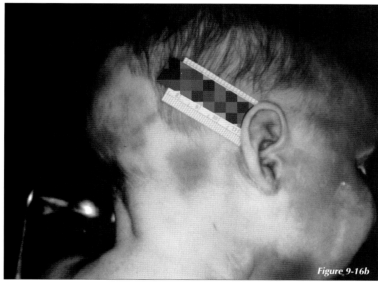

Figure 9-16b

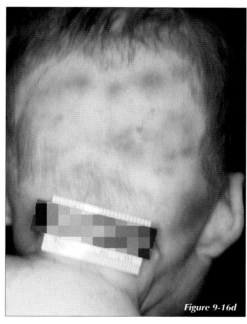

Figure 9-16d

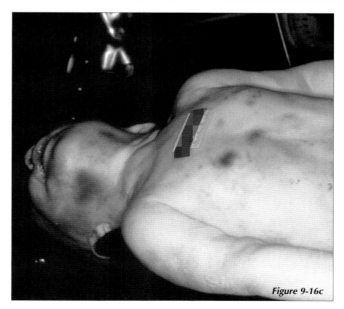

Figure 9-16c

Figure 9-17. Three different individuals. The first (**a**) is a child beaten with a cue stick. Note the characteristic pattern: two parallel erythematous areas bordering a blanched area. The second individual (**b**) is an adult beaten with a cane. By comparison, note the marks left on a child by a thin linear switch (**c**).

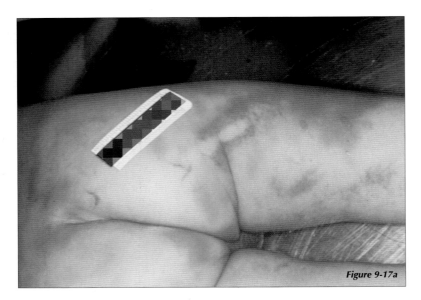

Figure 9-17a

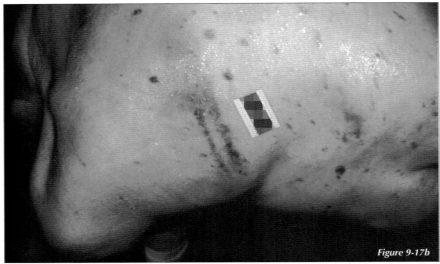

Figure 9-17b

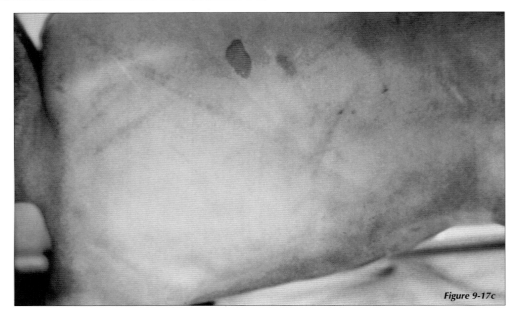

Figure 9-17c

Figure 9-18. *Self-induced scratching injuries to the forearm. They are not abuse.*

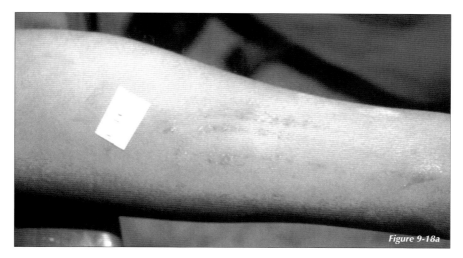

Figure 9-18a

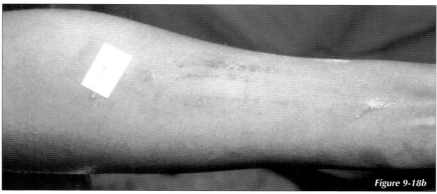

Figure 9-18b

Figure 9-19. *This is a teenage prostitute found dead. Her fingernails were broken in a fight. The circled wound on the abdomen occurred after death and was caused by a temperature probe.*

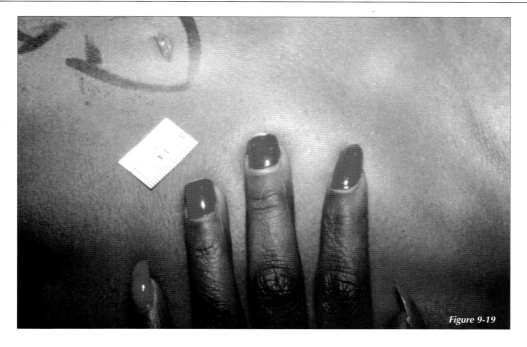

Figure 9-19

Figure 9-20. *This 9-year-old boy was killed by his mother's boyfriend. He was refusing to eat. The boyfriend force-fed him hotdogs and buns, using a hammer handle as a ramrod. Shown are the food bolus obstructing the airway at the glottic opening (**a** and **b**) and the stomach contents.*

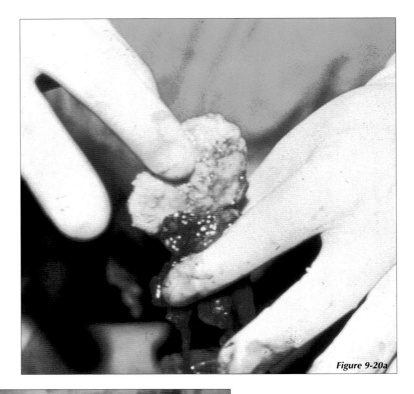

Figure 9-20a

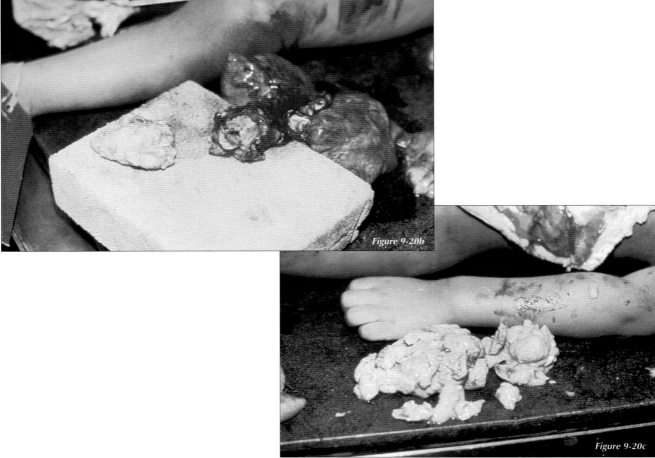

Figure 9-20b

Figure 9-20c

Figure 9-21. Same child as in Figure 9-17, who was beaten with a cue stick. He also sustained genital injuries.

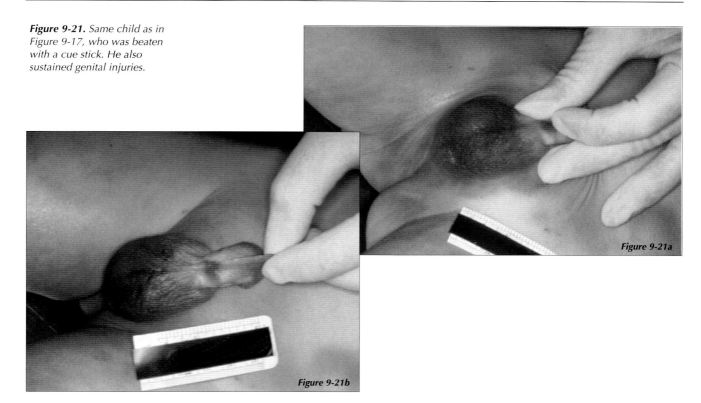

Figure 9-21a

Figure 9-21b

Figure 9-22. This older adolescent was the victim of a sexual assault. She sustained a perineal injury, anal bruising and dilatation, and abrasions on the backs of her legs.

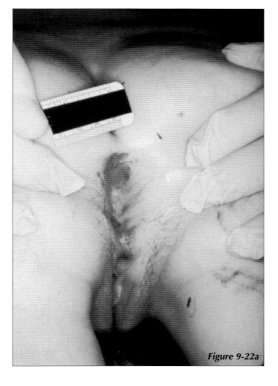

Figure 9-22a

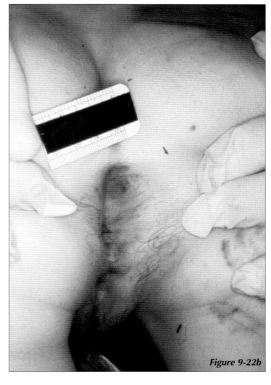

Figure 9-22b

Figure 9-23. *Victim of severe neglect. He was malnourished and found nearly dead in his bed, having been there, unattended, overnight. He had supposedly been ill for several days. He died from a ruptured retropharyngeal abscess. He had attended school earlier that week and was sent home because he could barely walk. The school did not report the case to the hotline. The lesions on the bottoms of his feet are abscesses. It took several washings in the hospital to remove the dirt from his soles in order to expose these lesions. This is the same child shown in Figure 11-5,* **a** *and* **b.**

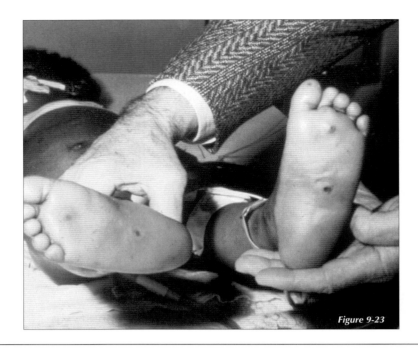

Figure 9-23

Figure 9-24. *These toddlers have severe soft tissue trauma. The extent of the deep bleeding is not visible until exposed.*

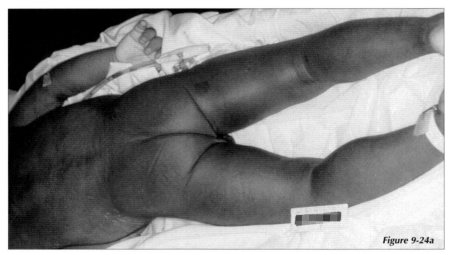

Figure 9-24a

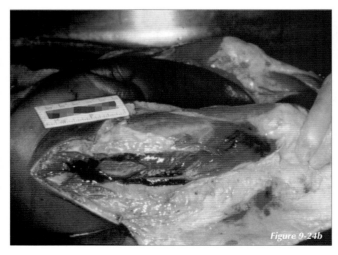

Figure 9-24b

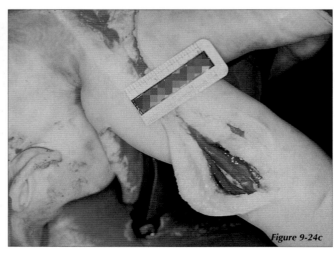

Figure 9-24c

Figure 9-25. *Fresh rib fractures in a 2-month-old child. Compare these with the rib fractures shown in Figure 9-5,* **e** *and* **f,** *which are healing and over 2 weeks old.*

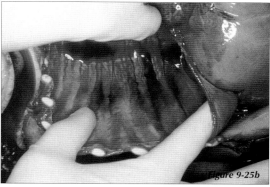

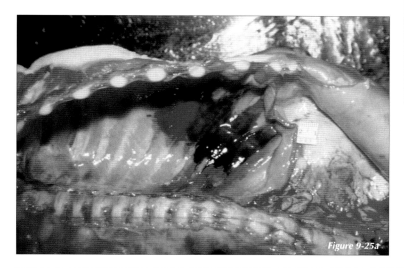

Figure 9-26. *This infant was found dead in his crib. He has a lacerated liver. His teenage father admitted to squeezing his abdomen in frustration to try to stop the child's crying. There were no external signs of injury. Parts* **c** *to* **f** *show four other cases with blunt trauma to the liver.*

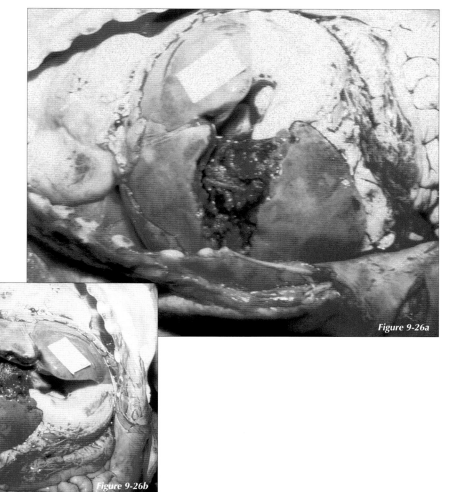

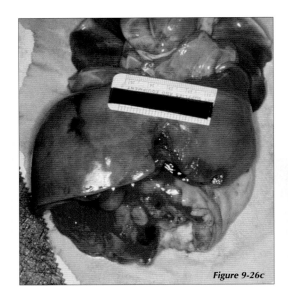

Figure 9-26c

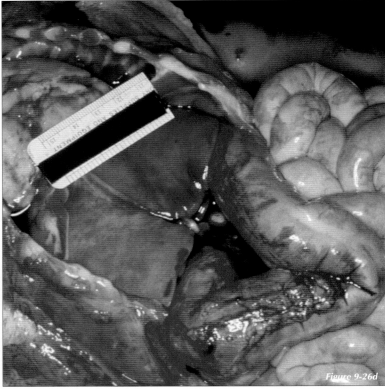

Figure 9-26d

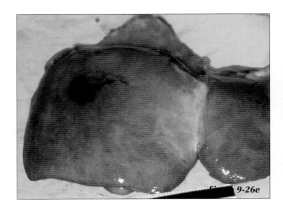

Figure 9-26e

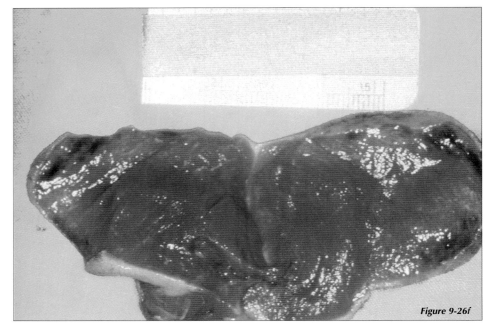

Figure 9-26f

Figure 9-27. Two cases of blunt trauma to the abdomen resulting in massive visceral bleeding.

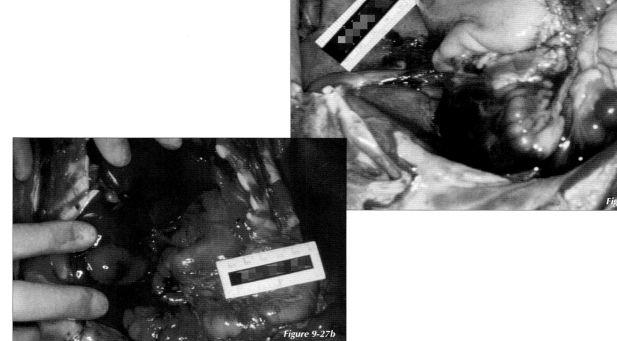

Figure 9-27a

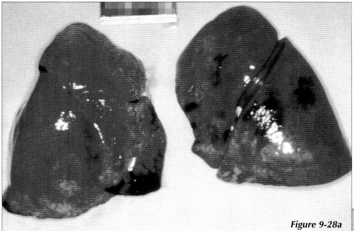

Figure 9-27b

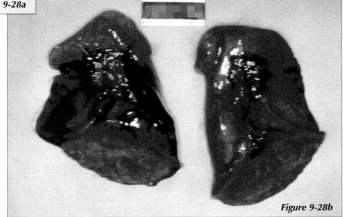

Figure 9-28a

Figure 9-28b

Figure 9-28. The lungs of an infant sustaining abusive blunt trauma to the chest, resulting in lung contusions.

Figure 9-29. *Two closed head injuries. The first (a) shows widening of the sutures secondary to cerebral edema and increased intracranial pressure in a case of shaken infant syndrome. There is no evidence of impact. The second (b) shows the result of impact. There is a fracture of the left posterior parietal bone. Note that the fracture stops at the suture line. Fracture lines do not cross over onto the adjacent bone in unossified sutures unless the blow is on the suture line. The suture line dissipates the force of the blow. A fracture of the adjacent bone would require a second blow.*

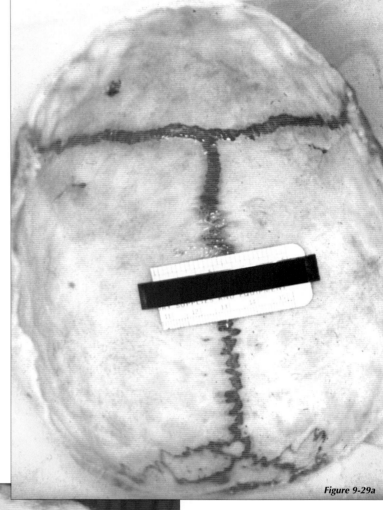

Figure 9-29a

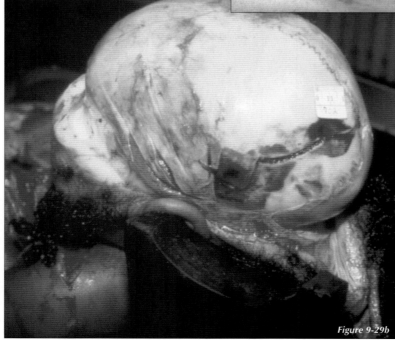

Figure 9-29b

Figure 9-30. *Subconjunctival petechial hemorrhage secondary to asphyxia. Children less than a year of age usually will not show this characteristic finding of mechanical asphyxia. They also may not show bruising of the neck when the pressure is applied there.*

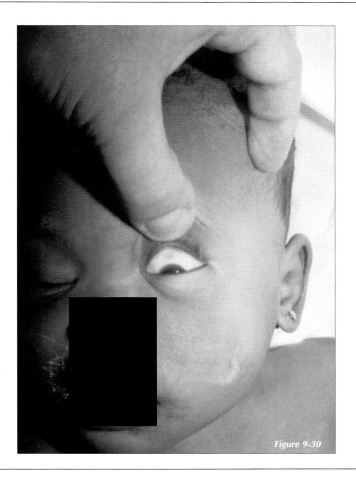

Figure 9-30

Figure 9-31. *This 9-year-old boy was playing with a loaded .38 caliber handgun. He placed it in his mouth and pulled the trigger. Emergency personnel thought the external perioral lacerations were caused by abuse. These are not abusive injuries, but are characteristic lesions secondary to the force of the gun blast. This death was determined to be accidental, but neglect on the part of the caregivers must be considered.*

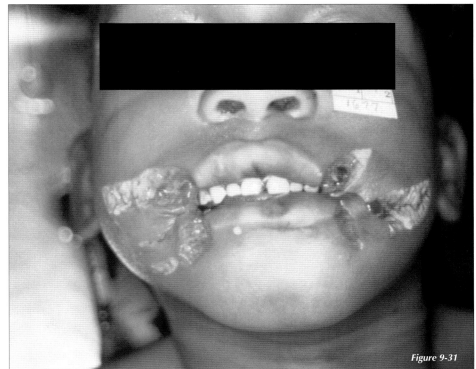

Figure 9-31

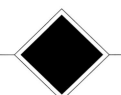

PART FIVE

Cases Involving the Police

POLICE INVESTIGATIONS

DET. GARY L. THOMPSON
DET. GARY W. GUINN
SGT. MILTON JONES, RET.
MISSOURI POLICE JUVENILE OFFICERS' ASSOCIATION
PHILLIP M. BURCH, M.D.
JANE B. GEILER

The involvement of law enforcement personnel is an integral part of all investigations into possible severe abuse. These situations require careful, methodical review of the circumstances, the individuals involved, and the physical evidence present in order to reveal the truth. Law enforcement personnel are trained to accomplish these tasks. The evidence gathered through photographs of the scene, interviews of witnesses and/or neighbors, and collection of physical data is needed to formulate an effective evaluation of the situation.

Ideally, special units should be formed within the police department comprising individuals who are sensitive to the special issues of children. In addition, these individuals should have expertise in dealing with child abuse and should work well with both social agencies and medical personnel.

The photographs in this chapter illustrate the environment in which police are called to work on these types of cases. Each involves child abuse or neglect.

Figure 10-1. The police were called to investigate the possible abandonment of nine children. They found a small apartment housing the children, ranging in age from 5 to 10 years. They were the children of two mothers who were living in a different, well-kept apartment with their boyfriends. The mothers were collecting welfare subsistence and occasionally dropped off food for the children. (**a** and **b**) The apartment housing the children was cold and had only one source of electricity, an extension cord that stretched down the hall and out of the bedroom window to another apartment. (**c**) There was little food in the house; the refrigerator was not working and was essentially empty. (**d**) The children were living on a combination of grease, potatoes, and pork and beans. (**e**) A frying pan, with no handle, had old lard still in it with evidence of rat prints in the grease. (**f**) The cupboard under the stove was full of rat feces. (**g**) Trash was strewn in one of the rooms. (**h**) Several of the mattresses were torn.

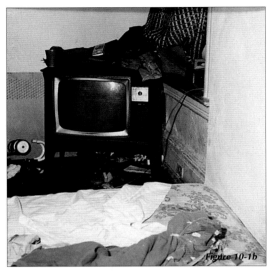

Figure 10-1b

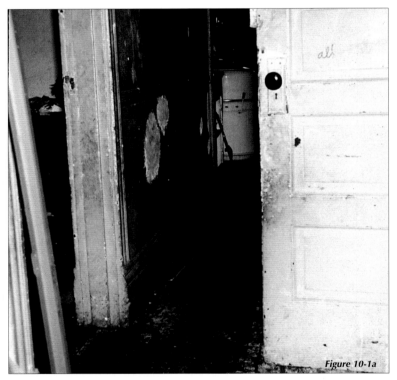

Figure 10-1a

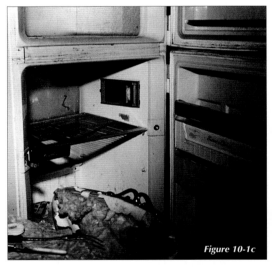

Figure 10-1c

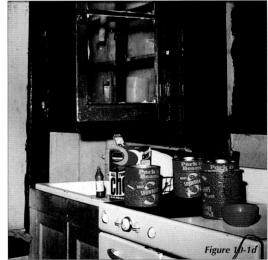

Figure 10-1d

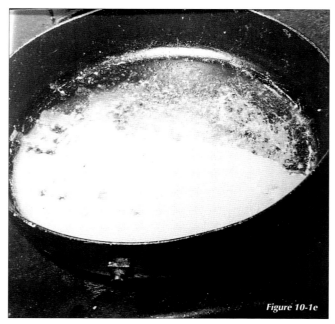

Figure 10-1e

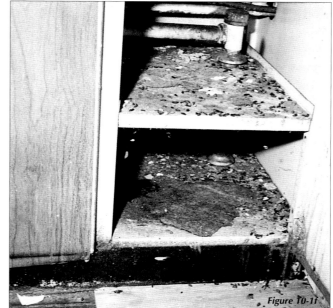

Figure 10-1f

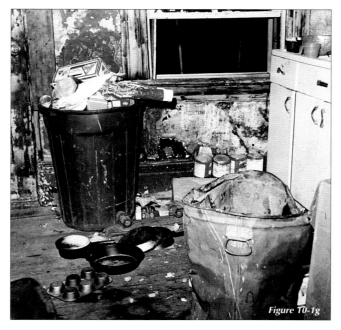

Figure 10-1g

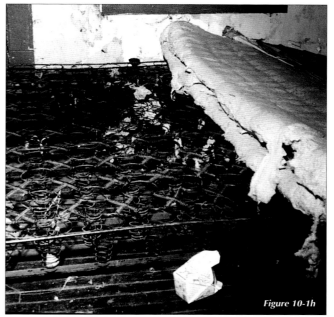

Figure 10-1h

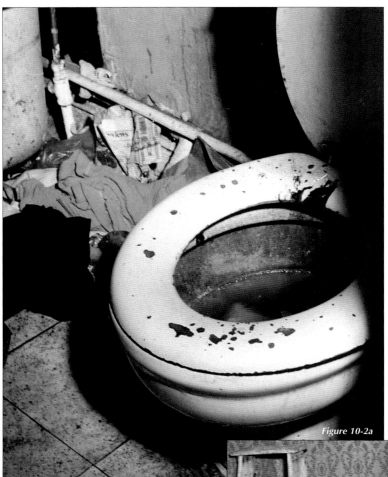

Figure 10-2a

Figure 10-2. *A worker from the juvenile court accompanied by the police went to remove two children from this home for parole violations. There were actually four children in the home, 9, 13, 14, and 16 years of age. When they arrived, they noted a strong, obnoxious odor. Dog and cat feces covered the floor and human waste was in the bathtub and on the bathroom floor (**a**). There were numerous trash bags (**b** and **c**). There was no heat, electricity, or water in the building. A full five-gallon gas can was used to fuel a portable stove which was sitting on the floor (**d**). All of the children had head lice.*

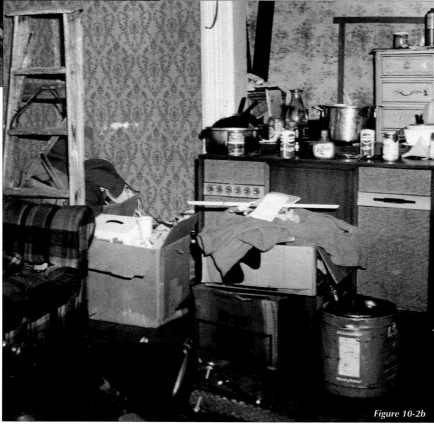

Figure 10-2b

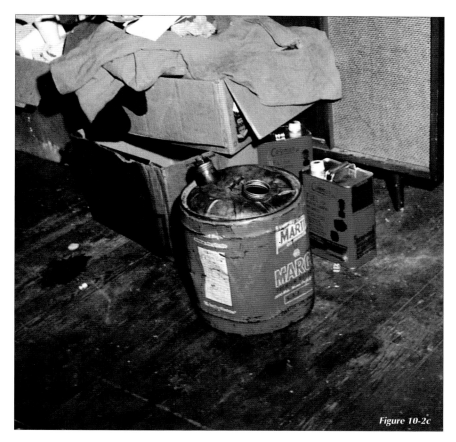

Figure 10-2c

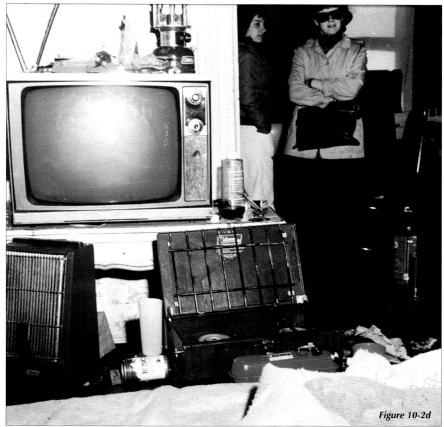

Figure 10-2d

Figure 10-3. *This case involved a drug raid. Five children, ages 2, 5, 7, 9, and 10 years, were found in the home along with six adults, who were arrested on drug charges. (a and b) The police found potent drugs as well as marijuana. (c) There was trash all over the house. (d and e) The tub was clogged and filled with waste, as was the toilet and a five-gallon plastic container under the bathroom sink. (f) Drug paraphernalia was in reach of the children, and an open, full gasoline can was in one of the rooms. (g) The crib was next to the space heater.*

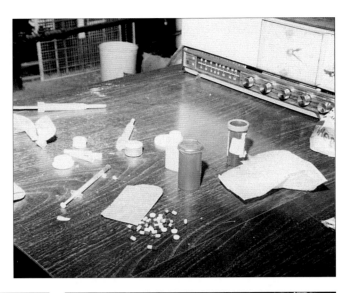

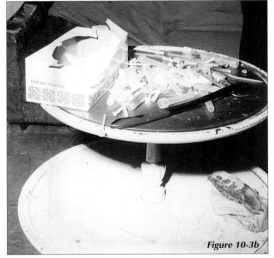

Figure 10-3b

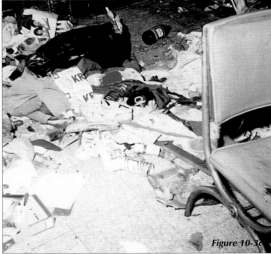

Figure 10-3c

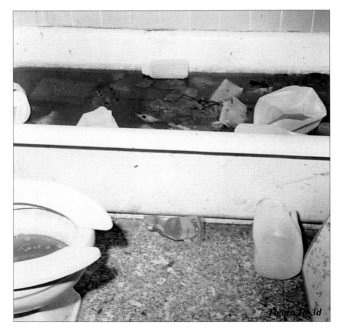

Figure 10-3d

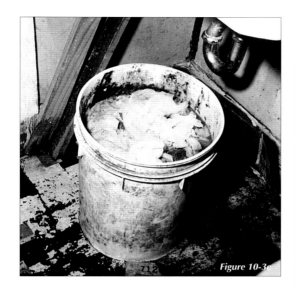

Figure 10-3e

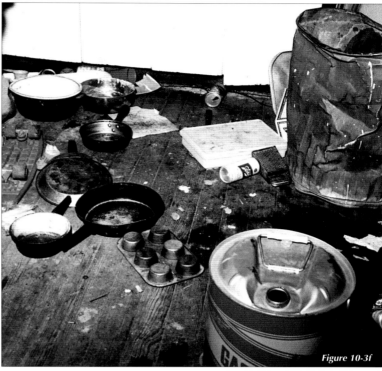

Figure 10-3f

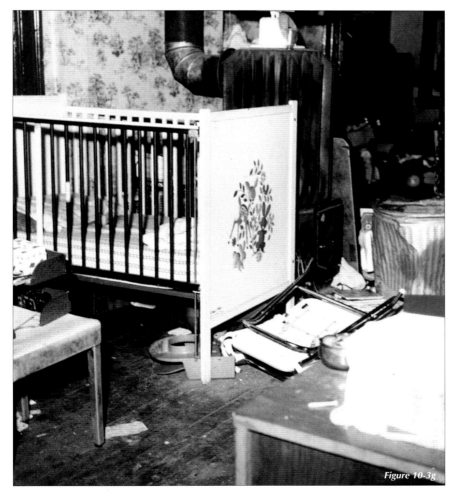

Figure 10-3g

Figure 10-4. *This 10-month-old boy was taken to the hospital with a severe head injury. He was found to have a right parietal fracture and a subdural hematoma. Emergency treatment was needed to evacuate the hematoma. The explanation for the injury given by the caregiver, who was the 21-year-old boyfriend of the mother, was that the child fell off of the bed. Because the explanation was incompatible with the severity of the injury, the case was referred to the Division of Family Services and the Police Child Abuse Unit was involved. The boyfriend admitted during further questioning that he had become angry with the child because he was a "momma's baby" and had hurled the child against the wall.*

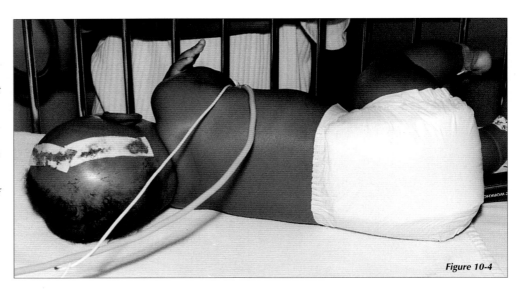

Figure 10-4

Figure 10-5. *This 3-year-old child was taken to the hospital with first- and second-degree burns to both feet (a) and the left elbow (b). The caregiver, who was the 31-year-old boyfriend of the mother, said that the child had walked into some hot water that had leaked from the hot water heater and puddled on the floor. The explanation seemed unlikely because the water would have had to be at least 2 inches deep to involve the dorsum of the child's feet. When asked how the child sustained the elbow burn, the caregiver stated that the child slipped on the wet floor and fell. There were no other burns noted, and the case was reported as suspected abuse. On questioning by the Police Child Abuse Unit, the caregiver changed his story several times and was subsequently arrested for second-degree assault.*

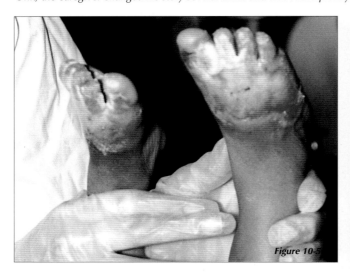

Figure 10-5

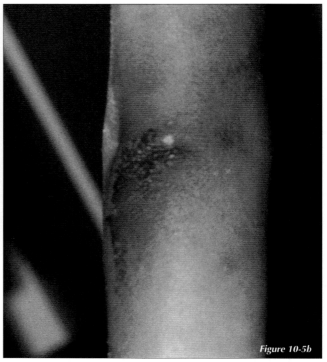

Figure 10-5b

Figure 10-6. This 4-year-old girl was taken to the hospital by her 22-year-old mother with second- and third-degree burns of the right hand (**a** and **b**). The mother said that the child had accidentally placed her hand into a gas furnace. With questioning by the police, the mother admitted that she had placed the child's hand into the furnace to teach her not to play with matches.

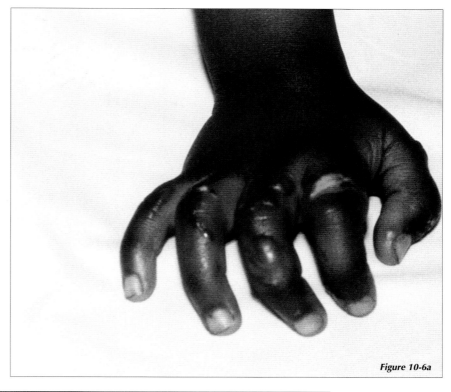

Figure 10-6a

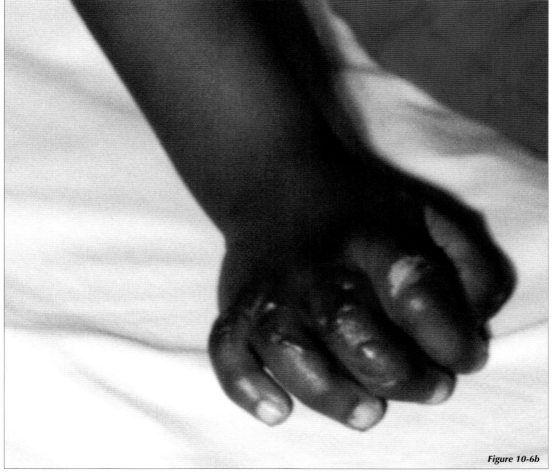

Figure 10-6b

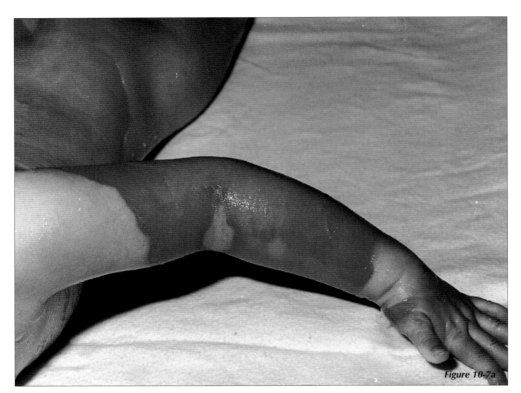

Figure 10-7a

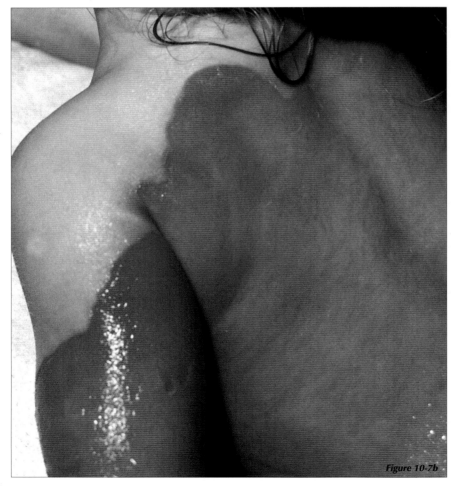

Figure 10-7b

Figure 10-7. *This 2-year-old girl was taken to the hospital with second-degree burns to the back of her arms (**a**), back (**b**), and buttocks, covering 30% of her total body area. The explanation given by the mother's 20-year-old boyfriend was that the child was bathing and accidentally turned the hot water on herself. The man later admitted that he became angry at the child after she had a bowel movement, and, as punishment, he forced her to lie in a bathtub of hot water.*

Figure 10-8. This 1-year-old girl arrived at the hospital with second-degree burns to both legs and arms, the genital area, and the buttocks. The explanation given by the child's 38-year-old mother was that she had her older daughter run bath water, hot only, to fill the tub. She had planned to watch television while the water cooled and then take a bath. The bathroom door was shut but not secured and the 1-year-old got into the room. She apparently threw her book into the tub and while trying to retrieve it, she accidentally slipped into the tub of hot water. A police investigation at the scene revealed that the child had attempted to get out of the tub by grasping the wall sink and breaking it. Clothing at the scene was found to have the child's skin attached. Based on these findings, the injury was determined to be accidental.

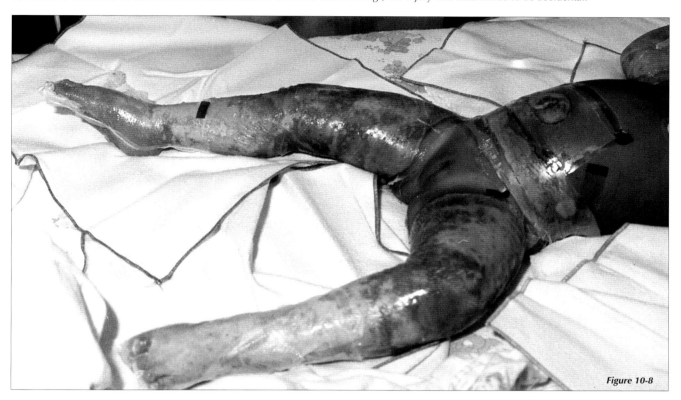

Figure 10-8

Figure 10-9. This 13-year-old boy stated that his father, while pinning the boy to the floor with his foot on the child's head, had beat him with a fishing rod numerous times. A neighbor noticed the marks on the boy's back (**a** and **b**) and reported it to the police. The father admitted to hitting the boy with a switch that was a three-foot section of a fiberglass fishing rod.

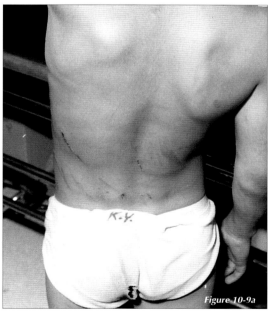

Figure 10-9a

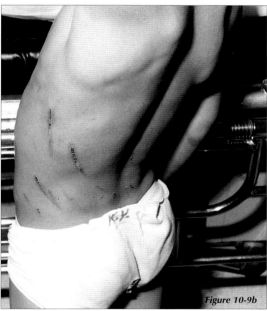

Figure 10-9b

Figure 10-10. *The police officers of the Child Abuse Unit were directed to a home by a witness who said that she had heard a child crying for a long period of time after apparently being injured. The mother and her boyfriend were at home when the police arrived and the mother stated that they were the only ones in the house. The police found this child hidden in a closet. She had been thrown against the wall of her residence, suffering a hematoma of the scalp and bruising to the face (a), right hand (b), and inner thighs.*

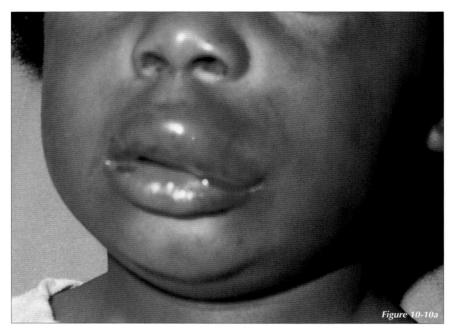

Figure 10-10a

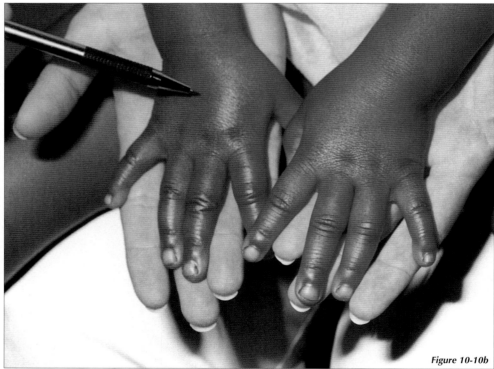

Figure 10-10b

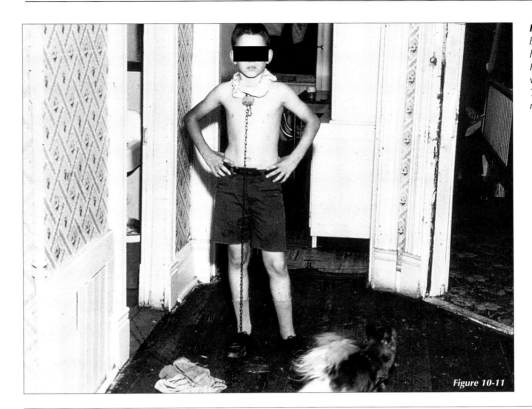

Figure 10-11. *This 9-year-old boy told a schoolteacher that he was chained at home. Police investigators found him with a chain around his neck. The dog in the foreground was running free.*

Figure 10-12. Child punished with a cigarette lighter.

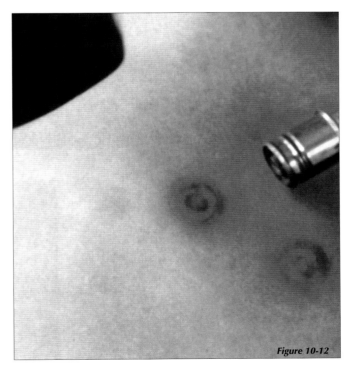

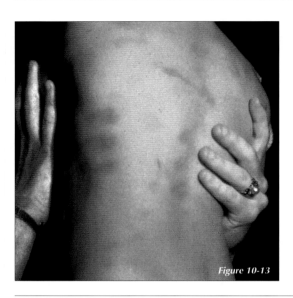

Figure 10-13. Bruising from excessive squeezing, leaving parallel finger marks.

Figure 10-14. Safety hazard—unsafe space heater. There is no safety glass in front.

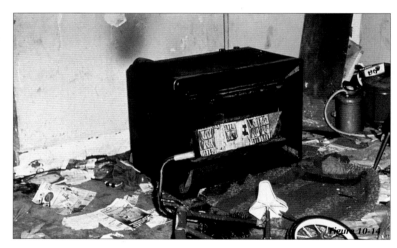

Figure 10-15. Dirty bathroom with no functional plumbing and unsanitary conditions.

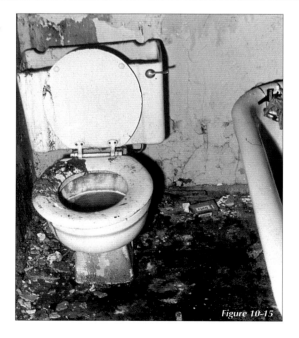

Figure 10-16. *Animal feces in unsanitary bathroom.*

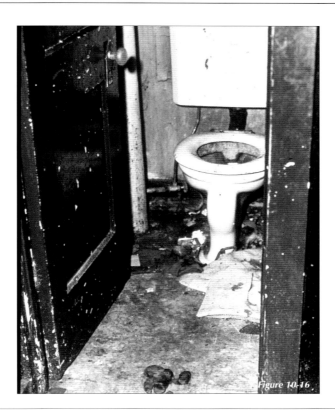

Figure 10-17. *Safety hazard— deadman bolt at the back door, making exit from that point impossible.*

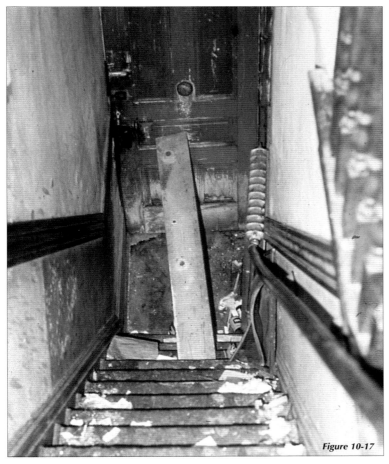

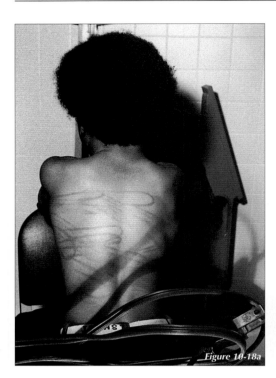

Figure 10-18. This 13-year-old child was whipped with a television cable (**a** and **b**). The cable is shown in the foreground of **a.**

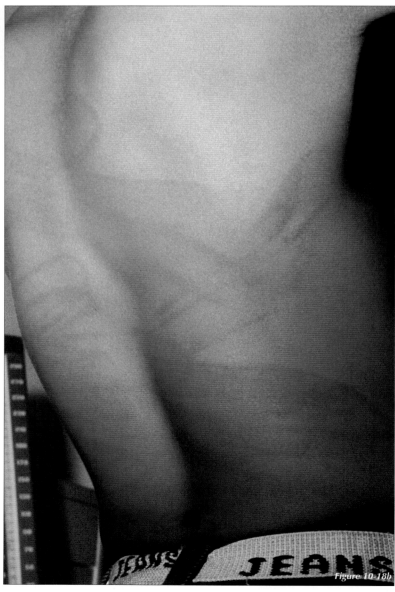

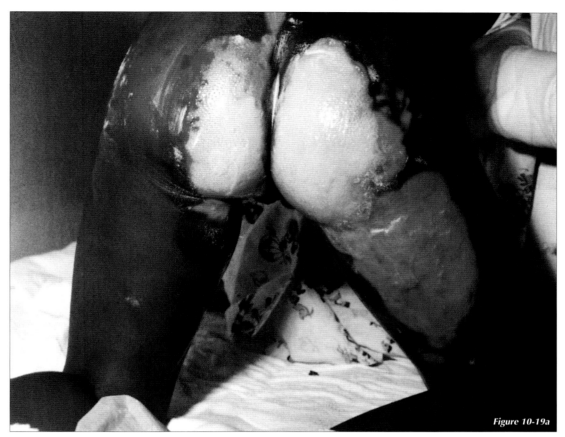

Figure 10-19. This 8-year-old boy "backed into a space heater" (**a** and **b**). The child said that he was set on the space heater as punishment.

Figure 10-19a

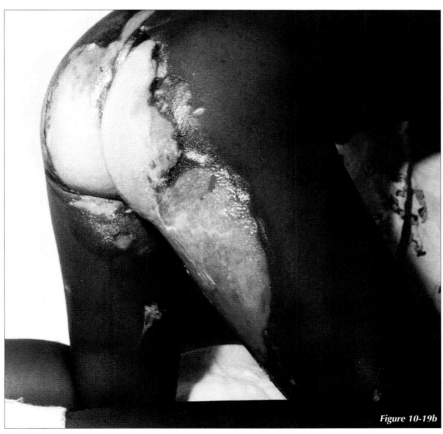

Figure 10-19b

Figure 10-20. *This 18-month-old boy was seen in the emergency room with a patterned burn to his abdomen **(a)**. The history given by the mother was that he fell off a rocker and landed on a heated floor grill. On inspection of the home, the rocker was found as described **(b)**, as was the grill in the floor. The grill was hot enough to have caused a burn, so the injury was determined to be accidental.*

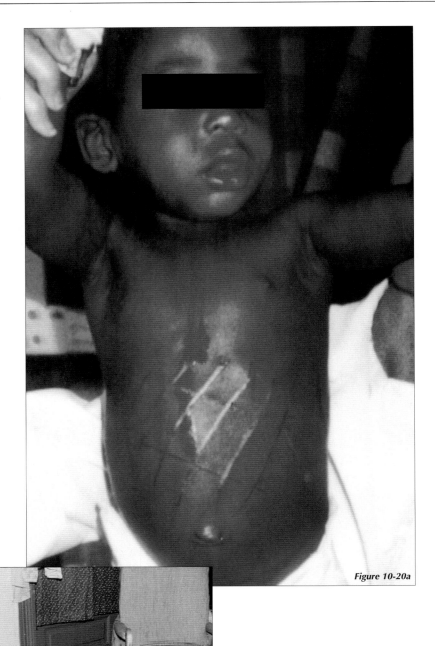

Figure 10-20a

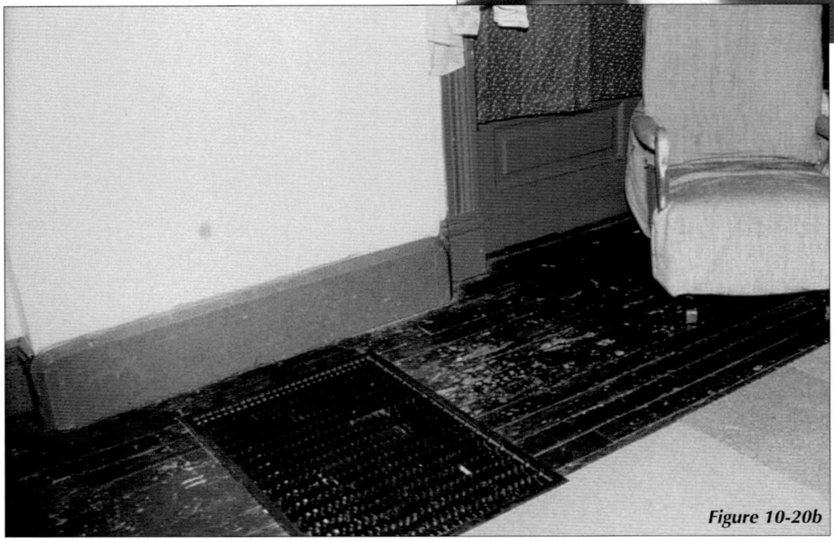

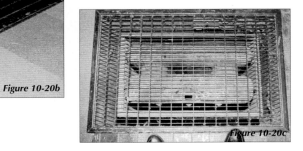

Figure 10-20b

Figure 10-20c

Figure 10-21. This 2-year-old boy was taken to the emergency room with second- and third-degree burns to his feet and legs. The child had been left in the care of two 10-year-old girls. They said that they had prepared a bath for him and, before they had a chance to check the temperature, he ran into the bathroom and jumped into the tub. Emergency room personnel felt that this was an immersion burn. There was a stocking-glove pattern at the right knee and above the left ankle. Note how distinct the line of the burn is. Also, the soles are severely burned. The pattern of the burn with the spared popliteal area and the burned area on the back of the thigh suggest that the legs were flexed when he was placed into the water. The incident took place at 1:00 AM, an unusual time for a bath. Police interviewed neighbors. Two witnesses in the house next door saw the two girls forcing the child to perform oral sex. Because he was resisting, they hit him with their fists and then held him down in a tub of hot water. (Courtesy Officer A. Doyle, St. Louis Police Department.)

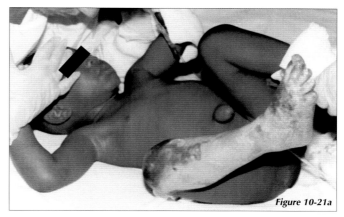

Figure 10-21a

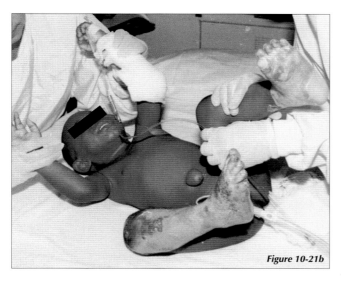

Figure 10-21b

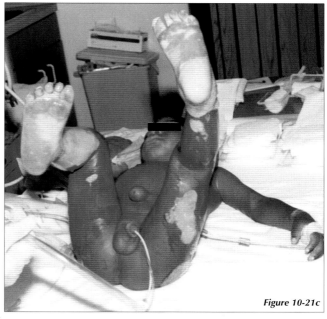

Figure 10-21c

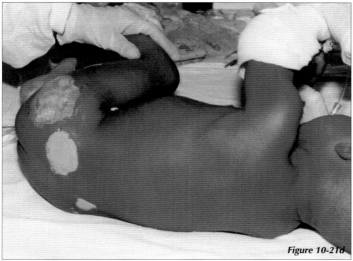

Figure 10-21d

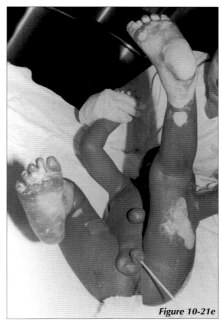

Figure 10-21e

Figure 10-22. Photographs taken during an investigation into the unexplained death of an 8-month-old child. The child was found dead on the couch after a nap. Dolls are valuable tools to demonstrate the position of the child when found. The child's head was buried between the seat cushion and the back cushion, both very soft. The cause of death was determined to be accidental, probably asphyxiation. Such deaths can be prevented by educating caregivers about the use of soft bedding for small children.

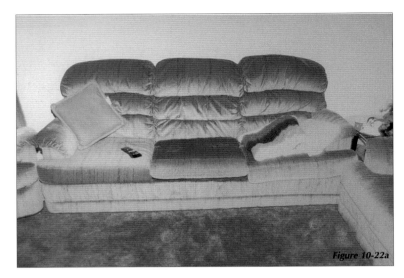

Figure 10-22a

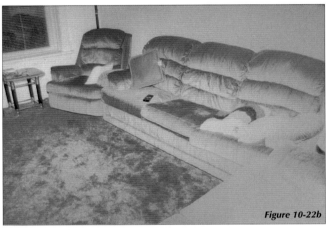

Figure 10-22b

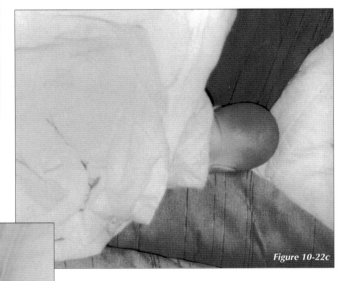

Figure 10-22c

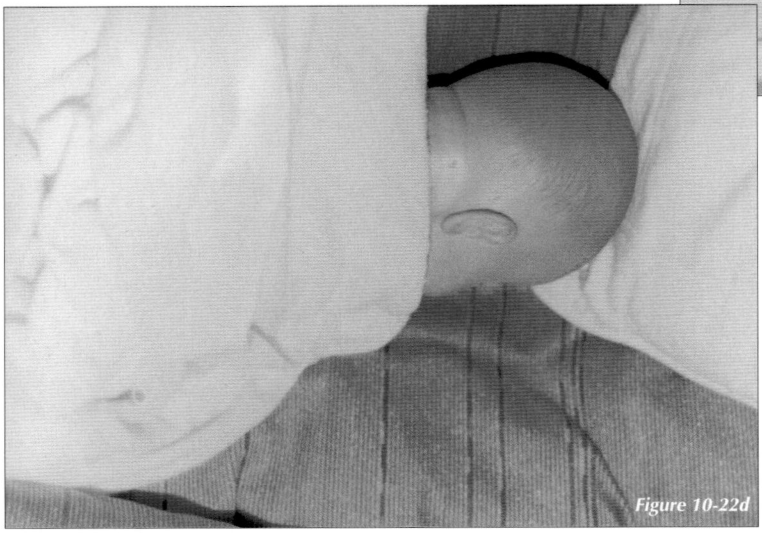

Figure 10-22d

Figure 10-23. *This 2-year-old girl was found dead in a portable playpen which also served as her bed (**a** and **b**). The cardiac leads were placed by EMS. It was learned later that the parents attempted to clean the area and the child, as well as the other children before calling for EMS and that the four children shared and were usually locked in the bedroom (**c**), a dank, austere, dirty space. Autopsy revealed a severely malnourished, dehydrated, dirty, wasted child, with dried, old feces in the diaper area, her head matted with dirt and old food (**d-f**). The cause of death was determined to be severe malnutrition and dehydration. The house was filthy with dog feces throughout (**g**). The bathroom was dirty, the toilet not working, and with only cold running water (**h**). Numerous empty beer and soft drink cans, infested with roaches, and empty beer cases were strewn throughout the house (**i-l**). There was no food in the house. There was ample dog and rabbit food. The parents stated that they could not afford baby food. They were well nourished, as were the dog and rabbit. The child, while alive, and her twin could not stand without support. They were severely delayed socially and physically. All of the children had been worked up for failure to thrive. There had been 14 calls to the hotline which were investigated and unsubstantiated, this due to manipulation by the parents and the grandparents. When the police arrived at the house, the parents were on the front stoop giving the twin sister water from an outdoor water hose, still running on the sidewalk (**m**). The police officer stated that the child voraciously consumed five bottles of water while he was there. The older children asked not to be sent back with their parents. All of the children thrived in foster care. The parents were found guilty of child abuse and sent to prison.*

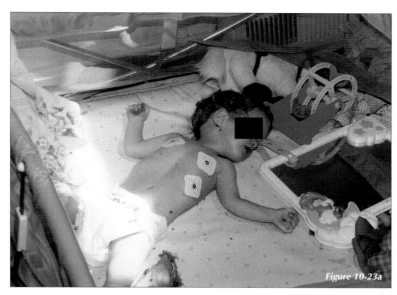

Figure 10-23a

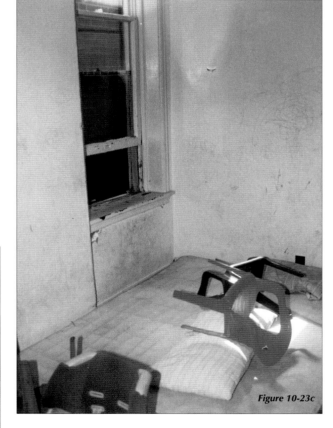

Figure 10-23c

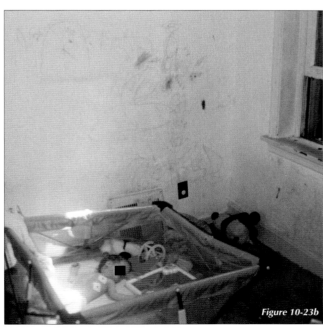

Figure 10-23b

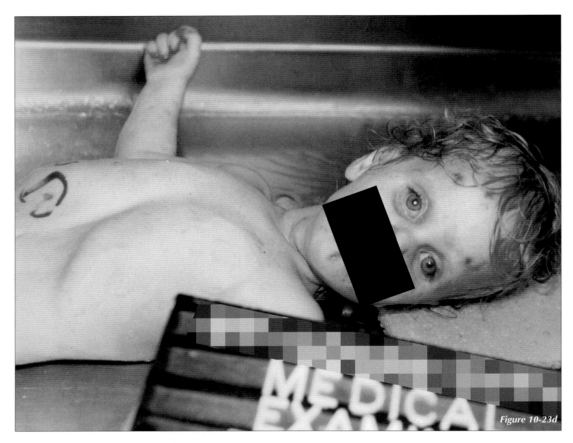

Figure 10-23d

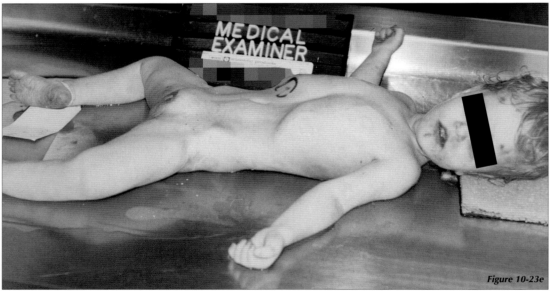

Figure 10-23e

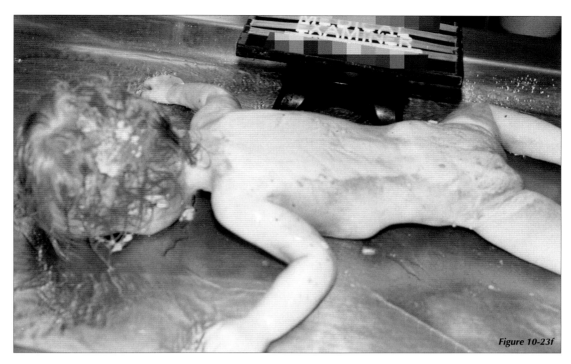

Figure 10-23f

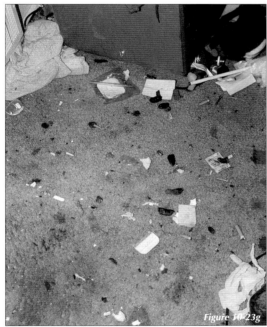

Figure 10-23g

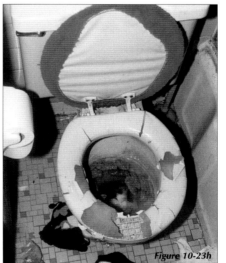

Figure 10-23h

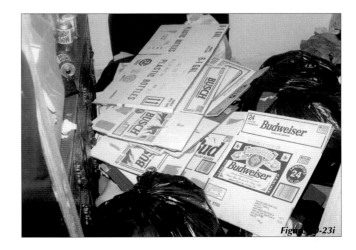

Figure 10-23i

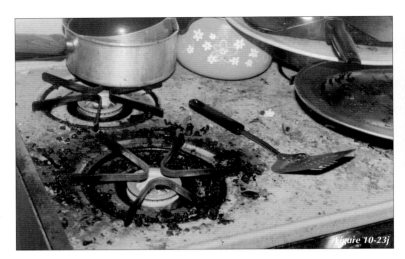

Figure 10-23j

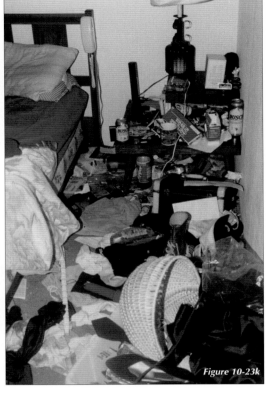

Figure 10-23k

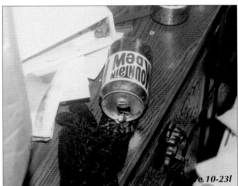

Figure 10-23l

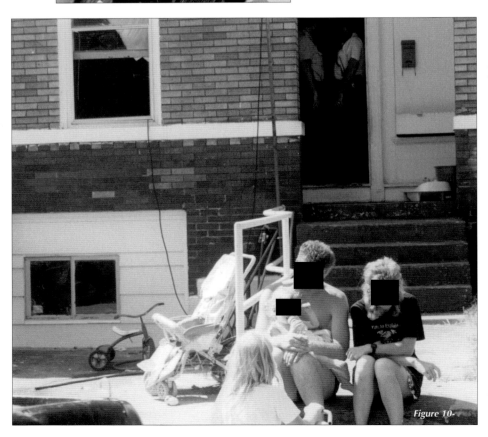

Figure 10-

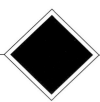

Part Six

Forms of Neglect

NEGLECT, ABANDONMENT, AND FAILURE TO THRIVE

JAMES A. MONTELEONE, M.D.

Neglect is a serious social problem concerning child maltreatment. Simply stated, neglect is the failure of a caregiver to provide for the basic needs of his or her child. Failure to meet the child's needs may vary in degree from minor to severe and can be short- or long-term in duration. While there is general agreement as to what constitutes extreme neglect, little concensus has been reached on what constitutes milder forms of neglect. In addition, the harm caused by neglect has yet to be quantified.

Abandonment is a legal term with legal implications that refers to the physical aspects of neglect and fulfills certain rigid criteria. It is defined as the caregiver's rejection of the child and the parental role. Another aspect of this attachment disorder is emotional abandonment, in which the caregiver completely withdraws from nurturing. In this type of abandonment, the caregiver does not meet the child's needs for physical security; therefore, these needs remain unmet or are provided for by others. Children may be abandoned with the intent to kill them (fatal or near-fatal abandonment). Other types of abandonment involve "throwaways," refusal of parental custody, and lack of supervision.

Nonorganic failure to thrive is an interactional disorder in which parental expectations, parental skills, and the resulting home environment are intertwined with the child's developmental capabilities. In some instances it relates to child abuse or neglect. It can be characterized by physical and developmental retardation associated with a disturbed mother-infant relationship. These children are slow to develop and learn, are physically puny, and have flattened emotional responses, even to pain.

Neglected, abandoned, and failure-to-thrive children suffer hurts in their bodies, minds, emotions, and spirits. The photographs included here illustrate the physical hurts. These can heal, but the hurts in their minds, emotions, and spirits have far-reaching ramifications. In addition to their own distress, they may become an abandoning parent in the next generation of the cycle of neglect.

Figure 11-1. *This 18-month-old girl had been seen in the well-baby clinic with a monilial rash but missed two subsequent appointments. In a telephone follow-up by the clinic nurse, the grandmother voiced concerns for the child's well-being. The grandmother stated that the mother never applied the medication given to her as a starter and did not fill the prescription. The mother was reported for medical neglect. The rash had progressed (**a** and **b**), and the child was found to have a healing ecchymotic area on the dorsum of the right hand (**c**). The Division of Family Services assigned a visiting nurse to check in on the home twice daily for the application of medication. The rash cleared promptly. A homemaker was also assigned to teach parenting skills.*

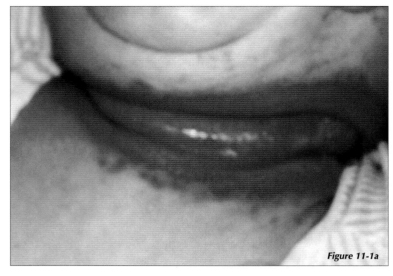

Figure 11-1a

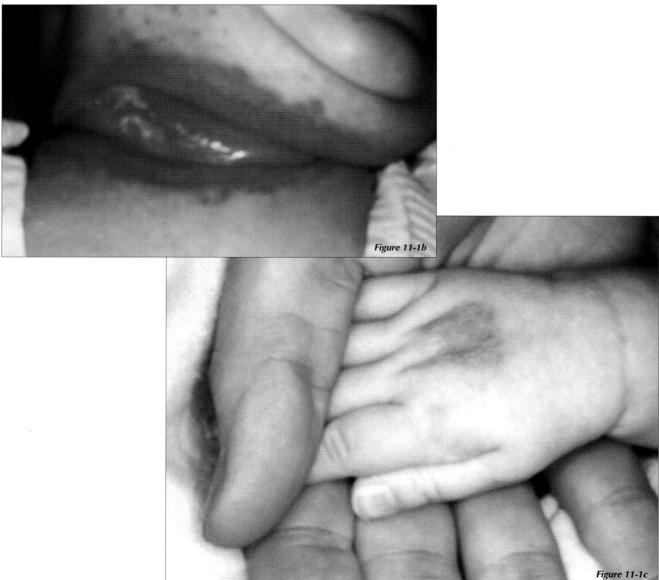

Figure 11-1b

Figure 11-1c

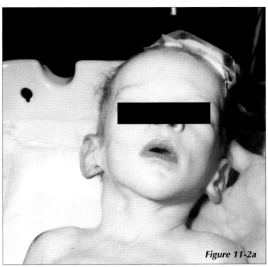

Figure 11-2a

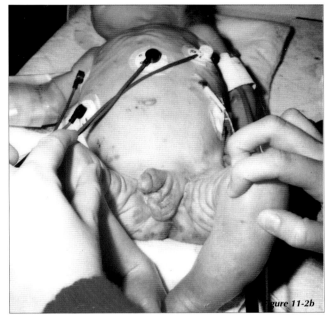

Figure 11-2. This 7-month-old boy was seen in the emergency room. He had had diarrhea for 2 days, was unresponsive, and could not eat *(a)*. The child was dehydrated and emaciated with no subcutaneous fat *(b)*. He was well below the third percentile in both height and weight. His abdomen was protuberant, and he had numerous cutaneous lesions *(c* and *d)*. Following rehydration and resolution of the diarrhea, he thrived while in the hospital. He was placed in a foster home and continued to thrive, with height and weight measurements 5 months later in the tenth percentile.

Figure 11-2b

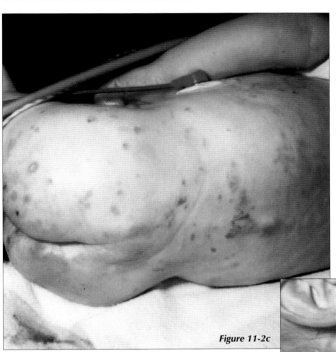

Figure 11-2c

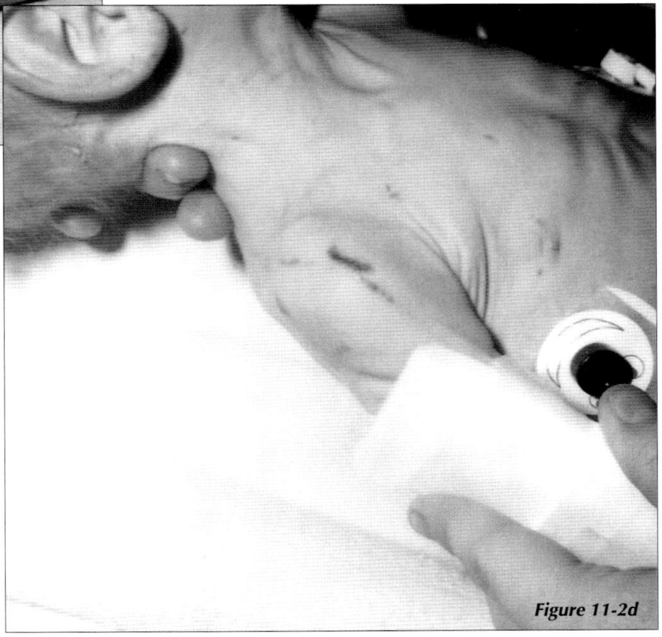

Figure 11-2d

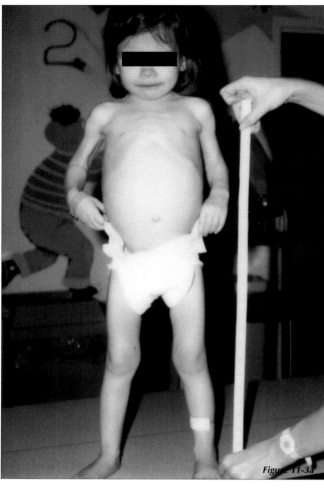

Figure 11-3. *Severely neglected 4-year-old girl. Note the lack of subcutaneous fat, protuberant abdomen, and passive, flat affect (**a** and **b**). She was still in a diaper and had diaper-area lesions (**c**). She thrived in a foster home.*

Figure 11-3a

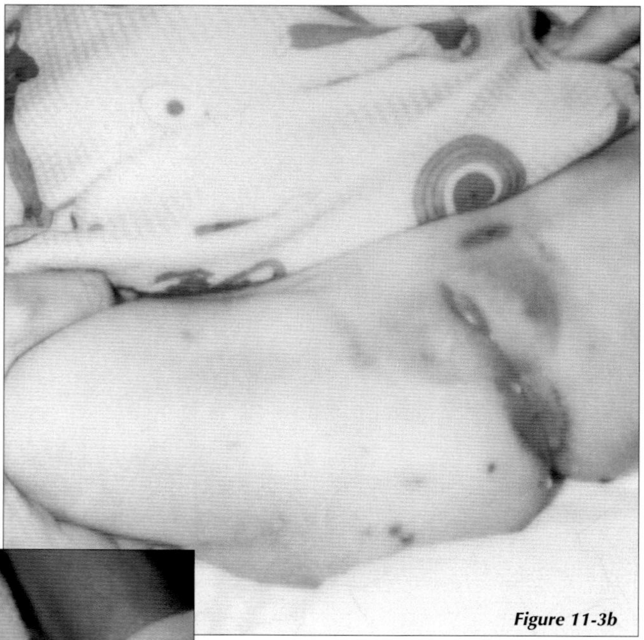

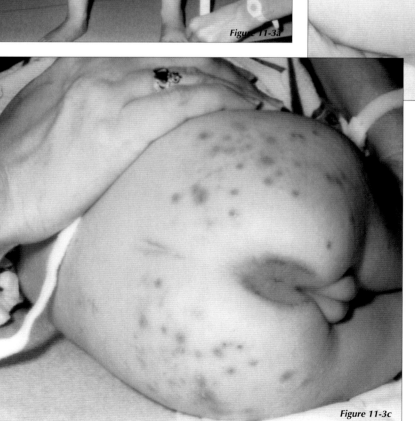

Figure 11-3b

Figure 11-3c

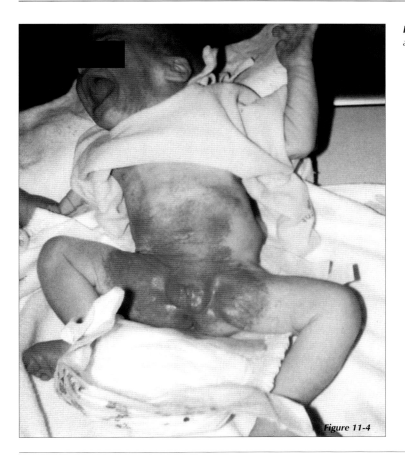

Figure 11-4. *Severe diaper rash in a 3-month-old girl.*

Figure 11-4

Figure 11-5. *This severely malnourished 7-year-old boy was taken to the emergency room by ambulance. The child's mother found him unresponsive in bed and not breathing (b). The mother stated that the child had had a cold for the past few days and appeared to be recovering. He was emaciated and dirty; the soles of his feet were encrusted with dirt that, when scraped off, covered several infected wounds, one resembling a cigarette burn (a). Attempts at resuscitation were successful and he was intubated and given fluids and antibiotics to treat severe bilateral pneumonia. After several hours in the hospital he suffered cardiac arrest and died. The three other children in the family were well nourished and healthy and the school reported that they attended school regularly. The 7-year-old had been absent a number of days, including the two weeks prior to his death, and teachers reported several instances when he had come to school in obvious distress, dirty, malnourished, and unable to work on his assignments. On one occasion, he was so weak that he could only crawl up the stairs. While it was suggested that the child be reported to the Division of Family Services, the principal decided that this was not needed since the siblings were doing well.*

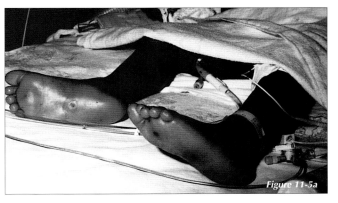

Figure 11-5a

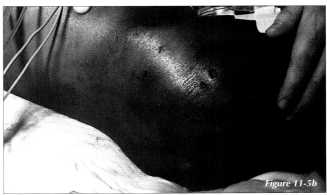

Figure 11-5b

Figure 11-6. *The growth grid of a 3-month-old boy referred for failure to thrive. He had a low normal birth weight. On a normal diet in the hospital, he thrived. The child's mother had lost a previous son and was determined that this one would die, too.*

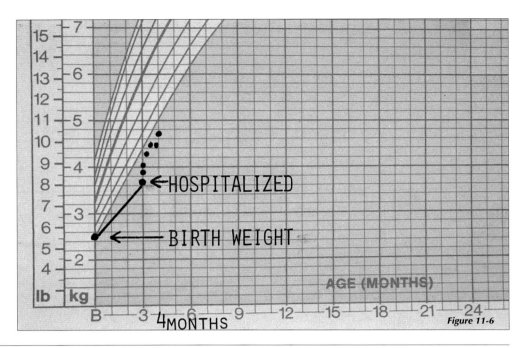

Figure 11-7. *The growth grid of a 5-year-old boy admitted for evaluation of failure to thrive and diagnosed as nonorganic failure to thrive due to maternal deprivation (a and b). (c and d) The growth grids of two siblings. (e) The growth grid of a normal child growing at the third percentile. (f) The growth grid of a child with organic failure to thrive resulting from hypothyroidism. The arrow marks the point about which the child's parents began to have marital difficulties. The child's mother was eventually hospitalized with schizophrenia. The R_x in f denotes the point at which therapy, thyroid replacement, was initiated.*

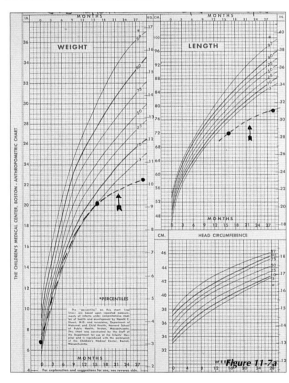

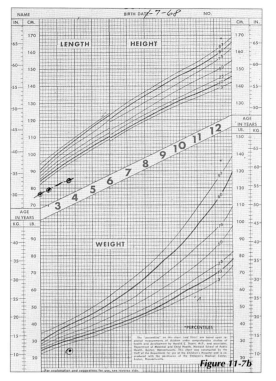

Figure 11-7b

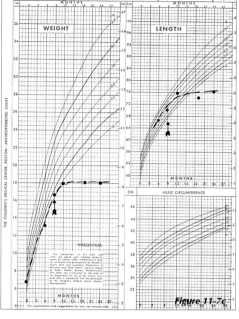

Figure 11-7c

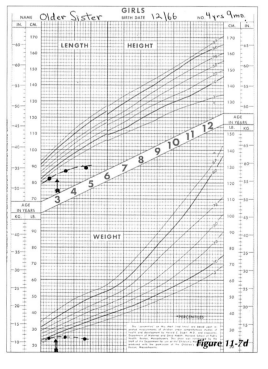

Figure 11-7d

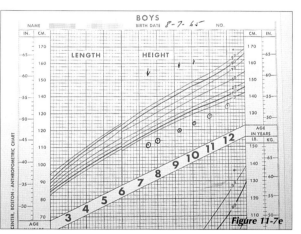

Figure 11-7e

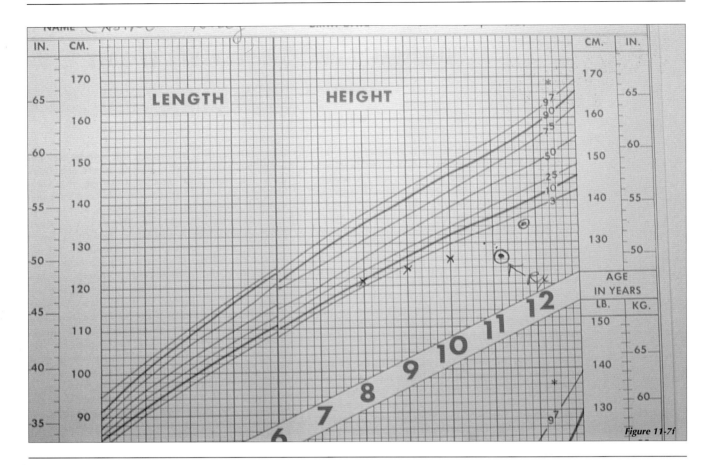

Figure 11-7f

Figure 11-8. *This 11-year-old boy with cerebral palsy was taken from a foster home. The foster parent ran a child daycare center. A second child, also with cerebral palsy, had been in the same foster care and was found dead with evidence of severe malnutrition. The foster parents initially denied neglect, stating that the child was difficult to feed because of the cerebral palsy. The boy's rapid weight gain in the hospital was attributed by the foster parents to the specialized care by an experienced nursing staff. Employees in the daycare center said the two children were kept in a secluded room alone all day. Feeding was done by the foster parents. The foster father confessed that the children were often poorly fed. He also admitted that when the boy was in the home, he was often locked in a closet. The boy is severely malnourished (**a** to **c**). Photographs were taken during his recovery (**d** and **e**). This illustrates severe nutritional neglect. It is important to document and plot old weight measurements and weight recorded during recovery to substantiate nutritional neglect (**f**). Also, in this case, it was important to document weight gain while the child was in foster care where the foster parent had no experience in feeding children with limitations. A picture of the child before he went into foster care (**g**) is of value in assessing the severity of the neglect. (Photographs published with special permission from the child's parents.)*

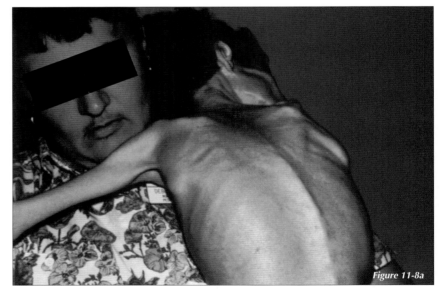

Figure 11-8a

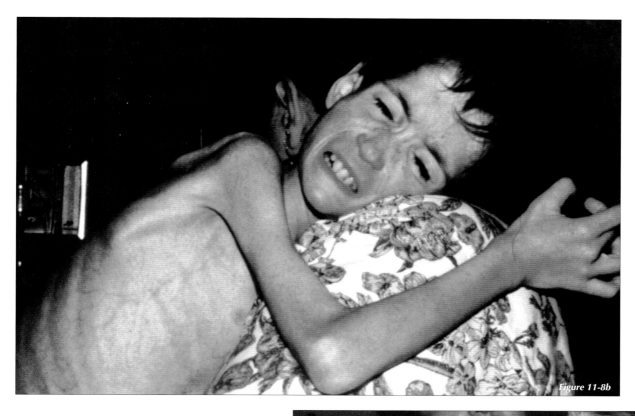

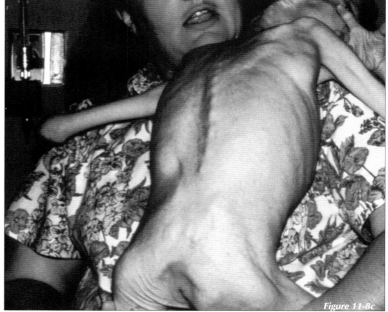

Figure 11-8c

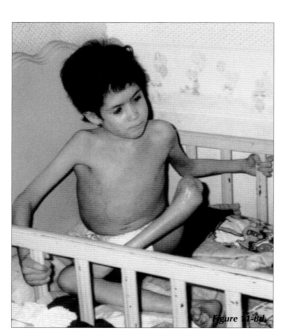

Figure 11-8d

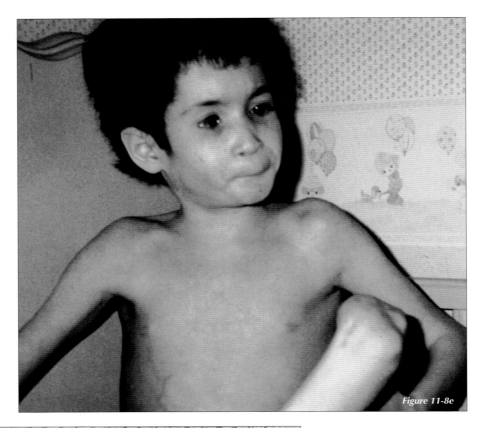

Figure 11-8e

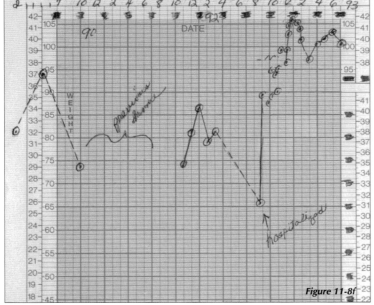

Figure 11-8f

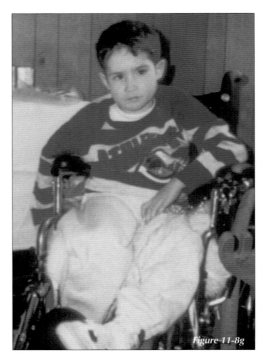

Figure 11-8g

Figure 11-9. *These two children, both less than 1 year of age and living in a multi-family dwelling, were left in the care of a psychotic adult who bit off the earlobe of the 11-month-old boy (a) and the distal end of the 9-month-old girl's fifth finger (b).*

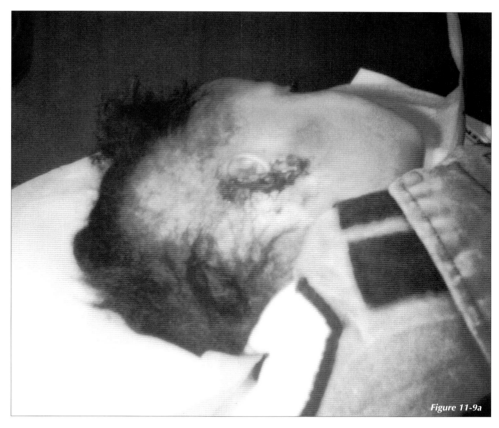

Figure 11-9a

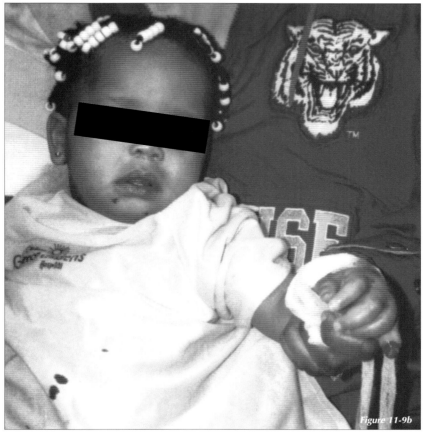

Figure 11-9b

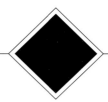

PART SEVEN

Drawings

Chapter 12

DRAWINGS IN ABUSE CASES

JOAN M. BOYER
JON C. BOYER
VICKI MCNEESE, M.S.
JAMES A. MONTELEONE, M.D.

Drawings can be a valuable tool in evaluating the abused child, revealing much about things the child will not or cannot discuss. They can be an ideal way to open and proceed with an interview with the child. The interviewer may ask the child to draw a man, draw himself or herself, draw a parent, or draw his or her house or any related subject. Children who have difficulty telling what happened to them often find it easier to draw a picture showing the event. Sometimes the interviewer can draw with the child. Drawings the child has made in the past can also be of value to art therapists in evaluating the child. It must be emphasized that drawings are a tool to aid in the evaluation of a child. They are not in themselves diagnostic.

Figure 12-1. *These drawings were made by a 5-year-old girl who was sexually abused by her grandfather. She was told to draw a picture of herself and her grandfather **(a)**. She told the interviewer that her grandfather had one leg. Then she stated that she had been abused on the couch. The interviewer drew a couch and asked the girl to show her what happened **(b)**. When asked what the object on the floor was, she responded that it was "grandpa's leg."*

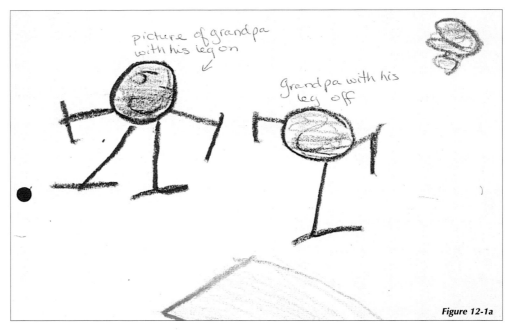

Figure 12-1a

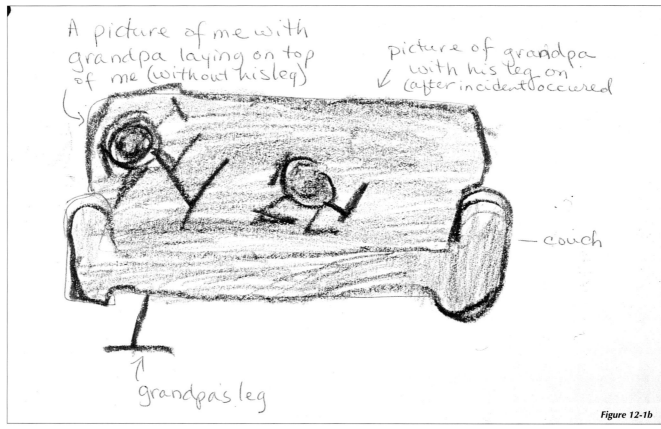

Figure 12-1b

Figure 12-2. This drawing was made by a girl to describe how she was abused. The interviewer related the story at the top of the page.

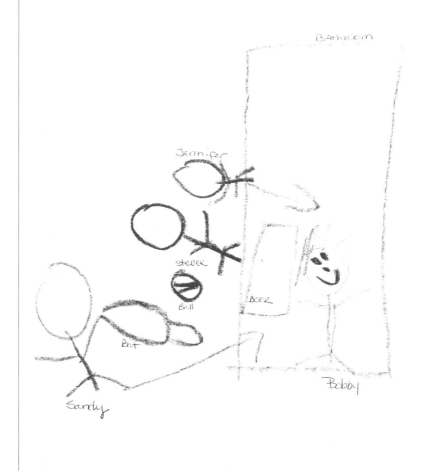

"We were playing ball in the basement. Then Bobby called my sister in the bathroom. After she was done then he told me to come in the bathroom. Then ~~Bob~~ Bobby pulled his pants down, then he pulled mine down. Then he sticked his weiner in The My front. Then we started playing ball again"

Figure 12-2

Figure 12-3. *This series of drawings were made by a boy who, as a grown man of 25, killed his father. His parents separated and divorced when he was 20. While visiting his father, following an argument, he shot his father and then tried to burn the body in a window well. He returned 3 days later, dismembered the body, and tried to dispose of the parts throughout the city. In the pretrial period, he disclosed that he had been sexually abused by his father beginning at the age of 3 years and ending just before puberty. His mother had saved all of his drawings while he was growing up, and the drawings were used at the trial, analyzed by an art therapist, to support his claim of abuse. These are just a sampling of the drawings, but they demonstrate fragmentation, intrusion, and encapsulation. Note the intensity of several of them and how chaotic others are. His age was not always noted with the drawings. Included at the end are several drawings he made as an adult in art therapy. (Drawings contributed by the artist's mother, Joan M. Boyer.)*

(a) A preschool drawing. Note the intensity and choice of colors. (b) An early drawing. Note the intensity, chaotic quality, and choice of colors. (c through g) Note the recurrent theme of encapsulation. (h and i) Self-portraits. These are fragmented, primitive, and diminutive. In i he drew a small sad face isolated in the corner of the page. (j through o) Latency age drawings. Again there is a more sophisticated demonstration of encapsulation and intrusion. Often the pictures are chaotic and primitive. (p through t) Art therapy drawings in which he depicted his family (p). Note the church and dove in the background. In q he describes the abuse. It began with fondling and progressed to anal sex in the bathroom, including enemas. He related that he would hide in the closet when his mother was out of the house and then sneak into his parents' room at night and sleep at the foot of the bed where he felt safe. In r and s he described his feelings about himself and his father and what had happened. In t he depicts his prison life.

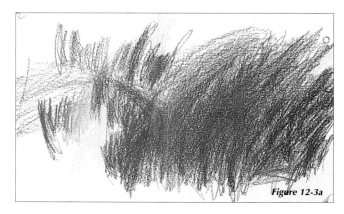

Figure 12-3a

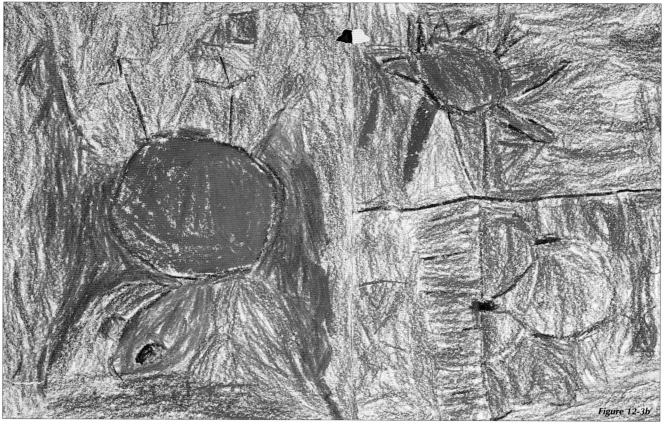

Figure 12-3b

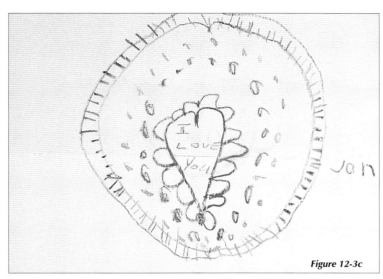

Figure 12-3c

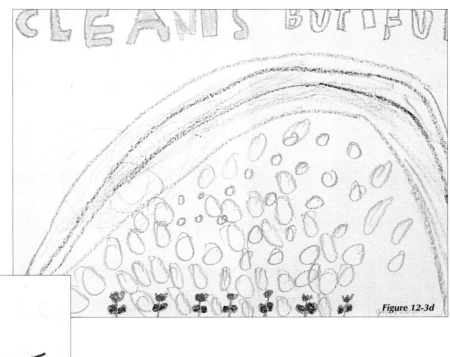

Figure 12-3d

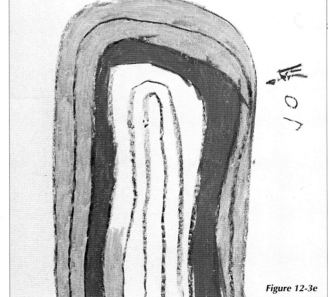

Figure 12-3e

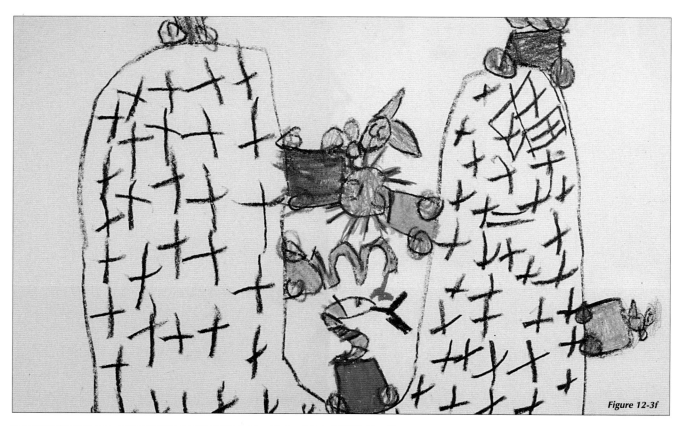

Figure 12-3f

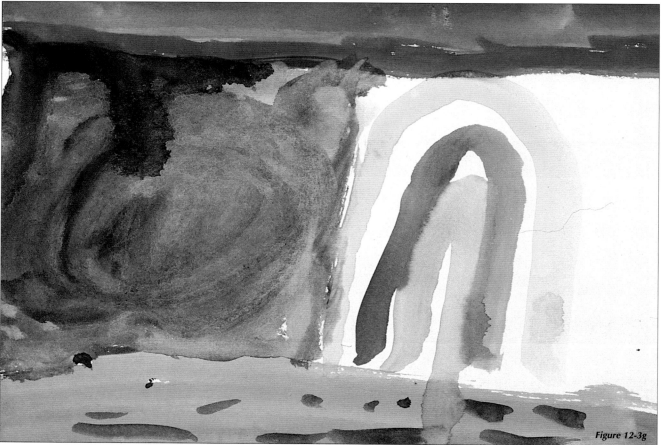

Figure 12-3g

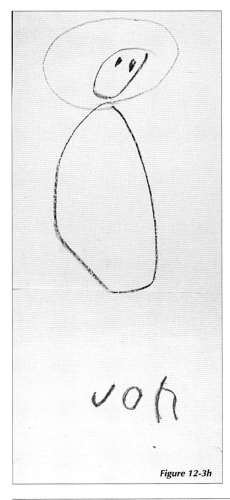

Figure 12-3h

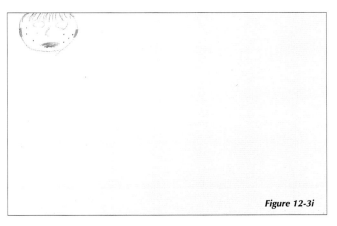

Figure 12-3i

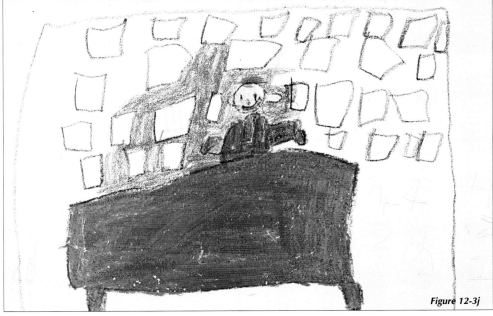

Figure 12-3j

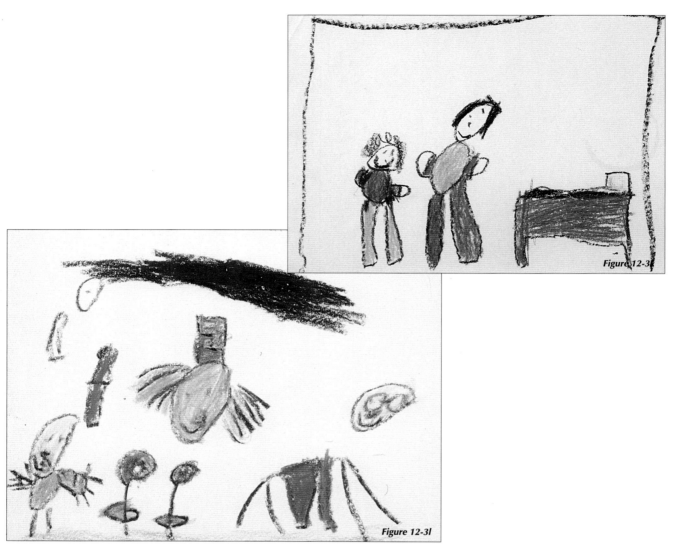

Figure 12-3l

Figure 12-3m

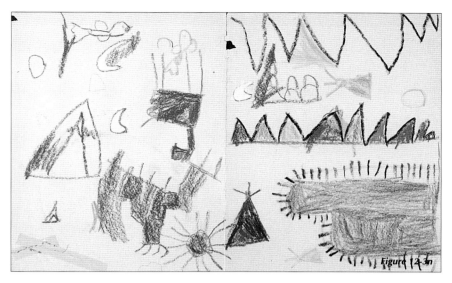

Figure 12-3n

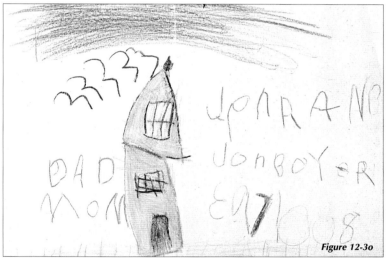

Figure 12-3o

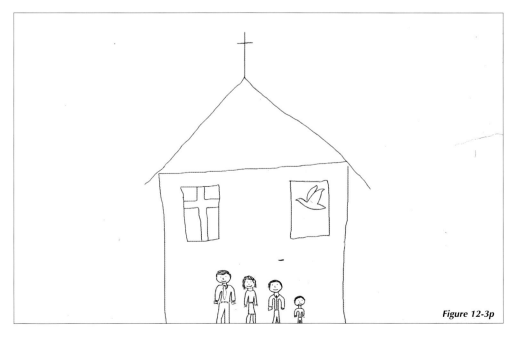

Figure 12-3p

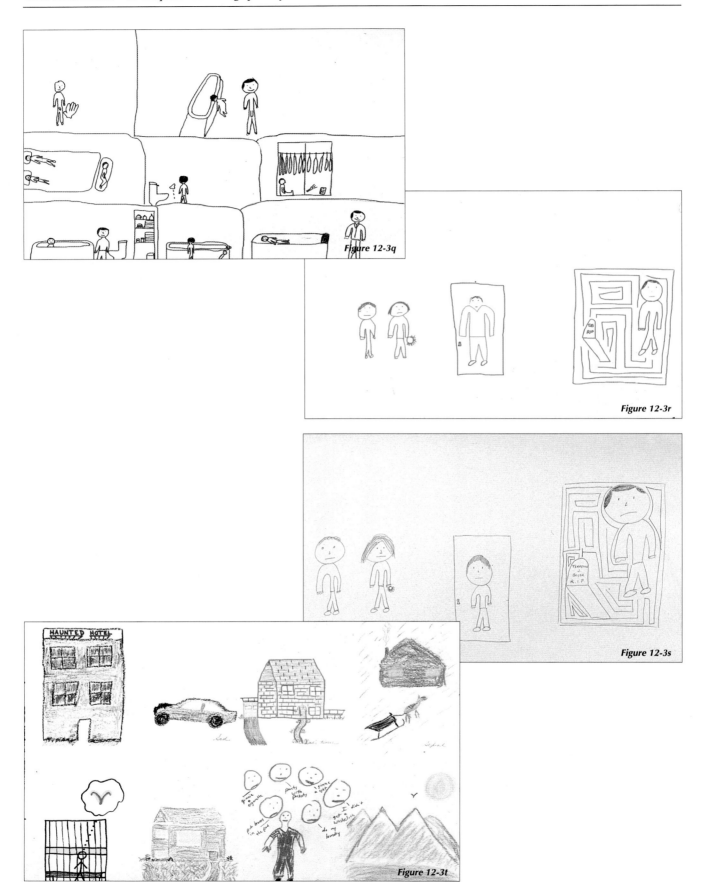

Figure 12-3q

Figure 12-3r

Figure 12-3s

Figure 12-3t

ART THERAPY

COLETTE M. RICKERT, LPCC, A.T.R.-BC

Art therapy is a human service profession that focuses on the process involved in healing. Each time a person creates a work of art, he or she moves a piece of himself or herself outside for the world to see. The individual is looking at the inner self and seeing a reflection of the true self in the art work. Art therapy can benefit almost anyone if the person is willing to more fully express inner feelings and thoughts.

The art therapist can and should be consulted when a child's or an adult's drawings consistently and significantly deviate from developmental norms. Issues that may be resistant to traditional therapy or those that are too difficult to talk about can be quite responsive to art therapy. Art therapy bypasses the criticism of technique and focuses on helping clients move toward integration by offering a way to express how they experience themselves, others, and events in a more complete way.

The rest of this chapter will present case studies showing how, through art therapy, abused individuals were able to communicate about their abuse. These studies also illustrate the thoughts and feelings of persons who have experienced abuse or neglect.

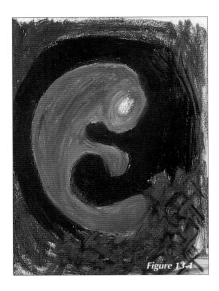

Figure 13-1. *This client stated, "The fires hurt the baby. She feels the fires." It represents a prenatal memory.*

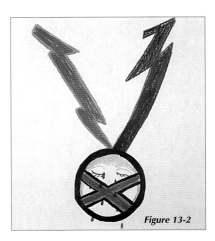

Figure 13-2. *This picture was drawn in response to a structured activity asking participants to make a drawing showing how they feel about art therapy. The client said that the red and orange X across the mouth came from her mother's messages to "shut up" and "quit complaining." The mother is shown as the red and orange lightning bolt at the top left of the picture. The brown and black X across the mouth came from her father's message to "never speak to me unless you have something decent to say." He is represented as the black and brown lightning bolt at the top right of the picture.*

Figure 13-3. (a) *Aspects chart, showing the various aspects of the personality.* **(b)** *This aspects chart was created by a child, age 12, who had been subjected to emotional abuse due to isolating, rejecting, and overpressuring during visits to a noncustodial parent. Although no overt sexual activities are known, age-inappropriate bathing activities occurred and covert sexual activities have abounded within the home. Note the lack of body-specific features in the physical areas, with colors surrounding the form. Although the mental aspect appears ordered with bricks neatly in place, the window could be broken. This child often dissociates during visits and reports experiencing a see-through barrier. In her words, In the top part of my chart (creative), I drew a plant with buds on it. To me that symbolizes my creative self really growing and full. I feel that at the present time I am trying to work more with that section and make it as big as the other parts have been. In the past I think that it has been smaller than some of the other parts, but now I think it is equal. In the right part of my chart (mental) I drew a clear window, with a brick wall around it. I think that that section is very strong and also very clear. Sometimes my mental side can be "out of it," (i.e., she dissociates) but it seems to always stay clear. In the bottom part of my chart (physical) I drew an outline of a human body with many colors. I think that I am starting to show how great I am on the inside as well as the outside. In the left part of my chart (emotions) I drew a heart with half of the background green and the other half blue. The heart symbolizes that I am starting to be able to show my emotions, but yet they aren't as sad and dreary as they have been in the past. The green and blue is to symbolize how much I love the earth and how happy I feel outside and on the earth. In the center part of my chart (integration) I drew scribbles, but I used all the colors that I used in the loops and I made them flow in a nice even circle that started in the center and worked its way out. I feel that this symbolizes all of them working together and making me "even." **(c)** This aspects chart was created by a woman during a deep depression. At the time of the drawing, she was aware of growing up in a home filled with physical violence, high degrees of emotional and verbal abuse, and general neglect. She was not aware of having been sexually abused until she began having recurring nightmares approximately 2 years later that eventually led her to uncovering abuse memories. Note that the physical area at the bottom is drawn with lines that appear fluid and blood-like. All of the areas contain circles that interrupt their areas. Boundary problems pervaded her home situation. Rectal intrusions were a regular part of her upbringing and "interrupted" her personal spaces and development.*

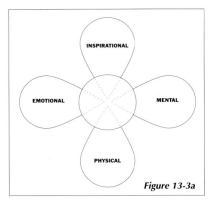

Figure 13-3a

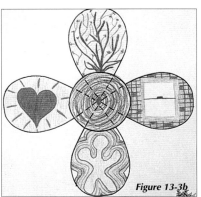

Figure 13-3b

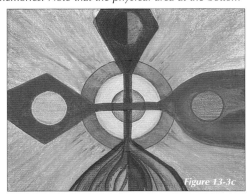

Figure 13-3c

Figure 13-4. This client attended group therapy sessions for a number of years and spoke very rarely in the group. When asked specifically if she preferred to discontinue therapy or be moved to another group, she stated that she wanted to stay. Eventually an art activity was suggested that she responded to with

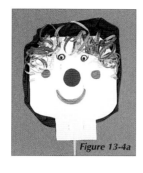

Figure 13-4a

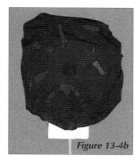

Figure 13-4b

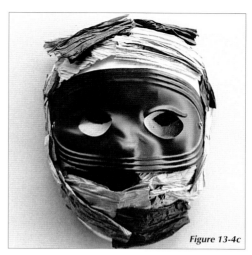

Figure 13-4c

noticeable interest. When asked to make an object that would represent her siblings, she created these masks (**a** and **b**), which have front and back images. This mask is of a brother she considered "two-faced." Her therapeutic journey became more fluid after these masks were done. She was raised in a family where children were never to speak unless spoken to first by an adult. She was supposed to sit still and not move whenever she was at home. If she did express herself or move, her brothers verbally assaulted her. She was isolated from other children and rejected and ignored by other members of her family. She cannot recall if she was physically or sexually assaulted. (**c**) Mask of brother who never spoke to the client.

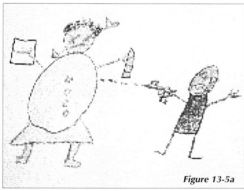

Figure 13-5a

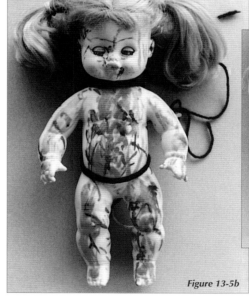

Figure 13-5b

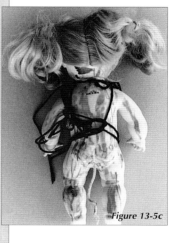

Figure 13-5c

Figure 13-5. This child was first brought to therapy because of behavioral problems at school. He appeared to have attention-deficit hyperactivity disorder with moderate indications of a learning disability in the area of reading comprehension. After initial resistance to coming to therapy, when he said, "There's nothing wrong with me. It's everybody else!" he became comfortable in the therapy setting and began doing art activities that were a blend of topics suggested by the therapist for assessment and diagnostic purposes (for example, **a,** where the child drew what he wishes he could do—kill his teacher) and spontaneous drawings he created based on the things that seemed to be worrying him at that time. During the process of treatment a prior sexual assault was depicted (**b** and **c**). The mother had known about it and proper authorities had been involved, so everyone thought that the experience had been resolved and the child was simply a behavior problem at school. During treatment he received medication for depression and difficulty paying attention at school. After therapy, moving to a new house in a different neighborhood, and beginning a different school, he was no longer considered a behavior problem. He seemed to adjust well, and medications were reduced significantly. Doll in **b** and **c** was a spontaneous creation wherein he replicated the rectal sexual abuse that he had experienced. Drawing in **d** was presented to his therapist as a going-away present, indicating that he was done with counseling. He stated that the therapist "no longer needed to know his private business" and that he did not need to come to therapy any more. This final picture shows a full-figured and colorful character, depicting the client when he chose to leave therapy—having set boundaries, full-figured, and richly colored.

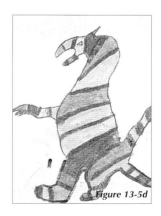

Figure 13-5d

Figure 13-6. This client grew up in a house with a violent and sexually abusive mother. Many times during therapy, she was completely unable to speak, aware that she was unable to speak, and frustrated with this condition. A person of extremely high intelligence, she was deeply distressed with her inability to understand why she drew seemingly inexplicable pictures of violence, enemas, sexual trauma, and cruelty. **(a)** Picture created during elementary school years. **(b)** After continued and repeated physical and sexual abuse, the client became aware of the presence of an angel who would watch over her. This painting reflects the client's sense of the angel weeping about what this woman was experiencing as a child. It was done 4 years before the client had any conscious memories of having been sexually assaulted. **(c** and **d)** These drawings depict a lack of boundaries or protective images; transparencies; X's; and distorted or missing body parts. They were drawn about 5 years apart and reflect abuse memories the client is still trying to sort out. **(c)** Shows the client at the age of 35 years. **(d)** Shows the client at about the age of 1 year. **(e** through **g)** These three drawings reflect the client's relationship with her mother and the abusive behaviors she experienced that led to her eventual dissociation at the age of 4 years. The client saw herself as having an evil companion who would deal with the mother while the client went to sleep crying. **(h)** Shows client feeling sad and locked in behind a glass wall as a child. **(i)** This drawing is an integration and awareness picture. It was done during a time when the client was first aware that she had been sexually assaulted both vaginally and rectally by her mother. She depicts her "child self" being taken into her own heart to love and protect. Although the tears of the woman flow down on the "child self," the client expressed an awareness that these were cleansing tears and that, in time, she was certain that the wounds would be washed clean.

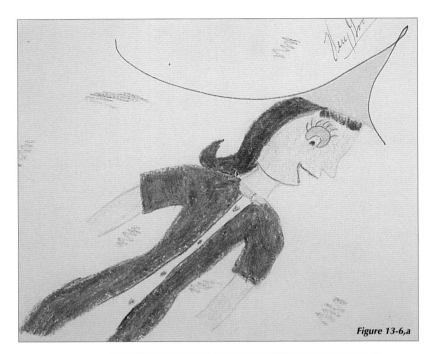

Figure 13-6,a

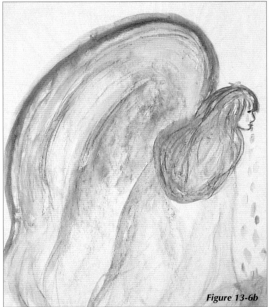

Figure 13-6b

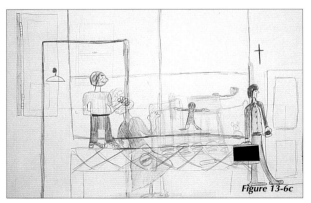

Figure 13-6c

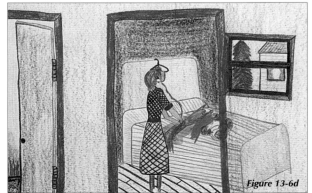

Figure 13-6d

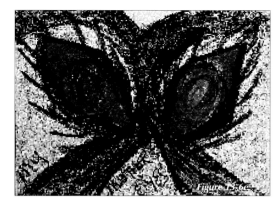

Figure 13-6c

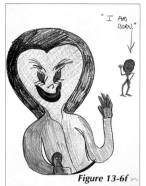

"I AM BORN."

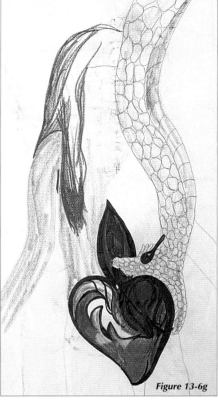

Figure 13-6f

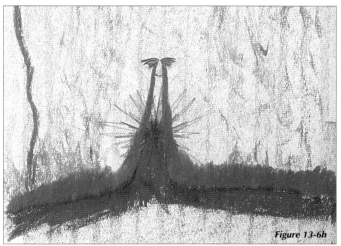

Figure 13-6h

Figure 13-6g

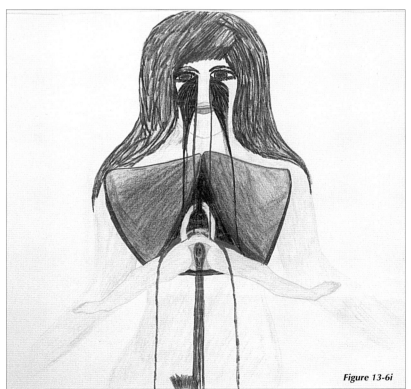

Figure 13-6i

INDEX

A

Abandonment, 266-267, 291-302

    emotional, 291

    fatal, 291

    near-fatal, 291

Abdomen

    acute, 146-147

    blow to, vomiting and, 137

    blunt trauma to, 45, 54, 259

    bruises on, 54, 150-151

    burn on, caused by cigarette lighter, healed, 98

    contusions on, 240-241

    ecchymotic area on, 26

    first-degree burn on, 100

    kick in, traumatic rupture of pancreas secondary to, 145

    linear marks on, 12-13

    pattern burn on, from floor grill, 282

    protruberant, 293, 294

    rigid, 140-141, 150-151

    second-degree burn on, 100

    severe blunt trauma to, ruptured hollow viscera and, 134

    squeezing of, 257-258

    third-degree burn on, 100

Abrasions

    on abdomen, 242-243

    on arm, 20-21, 242-243

    on back, 30-31, 242-243

    on chest, 30-31, 242-243

    on chin, 20-21

    corneal, 44

    on elbow, 20-21

    on face, 54, 242-243

    on head, 242-243

    on leg, 242-243, 255

    on neck, 20-21, 242-243

    from ring, 16-17

    on shoulder, 20-21

    on thorax, 20-21

Abscess

    on foot, 256

    retropharyngeal, ruptured, 256

Abuse

    child; *see* Child abuse

    physical; *see* Physical abuse

    sexual; *see* Sexual abuse

Accidental injuries, differentiating, from inflicted injuries, 3-56, 184

Acetaminophen, perianal and anal condyloma and, 115

Acid phosphatase, 184

Acute abdomen, suspected, 146-147

Acute increased intracranial pressure, 162

Acute vaginitis, 195, 201

Adhesions, labial, 183, 184, 194, 199, 202, 231

Adynamic ileus throughout small intestine, 150-151

Affect, passive, 42, 294

Age of injury, determination of, 133

Air, intraperitoneal, free, 134

Alcohol, elevated ethanol level and, 90

Allergic contact dermatitis, edema and, 114

Amblyopia, 125

Ampicillin, group B *Streptococcus* and, 219

Amputation of end of glans penis, 110

Anal bruising, 255

Anal canal, stool in, anal dilation due to, 224

Anal cellulitis, acute streptococcal, 226

Anal condyloma, 115

Anal dilation, 32, 184, 186, 221, 255

    due to stool in anal canal, 224

Anal fissure, 184, 221

Anal infection, 219

Anal laxity, 32

Anal pain, 32, 228

Anal penetration, 32, 186, 220, 222, 223, 225, 227, 228, 308-314, 316, 317, 318-319

    with broom, 210-211

Anal scars, 184

Anal spasm, 228

Anal tag, 184, 220, 226, 227

Anal tear, 30-31, 222, 224

    healing, 225

Anal verge, prominent, 184

Anemia, 22-23

Ankle, stocking-glove pattern of burn above, 91, 283

Annular hymen, 199, 205, 217

I

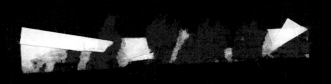